Practical Operating Theatre Management

Practical Operating Theatre Management

Measuring and Improving Performance and Patient Experience

Edited by
Jaideep J. Pandit
Oxford University Hospitals

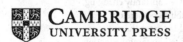

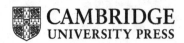

UNIVERSITY PRESS

Shaftesbury Road, Cambridge CB2 8EA, United Kingdom

One Liberty Plaza, 20th Floor, New York, NY 10006, USA

477 Williamstown Road, Port Melbourne, VIC 3207, Australia

314–321, 3rd Floor, Plot 3, Splendor Forum, Jasola District Centre, New Delhi – 110025, India

103 Penang Road, #05–06/07, Visioncrest Commercial, Singapore 238467

Cambridge University Press is part of Cambridge University Press & Assessment,
a department of the University of Cambridge.

We share the University's mission to contribute to society through the pursuit of
education, learning and research at the highest international levels of excellence.

www.cambridge.org
Information on this title: www.cambridge.org/9781316646830

DOI:10.1017/9781108164061

© Cambridge University Press & Assessment 2019

This publication is in copyright. Subject to statutory exception and to the provisions
of relevant collective licensing agreements, no reproduction of any part may take
place without the written permission of Cambridge University Press & Assessment.

First published 2019

A catalogue record for this publication is available from the British Library

Library of Congress Cataloging-in-Publication data
Names: Pandit, Jaideep J., editor.
Title: Practical operating theatre management : measuring and improving performance and
    patient experience / edited by Jaideep J Pandit.
Description: Cambridge, United Kingdom ; New York, NY : University Printing House, 2018. |
    Includes bibliographical references and index.
Identifiers: LCCN 2018022100 | ISBN 9781316646830 (pbk. : alk. paper)
Subjects: | MESH: Surgery Department, Hospital–organization & administration | Surgery Department,
    Hospital–utilization | Perioperative Care–economics | Efficiency, Organizational
Classification: LCC RA971.9 | NLM WO 27.1 | DDC 362.11068–dc23
    LC record available at https://lccn.loc.gov/2018022100

ISBN   978-1-316-64683-0   Paperback

Additional resources for this publication at www.cambridge.org/9781316646830

Cambridge University Press & Assessment has no responsibility for the persistence
or accuracy of URLs for external or third-party internet websites referred to in this
publication and does not guarantee that any content on such websites is, or will
remain, accurate or appropriate.

. . . .

Every effort has been made in preparing this book to provide accurate and up-to-date
information which is in accord with accepted standards and practice at the time of
publication. Although case histories are drawn from actual cases, every effort has been
made to disguise the identities of the individuals involved. Nevertheless, the authors,
editors and publishers can make no warranties that the information contained herein
is totally free from error, not least because clinical standards are constantly changing
through research and regulation. The authors, editors and publishers therefore
disclaim all liability for direct or consequential damages resulting from the use of
material contained in this book. Readers are strongly advised to pay careful attention
to information provided by the manufacturer of any drugs or equipment that they plan
to use.

Contents

List of Contributors

Cameron C. R. Buchanan, MB ChB, Dip Obs, FANZCA
Clinical Director, Department of Anaesthesia,
Clinical Unit Leader, Theatre and Perioperative
Medicine, Waikato Hospital, Hamilton,
New Zealand

Emily B. Goldenberg, MD
Clinical Instructor and Perioperative Management
Fellow, Department of Anesthesiology, Perioperative
and Pain Medicine, Stanford University School of
Medicine,
California, USA

Alex Macario, MD
Professor of Anesthesiology, Perioperative and Pain
Medicine,
Professor of Health Research and Policy,
Vice-Chair for Education,
Stanford University Medical Center,
California, USA

Peter H. J. Müller, MD
Operating Theatres Manager,
Medical Directorate,
University Hospital of Basel,
Basel, Switzerland

Yoshinori Nakata, MD, MBA
Anesthesiologist, Teikyo University Hospital,
Professor of Healthcare Management, Teikyo
University Graduate School of Public Health,
Director, Teikyo University Medical Information and
System Research Center,
Tokyo, Japan

Meghana Pandit, MBBS, FRCOG, MBA
Chief Medical Officer and Deputy Chief Executive,
University Hospitals of Coventry and Warwickshire,
Professor of Practice, University of Warwick,
Warwick, UK

Thomas Sieber, MD, MBA
Chairman, Department of Anesthesia, Intensive Care
and Emergency Medicine,
Hospital Graubünden,
Chur, Switzerland

André Van Zundert, MD, PhD, FRCA, FANZCA
Professor and Chairman of Anaesthetics,
Royal Brisbane and Womens' Hospital,
Queensland, Australia

Foreword

The successful management of operating theatres is essential to the success of a hospital. The challenges have always been to try to maximise the use of resources, whilst minimising any expensive and disruptive overruns, and preventing on-the-day cancellation of patients. This book, perhaps for the first time, explains how these three seemingly mutually exclusive goals can be achieved in a rational way. It does so using the language of mathematics, but presented in a way that makes it easily readable. Professor Pandit has considerable experience as a senior Consultant Anaesthetist, very familiar with the practicalities and environment of operating theatres, both in the United Kingdom and other parts of the world. He also has distinction as an academic leader. He has coupled his clinical insights with a scholarly and academic analysis that formed the basis of his own award-winning thesis. The result is an exceptional book that meets an important need and reaches out to all those involved in theatre management. Topics that might otherwise seem complex are made user-friendly through the use of simple toolkits and illustrations of practical examples using vignettes and scenarios. The international chapters underline the reality that healthcare challenges are broadly similar the world over – and if this is the case, then so too should be the solutions to meet those challenges. Professor Pandit has risen to the task of explaining core practical theatre management principles at a tactical level to all those responsible for managing operating theatres. The onus is now on managers to begin the work of translating those principles into reality, in a way that delivers real benefits to patients.

Professor Andy Hardy, BA, MBA
Chief Executive,
University Hospitals of Coventry & Warwickshire;
Professor of Practice, University of Warwick
Past President & National Board Member, the
Healthcare Financial Management Association

Preface

This book arose out of a series of papers I published focussed on the broad concept of 'theatre efficiency'. In turn, these were based on some very basic questions that occurred to me when I was appointed to an NHS Consultant post in the United Kingdom in 1999 (having been an Attending Anaesthesiologist in the United States for the previous year). I was tasked with a role of leading a new initiative based on improving preassessment of short-stay and day-case patients. Although our initial endeavours led to major improvements in patient care, it became clear that further improvements required more in-depth knowledge and analysis of concepts such as 'utilisation', 'efficiency' and 'productivity'.

I was struck by the dearth of information available to guide me in planning this new service. What relatively little there was largely originated from the United States and was not readily applicable to models of working in the United Kingdom. The existing literature was also presented in a way that was not accessible to those charged with managing operating theatres on a day-to-day basis, as it was rather academic in its approach. I therefore sought to fill this void and embarked on a long, continuous project using our own experiences from analysis of operating rooms in Oxford, as well as insights gained through official visits and collaborations internationally.

I presented my collected works as a doctoral thesis at the University of Oxford, where it was successfully examined by the Said Business School in 2015; in 2017 this thesis was also awarded the prestigious Emerald/EDRF Prize for Outstanding Doctoral Thesis in Healthcare Management. The idea of Cambridge University Press to help present these important ideas in a user-friendly format is very apposite, and I appreciate their encouragement and support throughout this project.

I sincerely hope that the principles presented in this book will create a new norm for how operating theatres should be managed, based on rational, data-driven principles. The notions of 'efficiency' and 'scheduling' presented are especially important. Moreover, the book will offer all parties involved in theatre management a common language and common understanding that they can use to communicate better with each other. I would like to see two rallying cries from theatre managers: '*Give us more data on timings!*' and '*Don't just use means; use variances!*' Not necessarily catchy phrases, but really essential ones nevertheless.

In summary the aim of this book is to disseminate the quantitative measures of operating theatre performance, already validated, that are useful and meaningful, presented in a simple way to improve patient care. I hope this book will achieve this aim.

Jaideep J Pandit St John's College Oxford

About the Author

Jaideep J Pandit has been Consultant Anaesthetist at the Oxford University Hospitals NHS Foundation Trust since 1999. He trained in Medicine at Oxford (Corpus Christi College) and obtained a Double First in Physiology and Medicine, with University prizes in Medicine, Cardiology and Clinical Pharmacology. After a Wellcome Trust Research Fellowship to support a DPhil in Respiratory Physiology at Oxford, he undertook anaesthetic training in the Oxford region. He was Visiting Assistant Professor of Anesthesiology at the University of Michigan, Ann Arbor (1998–9), and when appointed to his NHS Consultant post at the John Radcliffe was independently elected to a personal Fellowship at St John's College, Oxford, in 2000.

He has held several national and specialty roles. As the Academic Strategy Officer of the Royal College of Anaesthetists (2005–7), he published the specialty's *National Strategy for Academic Anaesthesia* – a policy document commissioned to help prepare the specialty nationally for changes in academic medical training. Since 2015 he has been elected Member of Council of the Royal College and its Director of Patient Safety (Chair of the Safe Anaesthesia Liaison Group). He served as member of the Court of Examiners of the Royal College of Surgeons of England (until 2010), examining the MRCS exams. For over 10 years he has been editor of the journal *Anaesthesia* and has served on roles at the Research Council of the National Institute of Academic Anaesthesia (United Kingdom) and as Scientific Officer of the national Difficult Airway Society (the largest specialist society in anaesthetics in the United Kingdom) until 2016.

In 2010 he was elected chairman of the John Radcliffe Medical Staff Committee (chairman of consultants) for a 4-year term and was the first consultant re-elected to a second term in 2014. In 2014 he published the international report (NAP5, United Kingdom and Ireland) on *Accidental Awareness during General Anaesthesia*, culmination of a 4-year Royal College project making over 60 recommendations for clinical practice. In 2016, he was appointed by NHS England to be a Clinical Associate, to advise on its New Care Models programme, a £50 million initiative designed to adopt new and efficient ways of working through selected 'Vanguard' sites. This work in part has included advice on topics related to theatre efficiency and management.

At the University Professor Pandit was the first Chairman of Examiners of the then new Graduate-Entry Medical Exams and has served several terms as Examiner for Oxford's Final Honour School in Medicine and Physiology. In post-graduate training he has served as Training Program Director for over 400 NHS consultants in Oxford, supervising their specialist registration as trainers with the General Medical Council (2014–17).

National and international awards include the Royal College's Gold (Jubilee) Medal (2000), Humphry Davy Medal (2006) and Macintosh Professorship (2012). He received the Spring Silver Medal (2012) of the College of Anaesthetists of Ireland. He has been visiting professor as follows: at the Mayo Clinic, Jacksonville, Florida, 2014; at Harvard University (the Massachusetts General Hospital), 2015; and at the University of Texas Southwestern, Dallas, 2016; Jobson Visiting Professor at the University of Sydney, Australia, 2017; USP Professor at the University of Michigan, Ann Arbor, 2017; Besokande Professor at the Karolinska Institute, Stockholm, Sweden, 2018; elected Difficult Airway Society Professor of Anaesthesia 2018. He is also an Associate Professor, Nuffield Department of Clinical Neurosciences, University of Oxford, and has delivered the invited Victor Horsley Lecture of the British Medical Association 2015 and the Spyros Makris Lecture of the Greek Society of Anaesthesia 2018.

Chapter

1

Introduction and Scope of the Book

Jaideep J. Pandit

This book is about managing operating theatres and leading teams that work in them. A great deal has been written about leadership and management styles, but almost all of it can be condensed to a simple idea. Leaders use styles that make them liked, respected or feared. In turn management is about the effective use of goodwill, money or power. These elements are used in different combinations, and successful leadership or management is about judging when to use which style or adopt which means, respectively, and in what relative proportions. This book is not directly about leadership or management, but readers will see in the examples and vignettes given, how these styles and means can be used to attain the wider objective of theatre efficiency. Arguably, successful leadership and management rely on one more factor: the effective use of information. Not in the sense of propaganda or image, but rather in the ability to analyse and communicate complex data clearly, to both the wider team and the consumer. In this way, the strategy and goals of the organisation can be best understood. This then is the prime focus of this book – describing the processes in operating theatres in an objective analysis that leads to rational, data-led solutions.

Hospital operating theatres represent a very large part of hospital activity (in some centres probably the largest part). It has been estimated that up to ~46% of patients discharged from hospital have undergone some form of surgery. In the United Kingdom (UK), about three million anaesthetics are administered annually, and operating theatres collectively have an annual NHS budget of >£1 billion. Yet, the long-held perception of many who work in theatres is that they can be an underutilised resource. Last-minute cancellations of procedures on the day of surgery are frequent and costly both to the patient and to the hospital. It seems appropriate, both in terms of patient care and financial investment, that theatres work as 'efficiently' as possible.

Although several authoritative reports over the years in the United Kingdom and elsewhere have attempted to describe how to best manage theatres and operating lists, they fall short of being practical manuals to guide those who actually manage the service. The recommendations of these reports are broadly similar and include measures such as: effective administrative systems, accurate records for analysis and audit, optimally managing staff time, and good preassessment of patients to optimise medical conditions. This list is not exhaustive. Collectively, these recommendations seem very reasonable and appropriate to implement.

However, what is lacking from any recommendation or from anything that has followed, is a practical tool to apply in the real world, usable by those working in the theatre environment, especially those in leadership roles. Little contained in those reports helps guide individual behaviour, especially of the consultant or attending surgeons or anaesthetists. Without engagement of these key staff, attempts to improve theatre performance are unlikely to succeed.

Yet, consultant anaesthetists and surgeons are – alongside other non-clinical managers – often asked to run operating theatre suites in a managerial capacity. What is their training? Where are the courses or additional qualifications? Topics like 'How would you schedule your operating list?', or 'Which patients would you prioritise on an operating list, and why, if time is constrained?', or 'How do you measure – and therefore minimise – the cost of operating?' are not asked during surgical or anaesthesia training programs, so the thinking is not embedded from an early stage of their training. Rather it is left to 'common sense' to manage after these doctors are qualified. Coupled with this, few healthcare management training programs deal with these issues at this level, focussing generally on the wider questions of strategy such as the problems of the ageing population, scarcity of funding, etc. (all of which are undoubtedly important, but few of which help make practical day-to-day decisions in an operating theatre suite). Operating theatre management at a practical level does not form the major part of any MBA (Master's of Business Administration) program.

Moreover, advice is lacking on what to measure during the process of improvement. How do we know if we are heading in the right direction, and how do we know when we have reached the goal of 'efficiency'?

The main purpose of this book is to fill these voids. This book is intended for a wide audience. Throughout the book we use the term *theatre manager*. This is used to denote a generic person being tasked to run theatres: it could be a clinician, a non-clinician, someone senior or junior. In essence, the theatre manager is the archetype of anyone who has some responsibility or desire to improve theatre performance. Theatre managers (from a variety of backgrounds) who are tasked with organising a theatre suite will find a ready-to-use manual, which they can reference, to help them make daily planning decisions. They can readily access the toolkits provided to solve practical problems. Those undergoing training for such roles will find the book useful as a learning guide, and the reference lists provide a rich source of further reading material. Medical and nursing staff of all grades – including medical and nursing students – will find this book indispensable for several reasons. First, if managers are applying the principles contained, they will need to understand how and why decisions around their working environment are being made. Second, as they themselves have some planning responsibilities, they can also use the principles contained directly. Third, they will find the book valuable for training, especially to learn the language of the theatre environment.

Core Principles

It is important first to understand some core principles underpinning this book. At time of writing there are very few similar books on the market and therefore, the first step is to understand some of the core terminology and approach (and therefore limitations) of what this book is about.

Strategy versus Tactics versus Operations

When we talk about 'policy' or 'planning' or 'achieving efficiency', etc., we can hold the discussion at several levels (hierarchies of organisation).

The *strategic level* concerns the big themes and philosophies underpinning the system as a whole. Examples of strategic questions related to healthcare would include: 'Should the health system be funded by general taxation or via private payments or via insurance?'; 'Should hospitals be organised as a few, large tertiary centres with smaller centres undertaking a limited range of surgeries; or as many broadly equal-sized units all doing similar work?' or 'Given an ageing population, should we invest scare resources into hospitals or into primary care?', etc. These are grand questions that set the envelope for the environment in which we all work. They are decided at senior governmental level, sometimes at regional or national levels, or sometimes through the ballot box in elections. These questions have nothing to do with this book. In the approach of this book, the strategic level is regarded as a given: i.e., we are where we are in the health service in which we work. We do not argue that the causes of any of the problems this book seeks to address are strategic ones.

At the other extreme, the *operational level* concerns the day-to-day matters that are often specific to a single centre. For example, achieving efficiency in a given hospital may require things to be done like ordering equipment or consumables in sufficient quantity and on time, making sure elevators work so patients can be physically moved, maintaining the temperature and lighting environment, etc. Again, this has nothing to do with this book; there is little need to write a book to remind readers of things that are self-evident (albeit important). In the approach of this book, the operational level is also regarded as a given: i.e., it can be assumed that all these matters are functioning well. The causes of any of the problems that this book seeks to address are not operational.

In between the strategic and operational lies the *tactical level*. These are the tactics to use, given the knowledge of any strategic envelope you are in and given any operational constraints. These tactics are often termed 'heuristics'. A heuristic is any approach to solving problems that uses a pragmatic method (not necessarily perfect) that is sufficient to attain the immediate goal. In other words, given (hypothetically) that we work in a health system funded wholly by taxation, and hospitals are structured in a certain way; and given that we have certain operational limits (a finite number of portering staff, elevators, etc.), what is the best way to maximise efficiency of a surgical list, or minimise costs? These are the issues that this book is about; because these are the questions that face a theatre manager on a daily basis (notwithstanding the fact that they may also have some responsibility for reordering equipment and making sure elevators are fixed, etc.).

A military analogy may help illustrate the distinctions. Strategic questions might include: 'Shall we go to war, when and with whom?' Operational questions might include: 'How many boots does a division need; how much food is required by a regiment, etc.?' The tactical question is: 'Given we are at war, and given a certain size of army with constraints on its supplies, how do we actually win the battles?'

Or, to use the language of leadership: strategy is the leader's vision and direction of travel; operations are the necessary elements required for the journey; tactics are the tools and skills employed to get there.

Quantitative Approach as Basis for Rational Discussion

Another core principle of this book is to assist the theatre manager by creating objective, *quantitative tools* that can be applied to dilemmas or problems. Only then can the ensuing discussion be *rational*. When faced with serious problems, such as a huge demand for surgery that creates very long waiting lists (patients waiting months or years for urgent interventions), the temptation is simply to conclude that staff are not working sufficiently hard. If only they worked harder, then there would be no waiting list. Unsurprisingly, such an analysis can lead to staff dissatisfaction and disengagement and a worsening situation. Instead, by studying the numbers underpinning the waiting lists, a more objective discussion can be had. This book shows how the objective principles can be used to defuse otherwise stressful situations.

Fundamental to a quantitative approach is an understanding of mathematics. All those running theatres have to be capable of numeracy – without exception. This is because the running of operating theatres requires mathematical knowledge and skills. We would not expect someone ignorant of anatomy to be employed as a surgeon. We would not expect someone ignorant of pharmacology to be employed as a physician. Similarly, we should not expect someone without some degree of numeracy and ability to draw and interpret graphs to manage operating theatres.

This does not mean that the theatre manager must always use advanced, abstract mathematics that

nobody else can understand. Rather, the mathematics in this book is quite basic – needing little more than Excel to solve most of the problems or a pocket calculator to perform any calculations. However, anyone who finds even the simplest of mathematical principles difficult should probably stop reading this book (and should also avoid becoming a theatre manager without further training in this domain).

'Time' as the Currency of Analysis: The Language of Probability

In the quantitative approach described earlier, the currency of our analysis is *time*. While 'patients' are undoubtedly important in a holistic sense – and we must never lose sight of that – erroneous conclusions result from calculations based simply on 'patient numbers'. This book recognises that a patient scheduled for surgery places defined *time* demands on the service. In turn, the capacity of the service to accommodate the patient is best measured in the hours or minutes of theatre *time* available.

In mathematical terms this distinction is important. The number of patients is a 'discrete variable' – one can have two or three patients, but no value in between. In contrast, time is a 'continuous variable' – one can have any value between two or three hours, measured in milli- or micro-seconds if needed. Using a continuous variable as currency of analysis in minutes or hours then facilitates calculation of *variance* (e.g., the standard deviation or range) of the relevant times. In turn, variance is easily linked to probability calculations. This instantly changes the language of debate. Rather than saying such-and-such will or will not happen, we can then say, using calculations based on variance, that there is a certain defined *chance* of something happening or not. As we will see, use of this mature probabilistic language to theatre problems is a very important aspect of this book.

The place of 'Lean Thinking' – and Its Limitations

Some readers may be surprised that a core concept of this book is not 'Lean' or 'Six Sigma' thinking. In fact, much of the book is indeed about Lean/Six Sigma principles, but is just not branded as such, for reasons explained later.

Lean has shown great promise in industry, by seeking reductions in variations of inputs such as raw materials or manufacturing steps. However, the success of applications to healthcare is still unproven (Vest & Gamm, 2009). Many individual Lean principles can be and are adopted, but really Lean is a whole-system way of thinking, and few healthcare systems are close to that – certainly not the NHS. It is not the purpose or intention of this book to change the whole-system culture from the primary care doctor's surgery all the way through a hospital to the care home – this is what a true Lean approach would seek to do.

Moreover, Lean/Six Sigma approaches are generally focussed upon processes within a patient's journey at an operational level, whereas the focus of this book is the tactical level.

Another difficulty is that the introduction of Lean within the NHS has been piecemeal, and it is not embedded into system culture. For example, there have been relatively few studies of the causes of large waiting lists (Martin et al., 2003), and it is readily appreciated that what might be called the 'productive capacity' of hospitals encompassing all their activities is hard to estimate and not standardised (Buhaug, 2002). Consequently when the NHS introduced hard targets for waiting times in the early 2000s, it was trying to solve a problem without fully knowing its fundamental cause or without establishing the necessary consensus around the measures of demand and capacity that were vital to make progress. Many anaesthetists and surgeons in the United Kingdom have by now experienced waves of initiatives concerning Lean. This is usually accompanied by armies of newcomers in suits observing theatres, carrying clipboards and then circulating 'fishbone diagrams' or simply suggesting everyone should start on time. What has never been disseminated are the basic mathematical concepts underpinning the Lean principles. An analogy would be for a health service (quite reasonably) to prioritise the treatment of sepsis, but then (unreasonably) decline to define what 'sepsis' was or to promote teaching of the basic mathematics of oxygen supply and consumption. In short, the way that the NHS has tried to introduce Lean into theatre management in the United Kingdom has probably given Lean a bad name.

Furthermore, there is a fundamental disagreement about the causes of variation in the system and if it can be eliminated. Gallivan et al. (2002) measured 'length of inpatient stay' as the key measure of demand on a cardiac intensive care service and used queuing theory (see Chapter 5, Capacity Planning) to conclude that, because of variability in this demand, they needed greater capacity to cope with admissions. However, several then-leaders of what was termed the 'NHS Modernisation Program' criticised the analysis, disputing that 'length of stay' was a correct measure of demand (but did not say what was preferable), and arguing that the variability in demand was caused by poor standardisation of procedures by specialists and poor coordination. In essence the NHS was disinclined to support a conclusion to increase capacity (as this would be expensive) and advocated instead measures to reduce variability in demand.

The broad concept of eliminating variation emanated from an influential analysis of Toyota's success (Womack et al., 1990). The ingredients were the principles of 'eliminating waste' (e.g., time and consumable); 'do it right first time' (no trial- or error-led behaviour); emphasis on 'value' (in both activity and product); 'flexibility' (e.g., staff roles and production line activities); and the notion that the customer (i.e., patient) 'pushes' the system rather than is sucked through it. One problem is that 'Lean' can be anodyne and unobjectionable – who can object to doing things right first time? Many principles like these are rather vague (e.g., how do we know if something is pushed or pulled through the system?) and impersonal (what about the patient who wishes to linger a while, and neither be pushed nor pulled?). Therefore they can be interpreted widely; there is no set of clear criteria or test of whether a system has achieved 'lean-ness'. The danger of a self-fulfilling prophecy is that 'Lean' is always the system that works.

As we will see later (Chapter 5, Capacity Planning), it is possible for a factory to control its input and have little or no variability because all materials used and end-units of production are alike. But in hospitals we have the unpredictability of patients' response to treatment, a constant uncertainty in diagnosis and indeed changing goals. The patient admitted with abdominal pain may in fact need primary cardiac surgery. It is as if a factory designed to make cars suddenly needed to make a boat. If patients are the greater part of variability for hospitals, then the only way to eliminate variability and become lean is to eliminate patients (Morton & Cornwell, 2009).

Proper Analogies for Operating Theatres

The fact that surgical operating theatres are not like factories or conveyor belts does not mean that we abandon quantitative analysis. The factory analogy fails because (a) the substrate of factories is fixed and unvariable (all the metal sheets, materials used conform to fixed sizes, shapes, etc.); (b) the same actions are performed on the conveyor belt to produce the output; (c) the output is also constant (all cars, trucks, cans, etc. that the conveyor belt produces are all alike, and designed to be so); (d) if time is lost by stopping the process for maintenance it can generally be sped up when restarted to catch up with production.

In contrast, the substrate for surgery and anaesthesia – our patients – are hardly ever alike; they are all different sizes, shapes, ages, with different morbidities. Second, our actions as doctors on the patients are hardly ever alike, even when directed to the same goal. Third, we do not seek the same result in all patients, but target the result to the needs of the patient. Fourth, if time is lost by cancelling a list, that time can never be regained.

In part, surgical operating lists more closely resemble professional service industries like law firms, accountancy partnerships or banks. An even better resemblance would be with a car repair shop (rather than a car manufacturer, like Toyota) or even antique clock restoration. Here the starting state of each precious clock is different. Although problems may fall into distinct patterns, the processes needed to fix the clock are highly specific to the clock. The time taken may vary greatly, but an experienced restorer will know broadly how long it will take, and this knowledge will underpin how much work is taken on. Unfortunately there is sparse literature on the economics of the antique clock industry or car repair shops. But nevertheless, this is the philosophy and approach guiding this book: to apply objective quantitative analysis to the processes by which we restore health to our patients.

Focus on the National Health Service: Language of Theatres

Readers will find that there is an emphasis on the National Health Service (NHS) in the United Kingdom, and the primary examples provided relate to the UK NHS. The reason for this is that much of the published experimental and observational work underpinning this book was undertaken using NHS data. Therefore we use the term *operating theatre* by default – but we also freely adopt the American term *operating room (OR)*. Similarly we use the terms *anaesthetist* and

consultant by default, but effortlessly switch to *anaesthesiologist* and *attending* when discussing US scenarios.

We focus much discussion on stereotypes of three patterns of surgical list: a 'typical UK NHS list', a 'typical US list' and a 'typical UK private list'. As explained in Chapter 2 (Defining Efficiency), these notions are useful shorthand to show the extent of applications of several principles.

A second reason for UK focus is that the only other related book on the market (Kay, Fox & Urman's *Operating Room Leadership and Management*) is already very US-focussed – in fact to the extent of having limited practical application in the United Kingdom. This book therefore provides a counterbalance and different perspective. The two books should be read in conjunction. Taken together they offer a comprehensive and complementary approach to operating room management. Indeed, one purpose of this book is to show how principles of management focussed on the United Kingdom NHS are nevertheless applicable to a wide range of countries in a wide variety of scenarios, including those encountered in the United States. Readers should constantly look for ways of adapting the principles to their own situation.

The chapters from international contributors take these principles further (Chapters 9–13). They demonstrate that many of the problems encountered by healthcare systems in the United States, the Netherlands, Belgium and Australia are common to those faced in the United Kingdom. The tariff structure in Queensland, Australia, discussed in Chapter 12, bears striking similarities (and shares deficiencies) with the NHS 'Payment by Results', discussed in Chapter 7 (Theatre Finances). The chapter on theatres in New Zealand (Chapter 9) shows how the principles in this book can be usefully adopted worldwide.

Patients

This book is a dispassionate analysis of the tactical methods available to maximise our use of operating theatre resources. This does not capture the patient experience. Yet the book often describes shortcomings or failures of the service. When this happens it is patients who are at the sharp end, and it is they, and not anyone else, who so often do the suffering. We must never forget that, however sophisticated our analyses or distant the mathematics in this book might seem from real life, its fundamental purpose is the improvement of patient care.

Bibliography

Ben-Tovim DI, Bassham JE, Bolch D, Martin MA, Dougherty M, Szwarcbord M. 2007. Lean thinking across a hospital: redesigning care at the Flinders Medical Centre. *Australian Health Reviews* 31: 10–5.

Brady JE, Allen TT. 2006. Six Sigma literature: a review and agenda for future research. *Quality and Reliability Engineering International* 22: 335–67.

Buhaug H. 2002. Long waiting lists in hospitals. *British Medical Journal* 324: 252–3.

Castille K, Gowland B, Walley P. 2002. Variability must be managed to reduce waiting times and improve care. *British Medical Journal* 324: 1336.

Chalice R. 2008. *Improving Healthcare Using Toyota Lean Production Methods*, 2nd edn. Milwaukee: Quality Press.

Chassin MR. 1998. Is health care ready for Six Sigma quality? *The Milbank Quarterly* 76: 565–91.

Coffey D. 2005. Matching strategies in car assembly: the BMW-Rover-Toyota complex. *International Journal of Automotive Technology and Management* 3: 320–35.

Coffey D. 2006. *The Myth of Japanese Efficiency: The Car Industry in a Globalising Age*. Cheltenham: Edward Elgar.

Gallivan S, Utley M, Treasure T, Valencia O. 2002. Booked inpatient admissions and hospital capacity: mathematical modeling study. *British Medical Journal* 24: 280–2.

Kay AD, Fox CJ, Urman RD 2012. *Operating Room Leadership and Management*. Cambridge: Cambridge University Press.

Martin RM, Sterne JAC, Gunnell D, Ebrahim S, Smith GD, Frankel S. 2003. NHS waiting lists and evidence of national or local failure: analysis of health service data. *British Medical Journal* 326: 188–98.

Martin S, Smith PC. 1999. Rationing by waiting lists: an empirical investigation. *Journal of Public Economics* 7: 141–64.

Morton A, Cornwell J. 2009. What's the difference between a hospital and a bottling factory? *British Medical Journal* 339: 428–30.

Rogers H, Warner J, Steyn R, Silvester K, Pepperman M, Nash R. 2002. Booked inpatient admissions and hospital capacity: mathematical model misses the point. *British Medical Journal* 324: 1336.

Silvester K, Lendon R, Bevan H, Steyn R, Walley P. 2004. Reducing waiting times in the NHS: is lack of capacity the problem? *Clinicians in Management* 12: 105–11.

Street A, Duckett S. 1996. Are waiting lists inevitable? *Health Policy* 36: 1–5.

Vest JR, Gamm LD. 2009. A critical review of the research literature on Six Sigma, Lean and StuderGroup's Hardwiring Excellence in the United States: the need to demonstrate and communicate the effectiveness of transformation strategies in healthcare. *Implementation Science* 4: 35–43.

Winch S, Henderson AJ. 2009. Making cars and making health care: a critical review. *Medical Journal of Australia* 191: 28–9.

Womack JP, Jones DT, Roos D. 1990. *The Car That Changed the World: The Story of Lean Production*. New York: Harper-Collins.

Worthington D. 1991. Hospital waiting list management models. *The Journal of the Operational Research Society* 42: 833–43.

Chapter 2

Defining 'Efficiency'

Jaideep J. Pandit

Surgical Operating Lists: The Different and International Scenarios

The purpose of this book, like the efforts of theatre managers and those who work in operating rooms (ORs), is to achieve an 'efficient' surgical operating list. But what is an 'operating list', and what is 'efficient'? Simple though it might seem superficially, it is necessary to define these terms so we can all agree on what we are talking about and what we are trying to achieve. Most of our discussion relates to 'elective' surgery. This is where cases are planned in advance, ideally at the time to suit the patient. In Appendix 2E, we consider issues pertaining to the concept of efficiency applied to emergency surgery, where cases require operating promptly.

A 'Typical' NHS List in the United Kingdom

We first consider what a 'surgical operating list' means in the United Kingdom (UK) National Health Service (NHS). An elective surgical list is a list of patients to be operated on within a given operating room, usually serviced by a single surgical–anaesthetic–theatre staff team. Thus on a certain Monday in OR6, Mr Smith (a consultant general surgeon, with perhaps a trainee resident surgeon) operates with his anaesthetist (Dr Brown, a consultant, who may also be accompanied by a trainee resident, and always assisted by an anaesthetic nurse or practitioner) and a surgical scrub team (whose individuals may change from week to week but are all suitably trained; Figure 2.1). The list will be scheduled to be of a certain known duration (e.g., 4, 8, 10 or rarely 12 hours), and the patients will be listed, on a physical sheet of paper matching any electronic records, by their name, identifiers (date of birth, hospital number, etc.) and the operation they are to have. There may be additional details relating to particular features (obesity, need for post-operative high-dependency care, special surgical instruments, need for X-ray, etc.). An example of operations listed may be: inguinal hernia, then varicose veins, then femoral hernia, etc.

For such a list, there will be a known start time, such as 08.30. Within the NHS it is not in fact universally specified whether 08.30 refers to the time the first incision is made, or to the start of anaesthesia, or something else. Local norms apply, and individual hospitals may have their own agreements or common understanding, but these are rarely strictly enforced. Commonly the agreed start time of 08.30 is taken to refer to the start of anaesthesia when the first patient of the day arrives in the anaesthetic room. In some centres the start time can be as late as 09.00. Consenting of the patients by the teams takes place before then, as does the WHO (World Health Organization) preoperative meeting. Given that the scheduled duration of length of the list is known (e.g., for an 8-hour list, the operations should all have finished by 16.30), at the end of the day there will either be an 'underrun' (if the list finishes before 16.30) or an overrun (if it finishes after 16.30). Of course, it might exactly finish on time at precisely 16.30, but that degree of precision is rare.

Because all NHS hospitals have such a high demand for surgery, there is always a waiting list; patients can wait weeks, months or even years to have the operation for which they were scheduled. This means that each surgical team or surgeon can be reliably allocated their list and can reliably fill it with cases, month after month, year after year. There is almost never an occasion when they do not have patients to fill the time allocated. This also means that individual surgeons can be allocated fixed operating days: e.g., Mr Smith every Monday, Ms Jones every Tuesday and so on.

This description may apply to patterns in many other countries. We will discuss later what 'efficiency' means in the context of such a list.

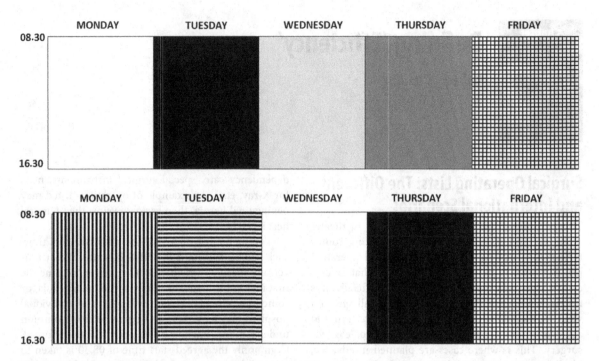

Figure 2.1 Illustration of organisation of a typical NHS list for a single OR over 5 days of a week. The times from 08.30 to 16.30 are shown on the side, with each day of the week, Mon–Fri shown for an OR. The top panel shows that, for each day, a different anaesthetist (along with different anaesthetic nurse and scrub team) are assigned to the OR. The bottom panel shows that each surgeon is also given their day in the same OR. This day-of-the-week assignment will not change (so Surgeon Black will always be on Thursdays, along with Anaesthetist Grey, and so on). In some centres, it is possible that anaesthetists will change the surgeon they work with week on week, but the surgeon assignment to a given OR will always be the same. Top panel: Anaesthetist allocations (different shade = different anaesthetist) Bottom panel: Surgeon allocations (different shade = different surgeon)

A 'Typical' US List

The US exhibits considerable variation in patterns. Some may be close to what was described earlier, for the NHS in the United Kingdom. However, there are several ways in which the situation differs. Because US surgeons have a more variable caseload, they cannot guarantee to fill a regular allocation of time with cases each week. Second, the US system is designed to provide access to surgery very quickly, as soon as is possible from scheduling the patient for an operation. Therefore, a surgeon may operate on three cases on a Monday, then do a clinic on a Tuesday where they book one patient for surgery and operate on that patient on the Wednesday. In other words, from the surgeon's perspective, a 'list' may vary considerably day to day or week to week in its size and duration (Figure 2.2, lower panel).

However, the surgeon will nevertheless be assigned to a certain (not always the same) OR (let's call it OR6 for this example), which will be staffed by an anaesthesiologist and scrub team (Figure 2.2, upper panel). This may be a trainee resident, or a nurse anaesthetist, supervised by an attending who in turn may be supervising more than one OR. (Note that UK anaesthetic consultants rarely if ever supervise more than one OR.) Therefore from the anaesthesia-scrub perspective, the 'list' is viewed as 'all the surgical activity in OR6 for the scheduled duration of operating', regardless of how many different surgical specialties use that OR.

It follows that from the perspective of the hospital, the particular OR will underrun if the operations are complete before the scheduled finish time and overrun if they are complete after the scheduled finish time. However, because the attending anaesthesiologist is supervising more than one OR, they will not finish their day until all their ORs are finished. Therefore, if they are supervising, say, four ORs and three

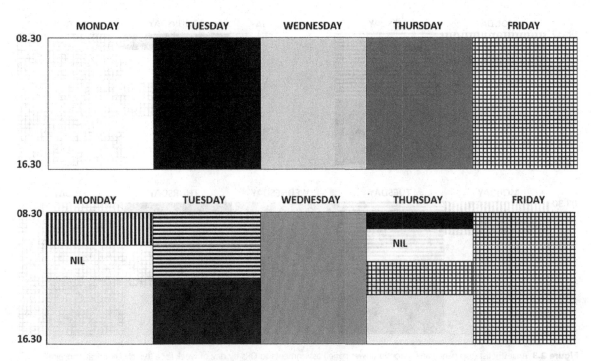

Figure 2.2 Arrangement of one type of a 'typical US list'. As for the UK NHS list in Figure 2.1, the anaesthesiologist and theatre staff team assignment is fixed for any given day to one OR (upper panel; the specific OR assignment may change week on week). However, while the block time for the OR as a whole is constant, different surgeons operate at different times (lower panel). Each shade represents a different surgeon, and the blocks marked 'nil' represent gaps where the OR has no scheduled cases.

underrun but one overruns, they – as an individual anaesthesia provider – have in fact overstayed their contracted time, even though the majority of their ORs were underused.

Consequently, perspectives of what is 'efficient' can vary across the staff groups, and between staff and the hospital. From the surgeon's perspective efficiency is likely to be related to measures like the speed of access to surgery from the time of outpatient clinic booking, or prompt start of cases so there is no in-theatre delay, or flexibility in accommodating a highly variable surgical schedule, enabling access to an OR any day of the week. From the hospital perspective, the efficient state is one where all the ORs made available to surgical faculty are as fully used with cases with no over-running. From an anaesthesiologist's perspective, efficiency may be being fully engaged in activity throughout the day (i.e., with no downtime where there is no surgery), and finishing on time without overrun.

A Typical Small Private Hospital List in the United Kingdom

In the United Kingdom, hospital consultants are allowed to undertake private practice so long as it does not interfere with their NHS work. Private work is often located in smaller hospitals that do not generally have an intensive care unit; the cases tend to be day cases or short-stay cases in a fitter population than is encountered in the NHS. Consultant surgeons and anaesthetists are not employed by these private hospitals, but have 'admitting rights'; i.e., rights to practise there. Whereas patients are not charged for NHS treatment, they are for private health care, with fees paid to surgeon, anaesthetist and private hospital either directly or via an insurer. The perceived advantage is that private treatment guarantees treatment by a consultant, whereas in the NHS care may be given primarily by a trainee resident, albeit one supervised by a consultant.

Because overall, private health care forms only a small proportion (~10%) of the overall market,

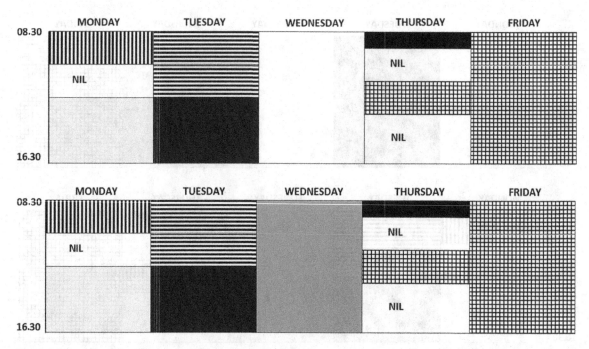

Figure 2.3 Anaesthetist (top panel) and surgeon (lower panel) assignments to ORs by day of week for a 'typical UK private hospital'. Note that each surgeon works with their own anaesthetist, so the shades for surgeon correspond to those of anaesthetist (e.g., Surgeon Grey always works with Anaesthetist Grey) etc. Of course, depending on availability, Anaesthetist Grey may ask a colleague to cover (e.g., during vacation) or in turn cover another anaesthetist's work, by mutual agreement (e.g., on Wednesday Anaesthetist White is covering Anaesthetist Grey's normal work). Sections marked 'nil' represent no activity.

a typical surgeon's caseload in a private hospital is likely to be very variable week on week, similar in that regard to the typical US list described earlier. Moreover, a consultant surgeon will generally work with the same consultant anaesthetist (in part because, as they both arrange their schedules so as to avoid conflict with NHS duties, they are available for private work at similar times). A given private OR may therefore facilitate Surgeon A accompanied by Anaesthetist A for an hour, followed by Surgeon B accompanied by Anaesthetist B for 4 hours, and so on (Figure 2.3). The private hospital will need to provide the OR and associated staff, including an anaesthetic nurse/practitioner, but the dilemma for the hospital will be whether to make these resources available for the whole day, or only for part of a day. If employed for a whole day, then on many days there may be very little work for these staff to undertake. Sometimes, therefore, these private hospitals make use of contractual arrangements that ensure a minimum hours commitment, with additional payments made at

more premium rates if staff make themselves available when needed. These aspects of the 'small UK private hospital' are therefore very different from both the typical UK NHS hospital and the typical US hospital described earlier.

Consequently there are different perspectives on what is 'efficient' in this context. Broadly from the surgeon/anaesthetist perspective the efficiency relates to how quickly from booking a patient can receive the operation and how flexible the hospital is in accommodating the surgery on any given day at any given time. From the hospital perspective, the challenge is to accommodate as many surgeons as possible reliably into one OR (rather than, say, staff several ORs in parallel for only a few hours each day).

The Emergency List

In many hospitals, emergency cases (unwell or critically ill patients who are not scheduled for surgery, but who arrive via the emergency department or as casualties) are undertaken on a dedicated list. This emergency list (there may be several such lists on any given day) is fully staffed by the required anaesthetists and nursing staff, 24 hours round the clock. Patient access to these lists is purely by urgency of the case and demand, and the relevant surgical subspecialties determine the order of the cases where several are booked at similar times.

By definition, the emergency list can be regarded as a 'stand-by' resource. Even if there are no emergency cases, the same provision of staff and resources will be needed. If there is a huge influx of emergency cases, and this is something known in advance or a regular occurrence, more than one emergency list may be required. For these reasons, it is difficult to assess whether or not an emergency list is being used 'efficiently'. However, these concepts have not been studied meaningfully to date, and the management of the emergency list is not a specific focus of this book. We discuss some considerations in Appendix 2E at the end of this chapter.

Summary Remarks on Types of 'Surgical List'

It should be apparent that the scenarios outlined earlier are stereotypes of 'extremes' of patterns that may be encountered. Hybrid patterns may also be possible. The point is that the theatre manager should become familiar with the system that operates within their particular environment and appreciate that definitions of 'efficiency' might differ accordingly, and also that notions of efficiency might vary from the different perspectives of surgeon, hospital, anaesthetist or theatre staff.

We discuss later the notion of efficiency in relation to the UK NHS surgical list model. We first outline flawed or erroneous measures of efficiency and then present a more accurate and workable measure that can be applied in practice.

Misleading Measures of Surgical List Efficiency in a Typical UK NHS List

In this section we discuss several erroneous potential measures of 'efficiency' of a surgical list. These fallacious measures include: utilisation, preventing cancellation, start times and profitability. We discuss why they are wrong, and in the next section introduce an unbiased measure of efficiency.

The Fallacy of 'Utilisation' as a Measure of 'Efficiency'

The typical UK surgical list as described earlier can be classed as a 'block time' list, where the surgical team is allocated on a particular day a fixed number of hours for operating. Some individual hospitals and even the United Kingdom's Department of Health suggest that the measure of maximally utilising the allocated time on the list is a good measure of efficiency (i.e., 90% utilisation of time means only 10% waste of time). Superficially this makes sense: if a team is allocated 8 hours but only uses 6 hours, this represents 25% wasted resource and if replicated across all lists would be a massive drain on the system. Consequently, the majority of UK NHS list performance is described using the metric of 'utilisation', expressed as a percentage of the scheduled list time.

However, the fallacy of doing this is readily explained. High utilisation can be easily achieved (and often is) by the simple expedient of overbooking the list with cases that could not possibly be completed within the allocated time. When the scheduled list time is utilised (100% utilisation), the remaining cases are cancelled. Thus although utilisation is high, this is at the expense of cancellation. This may not matter, if perversely the performance managers or health department are focussing only on utilisation. Clearly, though, this tactic is unhelpful and distressing to patients, and expensive for the organisation (for reasons we shall see later).

Second, high utilisation can be achieved through perverse behaviours such as working more slowly. If, say, a surgical team finds they have underbooked their list and fear repercussions of underrunning, they simply operate very slowly and reach their 'target' finish time. This helps no one.

Third, high utilisation can only consistently be obtained by overrunning. No planning is ever perfect, so precisely 100% utilisation of a list is unlikely. For any given team, some lists will have <100% utilisation and therefore, if the team is to average high utilisation then at least some of the lists must overrun with >100% utilisation. But does overrunning one list yield benefits that 'compensate' for the detrimental effects of underrunning another? Modest degrees of overrunning might be necessary to prevent cancellation of some of the remaining patients on that same list. Completing as many surgeries as possible also potentially accrues more income to the organisation.

However, on the other hand there are potent reasons why overrunning is so detrimental as to eliminate any possible gains.

First, there is a powerful logical argument. If overrunning were always advantageous then we should always do it. And if we should always do it, then why bother scheduling anything at all? Simply book whichever cases we like, in whatever order or manner and work until they are all complete. It is self-evident that this is a recipe for organisational chaos. Indeed, it is impossible to employ staff or organise a service on this basis. Occasional overruns are inevitable (as are underruns), for example, when something unforeseen happens that causes delay (or of foreshortening of the list, in case of underrun). But consistent overrunning undermines the very purpose of scheduling anything in the first place.

The reason why hospitals need to schedule lists to certain published times is that (regardless of their funding arrangements, public or private), they need to budget for them. This includes the employment and contracting of staff to those stated times. Thus, a surgical list starting at, say, 08.00 hours and ending at 16.00 hours will have the associated cost of 8 hours of staffing, lighting, heating, equipment and so on. The hospital finance department will register this cost as a recurrent expense in the ledger, and so they will know that any income from surgeries performed will offset this degree of expenditure. An overrun will accrue unplanned, unbudgeted expenditure (staff overtime, additional equipment, consumables, heating, lighting, etc.). The finance department will need to find additional income (not part of its original plan) to cover this unforeseen expense.

Moreover, staff overtime always costs more than fully utilising staff within their contracted hours. If it did not, then it would, of course, make sense for the employer to do more work in overtime (at the putative cheaper rates of pay) than within contracted hours. In other words, overtime pay forms an incentive for staff to stay late if they need to, and a disincentive for the employer to create situations where work overruns its scheduled time. It is less likely that an employer will gain a profit from work in overtime. The pay in an overrun is compensation for workers, rather than an incentive to work late, because there are other costs to employees in the form of physical exhaustion, disruption to personal lives, additional costs of childcare, etc. That said, there has historically been one curious situation where overtime pay was

less than within-contract rates. In the UK NHS, trainee doctors up to the 1990s were paid only one-third the hourly rate of their regular income for overtime. This created an incentive for NHS employers to disregard other regulations on working time limits and led to overwork of this staff group. The service was therefore built upon cheap labour. Its fundamental unsustainability became evident when, in the mid-1990s, robust employment legislation emanating from the European Union (the Social Chapter and European Working Time Directive) introduced strict limits on working hours, with harsh penalties for transgression. In large part, this is the cause of the strains currently faced by the NHS in recent years. It has also led to national strikes by junior doctors in the United Kingdom that have been deeply damaging to morale and destabilising to running the service. In summary, planning a service around overruns is unwise and counterproductive. Measuring surgical list performance by utilisation – and therefore regarding >100% as beneficial – is wrong.

The Fallacy of 'Preventing Cancellations' as a Measure of 'Efficiency'

If utilisation is a poor measure of efficiency and cancellation so important, it would seem a simple matter of using operation cancellation rate as the relevant single metric of efficiency. Yet this leads to its own fallacy.

First is the question of whether cancellation of a major case expected to last several hours for which support services like post-operative high dependency care or intensive care have been booked (e.g., oesophagectomy) is equivalent to cancelling a short day case (e.g., diagnostic staging laparoscopy). For two hypothetical lists consisting of one each of these cases, the measured cancellation rate will be 50%, regardless of which is cancelled on the day of surgery. Notwithstanding the fact that the emotional upset of the two patients may be similar, intuitively, we feel that the major case is somehow more 'important' than the smaller case. This importance is not reflected in the crude cancellation metric.

Second is the question of when cancellation 'counts' in our performance measure. Most often, analysis in the literature has focussed on cancellation on the day of surgery, or sometimes only after the patient has entered the hospital. Yet, from the patient perspective plans need to be made from the time they are told to arrive for surgery, which may be weeks before the surgery date. Any change to plans from the moment they are told is disruptive and should be counted as a 'cancellation'. Or perhaps classed as a lesser category of 'change of plan'.

Third is the issue that several factors can lead to cancellation, not all of which are under the direct control of the surgical–anaesthetic team on the day of surgery. While factors such as poor scheduling of the list can be regarded as the responsibility of the surgical team, poor preoperative preparation cannot (resting as it should with the separate preassessment team; see Chapter 8). Communication errors leading, for example, to patients not being starved or arriving on the wrong day may be the fault of other hospital departments. Table 2.1 lists some of the reasons for cancellation documented in extensive literature. Thus cancellation might be a useful measure of the overall hospital performance in respect of surgery, but less useful as a marker for performance of any individual team.

Fourth, introducing cancellation as a performance measure can lead to perverse behaviours. Teams might then underbook their lists, to avoid overrunning as a cause of cancellation. Or they might be highly selective in cases, i.e., operating only on the very healthy, so as to avoid cancellation due to poor preoptimisation of medical conditions. Or, even where key results are absent or the patient is not optimised, they might operate anyway knowing that it is the cancellation metric, not any patient outcome metric, by which they are judged. All of these behavioural responses are undesirable.

The Fallacy of 'Starting on Time' as a Measure of 'Efficiency'

Late departures are a relatively good metric for buses, trains and aeroplanes, so why not for surgical theatres? Prompt starts of the day to operating lists would seem important. If a list starts late, it should be expected to finish late, causing an overrun, which, as we have discussed earlier, is bad. A late start is also akin to underutilisation of resources as no work is being done. There are several reasons why, in fact, late starts are also a fallacious measure of overall efficiency.

A prompt start is important if – and only if – the operating list is scheduled properly in the first place and can be expected to finish to time. In the case of a train or plane travelling at a generally fixed speed between two points, a delayed start will inevitably cause a delayed arrival. However if, akin to an overbooked surgical list, the train or plane is asked to double its travelling distance then a delayed start will not matter: it will always arrive late at its now further destination because it cannot or should not travel faster than is safe or possible . Equally, an underbooked surgical list will always finish early, almost regardless of the start time.

In other words, if there is a hypothetical surgical list scheduled for 8 hours duration on which ~12 hours of surgery has been booked, there is no reason (other than adherence to their personal professional standards) for staff to make undue effort to start on time; this list will finish late, regardless. Equally if this same list is booked with just ~4 hours of surgery, then

Table 2.1 Causes of cancellation on day of surgery

Patient does not arrive for surgery
Patient declines consent for surgery
Operation no longer needed
Key members of staff not available, off sick or staff shortages
Equipment unavailable
Patient not optimised for surgery (missing results, treatments, case notes, medications taken that should have been omitted)
Operation deemed no longer necessary
Surgical list overrunning
High dependency or intensive care bed (if needed) unavailable
Funding for surgery unavailable (for private/fee-paying patients)

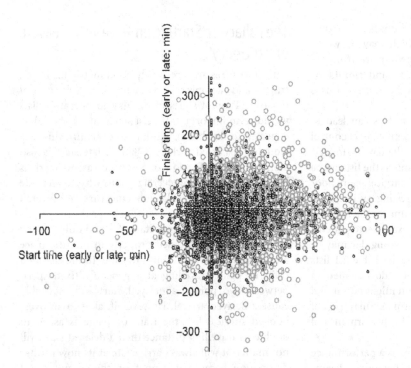

Figure 2.4 Lack of correlations between start time (*x*-axis) and finish time (*y*-axis) for >7,000 surgical lists studied at two large hospitals in the United Kingdom (white and grey dots, respectively). Each dot is a list. Note that a delayed start does not lead to a late finish, or an early start to an early finish.

again, why bother to rush to start on time, as either way the team will finish early?

In this way, delayed starts can be viewed as we might regard a fever in clinical practice. Treating the fever alone does not make the patient better as there is some other underlying cause that must be addressed (e.g., an infection). Delayed starts may be a thermometer that indicates some other process problem, but simply forcing a prompt start will not cure the service of its ills (just as merely bringing down the patient's temperature will not cure the infection).

Several large studies have shown that, in large part for these reasons there is no relationship between a late start and a late finish: see Pandit et al. (2012) for a detailed analysis. Figure 2.4 illustrates data from two large hospitals, to emphasise the point.

Start times can be difficult to define and, hence, to enforce at the local level. This is because different staff groups can have a different understanding of when a list 'starts'. The scrub staff's theatre day in reality starts early (e.g., 07.30 in a hypothetical hospital) as they have morning coordination meetings, they turn on the power, check the equipment, start to obtain the surgical trays, etc., needed for the day's operating. If they turn up later than 07.30, then other things will be delayed. The anaesthetists' day in this same hospital starts at, say, 08.00, when they visit and consent the

first patients on the ward. Then, anaesthesia induction may commence at 08.30. Again, any delay to their visiting the patient or commencing induction leads to later delays. The surgeons' day might begin with a short visit to the first patient anytime before anaesthesia induction. This visit is not time-critical because the patient would already have been seen and consented in surgical clinic, days or weeks before, but let us suppose it occurs also at 08.00. Then there is a gap to the surgeon's work until anaesthesia is complete and the patient is on the operating table – only then is the surgical team actually required (e.g., 09.00). Only if the surgeon is late at that point will things be delayed. Even then, it may take over 30 min to position the patient correctly, and then perform any preoperative checks that can only be done in sterile conditions, such that 'knife to skin', the start of surgery, may occur at 09.30. Which of all these times should be the hospital's reference 'start time'? (In this example we have overlooked the time at which the team needs to perform the WHO premeeting, which is usually after surgeon and anaesthetist have seen the patient, but before patient is brought to theatre for surgery).

Within this complex scheme, let us label the start of anaesthesia induction the 'anaesthesia start time', and label the start of surgery 'knife to skin' as the 'surgery start time'. It can readily be seen that the 'anaesthetist start time' and 'surgeon start time' are intimately linked. Fixing an anaesthesia start time automatically means that surgery start time is variable because it depends upon how long anaesthesia takes. Longer anaesthesia times can occur with high-risk patients (e.g., airway management difficulties) or major surgery (insertion of invasive monitoring lines) or operations requiring specific post-operative pain management techniques (e.g., insertion of regional blockade). Conversely, fixing a surgical start time automatically means that the anaesthesia start time must be variable, dependent upon the estimated time anaesthesia will take for the first patient. This underlines the fallacy of using start times as a measure of efficiency.

For any hospital to say 'we always start surgery at fixed time X' ' means that someone else (anaesthesia) is starting much earlier and has no fixed start time. For another hospital to say 'we always start anaesthesia at fixed time X' ' means that someone else (surgery) is waiting for a variable length of time to start. Appendix 2A outlines a case study related to managing start times.

The Fallacy of 'Financial Efficiency' as a Measure of Surgical List Efficiency: A Typical US List

It has been suggested by Dexter and colleagues, focussing on US work (McIntosh et al., 2006), that efficiency for a surgical list can be described very simply by a formula:

$$\text{Efficiency} = [\text{cost of underrunning}] - [\text{cost of overrunning}]$$

Equation 2.1

Where costs in this formula are measured in the prevailing currency ($ or £ or €). Because the cost per minute of overrun is generally 1.5–2 times as expensive as the cost per minute of scheduled time, the simplest strategy for any theatre manager to adopt to achieve surgical list efficiency, is to prevent overruns. This might be achieved, for example, by moving cases from potentially overrunning ORs to currently underrunning ones, or by amending schedules for persistently overrunning lists such that these are scheduled to last longer (e.g., 10 or 12 hours instead of 8 hours).

While this formula is superficially simple, and also true to the extent that ultimately efficiency ought to be related to costs, there are shortcomings.

The first and most obvious limitation is are that 'costs' in the formula must be known. If costs are not known, then the formula is useless. Knowing costs is not always easy, as we will discuss in Chapter 7. In essence, it can be very difficult if not impossible to disentangle 'costs of the theatre' from other hospital- or surgical-related costs, and how costs are apportioned within an organisation makes a great deal of difference to the outcomes yielded by Equation 2.1.

Second, the formula makes no acknowledgement of the fact that cancellation is one potential consequence of a late-running list and carries a cost independent of overrunning. Equation 2.1 only factors in overrunning. If two parallel lists overrun equally they are regarded in Equation 2.1 as equally inefficient. Yet if one of these lists cancels a patient, we would instinctively regard that list is more inefficient for the same degree of overrun.

To take this point further, cancellation can be a tactic to prevent overrunning. Consider two parallel lists: one overruns but completes its cases; the other finishes on time because it cancels the last case. Equation 2.1 regards the first list as more inefficient – but should it not be the second list, because this list completed fewer cases?

Cancellation not only carries a separate tangible cost (lost revenue), but it also carries intangible cost (inconvenience to patient, reputation damage to organisation, etc.).

Finally, the overall efficiency as calculated by Equation 2.1 depends upon the actual costs involved. Let us suppose that there are two identical lists based in different healthcare settings. In one the cost of overrunning is 2.5 times that of underrunning; but in the other the cost of overrunning is just 1.01 times that of underrunning. An equivalent overrun will yield a result of extreme inefficiency in the first instance, but a trivial inefficiency in the second. Therefore, the formula is not unbiased, but very dependent upon a single factor (namely, absolute cost).

Unbiased Measure of Efficiency, ε

The dilemma appears to be that each of the superficially intuitive measures of efficiency are mutually exclusive. Aim for full utilisation, and this can lead to overbooking to achieve this and high cancellations. Aim to reduce cancellations, and this can lead to underbooking to ensure all the cases can easily be done. Aim to minimise overrunning, and this can also lead to underbooking. And so on. Any potential measure will need to take all these elements into account, whilst not creating perverse incentives.

A starting point is a statement we can all agree on as a definition of an efficient surgical list is:

A surgical list is most efficient when all the scheduled time is utilised, without overrun and without cancellation.

This incorporates the three key elements: 'utilisation', 'cancellation' and 'avoidance of overrun'. It is possible to convert this sentence into a mathematical equation as follows:

$$Efficiency, \varepsilon = \left[\left(\begin{array}{c} fraction\ of \\ scheduled\ time \\ utilised \end{array} \right) - \left(\begin{array}{c} fraction\ of \\ scheduled\ time \\ overrunning \end{array} \right) \right] \times \left(\begin{array}{c} fraction\ of \\ scheduled\ cases \\ completed \end{array} \right)$$

Equation 2.2

By converting quantities to fractions, this formula enables us to factor in both utilisation and overrunning in an unbiased way. The 'fraction of scheduled time utilised' means that if a list scheduled for 8 h finishes in 6 h, this quantity is ¾, or 0.75, and the 'fraction of scheduled time overrunning' for this list is zero. The 'fraction of scheduled time overrunning' means that if a list scheduled for 8 h overruns by 2 h, this quantity is ¼, or 0.25, and the fraction of scheduled time utilised for this list = 1. Thus the first two terms operate in a mutually exclusive manner: i.e., a single list cannot be both under- or overutilised at the same time. The 'fraction of scheduled operations completed' means that if four of five of the patients booked onto the list have their operations (i.e., one patient is cancelled), this quantity is 4/5, or 0.80.

The formula theoretically yields a result for efficiency ranging from 0 to 1.0 (or 0–100% if this result is multiplied by 100). The value of 100% is obtained when all booked cases are complete at the scheduled time. The formula can also give 'credit' for a list that completes its own booked cases early (e.g., four cases) and accepts and completes extra cases (e.g., a fifth case from another list). Thus a number >1 in the last term

(i.e., the fraction of patients completed = 1.25 for this example) could translate as an efficiency >100% for that particular list.

Clearly, an efficiency of 100% is the ultimate goal, but in practice is unlikely for every list. An efficiency of 80% is equivalent to one patient in five being cancelled on a list and seems unacceptable. An efficiency of 90% equates to one patient in 10 cancelled and is better. Such considerations lead us to suggest that 85% efficiency is the very minimum that should be attained, with > 90% being highly desirable.

The ε calculator tool yields the relevant statistics for minutes of late start, minutes late finish, % cancellation and efficiency, ε (see: www.cambridge.org/9781316646830).

Can Efficiency ε Ever Be > 100%?

Although it seems odd to imagine what efficiency more than 100% might mean, Equation 2.2 allows for it in the specific circumstance that a team not only completes their own work but also takes on additional cases from neighbouring ORs, or from the emergency list, whilst still completing its work in a timely manner. Thus, the proportion of scheduled cases completed in such a case would be >100%, and even if there is a modest overrun, or underrun, ε would be >100%.

Taking on extra cases is also one means of mitigating deleterious effects on ε of over- or underruns, or by replacing one's own cancelled cases. So Equation 2.2 demonstrates considerable flexibility in its application.

Equation 2.2 has been embedded into the ε Calculator – an Excel tool – for use with this book. Appendix 2A explains step-by-step how to use it (see: www.cambridge.org/9781316646830).

Advantages of Efficiency ε

The advantages of ε are self-evident. As a balanced measure incorporating the key elements contributing to a universal understanding of efficiency, it does not favour one element over another. A team seeking to improve its ε score by overrunning will only find ε declining; a team underbooking cases to minimise cancellation will find its ε lower if it then underruns. And so on. In other words, there is no ready means of 'gaming' behaviours artificially to maximise ε. The only way that teams can achieve high ε is by trying to utilise their list maximally, whilst avoiding overruns and cancellations.

Furthermore, the ε equation can be easily modified to take into account local factors or strategies that inherently (dis)favour one element over another by adding constant a, b and c to each of terms. These constants can have any values 0–∞ depending upon the weight to be given to that factor:

someone argues that each of full utilisation and preventing overruns and avoiding cancellation are all extremely and equivalently important and therefore constants a, b and c should each be assigned a value of 10 in Equation 2.3, then that is the same as each of these factors having a value of 1 (i.e., the same as Equation 2.2). Second, excessive weighting of one factor essentially negates or eliminates the others and makes the formula as a whole redundant. Thus, if someone argues that avoiding overruns is the only thing that really matters and so assigns constant b a value of 100 (constants a and c being 1), then there is little point in having a formula at all to influence tactics; one might as well simply say 'never overrun'.

$$Weighted \ efficiency, \varepsilon = \left[a \begin{pmatrix} fraction \ of \\ scheduled \ time \\ utilised \end{pmatrix} - b \begin{pmatrix} fraction \ of \\ scheduled \ time \\ overrunning \end{pmatrix} \right] \times c \begin{pmatrix} fraction \ of \\ scheduled \ cases \\ completed \end{pmatrix}$$

Equation 2.3

For example, we can imagine a system in which it is really important to avoid overrun, even if it means tending to underrun. Then, constant b in Equation 2.3 might be assigned a value of 2. Thus, a 2-hour overrun on an 8-hour list becomes a fraction of ½, or 0.5, rather than ¼, or 0.25, in the original formula in Equation 2.2. Efficiency ε is thus influenced more by the overrun than by other factors. Or, if cancellations are to be avoided over other elements, constant c in Equation 2.3 could be duly weighted.

There are several rationales for such weighting. For example, if overrunning costs twice as much as underrunning (due to overtime costs) and achieving financial balance is an overriding priority, then weighting constant b by assigning it a value of 2 seems rational. This discussion underlines the distinction between 'strategic' and 'tactical' considerations outlined in Chapter 1. The questions of achieving financial balance as an overrising priority – or instead above all else, avoiding cancellations – are strategic questions, and therefore not of relevance to this book. It is up to each organisation or health system to set its own priorities. The efficiency formula ε describes the appropriate, objective, quantified tactics to achieve whichever strategic objective has been decided.

It is worth making two comments on weighting. First, there is, of course, no point in weighting everything; then nothing is really weighted. Thus, if

A further advantage of ε is that it is related to financial balance of the surgical list. We explore finances in more detail in Chapter 7. Briefly, as we earlier discussed, hospitals budget for the given list schedule: anything that runs over this time is an added unbudgeted expense; anything that underruns this time wastes the invested resources. Therefore, the point at which the invested budget is met or recouped must by definition be at the maximum ε of 100%.

Limitations of ε

Although we stated earlier that ε cannot be 'gamed', there is one potential way that a high ε might be achieved through little utilisation of the list. The efficiency score ε does not explicitly take into account 'gaps' within a list. Gaps are the non-productive periods between cases, when no anaesthesia or surgery takes place, or when theatre staff are not checking equipment, opening packs, etc. In other words the whole team is perhaps sitting drinking coffee. Thus, it is theoretically conceivable that an anaesthetic-surgical team could start a list scheduled for 8 hours with two patients. The team starts on time with one patient whose operation takes just one hour. Then, for whatever reason there is a gap of 6 hours in which the team drinks coffee, and the next (final) patient's operation is commenced, which also takes one hour. So on the face of it, this list has started on time, finished on time, and suffered no cancellations. Yet, ascribing it to be 100% efficient seems inappropriate. For example, another parallel list that had the same two cases but finished just 2 hours after a prompt start would be ascribed an efficiency of just 25%, because it would be deemed to have finished 6 hours early. However, this scenario is extremely rare, for the simple reason that human behaviour is such that teams do not simply wish to stay late when they can finish early, and also because the pressures on the system are such that 'open' theatres are commonly filled with cases from other theatres, including emergency cases, regardless of whether that 'open' time is in the middle of the list or at the end. That said, Chapter 3 on *Productivity* shows how even this rare factor can be taken into account.

Using Efficiency ε in Practice: Graphical Displays

Isogram Plots

An isogram is a line on a plot joining points with equal values. The efficiency Equation 2.2 can be plotted as a graph, with the *x*-axis being the list utilisation (or time since start of the list), and the *y*-axis is ε. For any prevailing level of cancellation, the result of a list's performance will lie on a line that forms a triangle (Figure 2.5).

Let us suppose there is no cancellation on the day of surgery. The team starts to operate, and as it does so, its performance rises (point a, Figure 2.5) on the ε plot. If all operations are complete by the scheduled time, then the team finishes its work at the peak of the triangle (point b, Figure 2.5). If, however, by this time the work is not complete and the list overruns, then it ends the day along the descending part of the triangle (point c, Figure 2.5). If there are cancellations, then the result of the list will lie within the largest triangle (e.g., point d, Figure 2.5, if only 80% of cases are completed).

The position of any single list plotted on the graph displayed in Figure 2.5 indicates approximately its performance in terms of utilisation and cancellation (Figure 2.6).

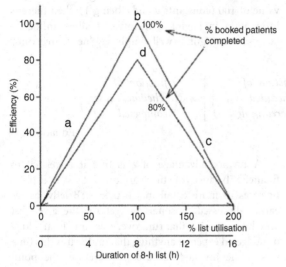

Figure 2.5 Graphical representation of Equation 2.2. Efficiency ε is plotted in % either against the percentage list utilisation, or a parallel *x*-axis indicating the corresponding actual hours completed (that for an 8-hour list is shown). The percentage of booked operations completed (rates of 100% and 80% are shown, corresponding to cancellation rates of 0% and 20%, respectively) form 'isograms' for the relationship. Points a–d discussed in text.

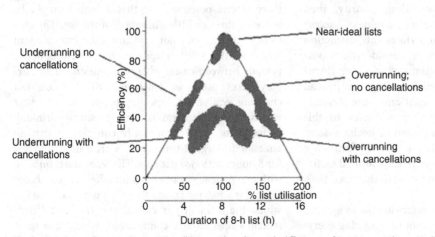

Figure 2.6 Same plot as in Figure 2.5 to illustrate where lists with different performances might generally lie.

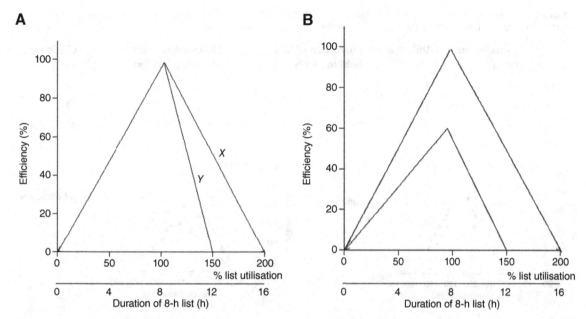

Figure 2.7. Panel A: ε in Equation 2.2 is weighted for overruns (slope *y*) such that there is a steeper decline in ε than in the unweighted formula (slope *x*). Panel B: in the inner isogram, ε is weighted both for cancellations, such that a 20% results in ε of 60% even when the list finishes on time (rather than 80% for unweighted formula; see Figure 2.5, point b); and also weighted for overrun such that there is a steeper decline in slope with overrun (see Panel A).

The isograms plots may also be adapted for the 'weighting' to the efficiency equation as discussed earlier. Thus, Figure 2.7A shows a weighting applied to overruns (i.e., overruns considered twice as adverse as underruns). The effect is a steeper downslope to the triangle than the upslope, such that a 4-hour overrun results in an ε score of zero, rather than 50% in the unweighted formula. Figure 2.7B shows weighting applied to both cancellation and overrun. Thus, a cancellation rate of 20% results in just 60% efficiency (not 80% for unweighted calculation). This is coupled with a weighted overrun.

Using Isograms Plots to Monitor and Influence Performance

Monitoring single teams. An isogram plot can be used to monitor the performance of a single team over time, as each of its lists is sequentially plotted on the same diagram. After a suitable period of monitoring, a picture might emerge of the team's performance and where problems might lie.

Table 2.2 shows some key performance data for three hypothetical lists. It is not clear from these – or perhaps only to the expert eye – which of these is the most efficient, or the precise reasons for any inefficiencies. It is only by then drawing the isograms' plots that a picture emerges of team performance (Figure 2.8). The characteristic of Team A is that it overruns: the main cluster of data points is at the downslope of the isograms (Figure 2.8A). There are some cancellations, but the prevailing ethos is one of completing the cases that have been scheduled. Further investigation reveals that the fundamental problem leading to this team's very low ε score is overbooking of cases. The schedulers are just too ambitious and optimistic. Although patients are not generally inconvenienced through cancellation on this list, because Team A works late to complete as much as is booked, there is organisation chaos (as the overruns impact on after-hours emergency operating) and additional expense (as staff claim overtime, and there is unbudgeted use of consumables). It is also unclear that this situation is sustainable in the long run, with staff exhaustion, or where current staff leave and new staff are unable or unwilling to meet the unexpected demands of this list. The theatre manager needs to focus on better scheduling to improve team performance.

Team B has a similar overall low efficiency as Team A but the isogram in Figure 2.8B reveals that it is for very different reasons. Here, the cluster of points lies well within the triangle denoting the 100% isograms: this means there is a high incidence of cancellation on each list. (For added clarity, the 70% isogram is also

Table 2.2 Key performance data for three hypothetical lists (*n* >20 for each team). For any given team, some data are striking but the picture is not revealed until the isograms plots are drawn (see Figure 2.5).

	Cancellation rate (%)	Utilisation (%)	Proportion of lists finishing early (%)	Proportion of lists finishing late (%)	Efficiency ε (%)
Team A	8	110	25	30	72
Team B	15	108	20	50	73
Team C	6	96	20	10	90

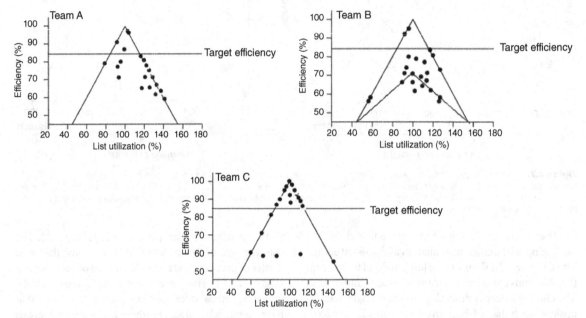

Figure 2.8 Isogram plots for the data in Table 2.2. There is an overlay of points, but the data represent *n* > 20 for each team. The different patterns exhibited by Teams A–C are discussed in text. A target efficiency horizontal line of 85% is drawn, and for Team B, a 70% isogram is also shown. Compare interpretation of team performance with Figure 2.6.

drawn in Figure 2.8B.) Overruns do occur, but are modest, and the prevailing characteristic is 'cancellation'. The fundamental reason, as it turned out after analysis, was poor preassessment of patients. The theatre manager's solution for this team should be a focus on improving preoperative preparation.

Team C represents a pragmatic ideal. The data points here are clustered around the top of the 100% isograms. Naturally there are inevitable cancellations, etc., but given the variation in performance that is expected, this is a well-performing list. If any intervention is to be made, it might be an exploration of productivity – adding more cases to the list (see Chapter 3).

Monitoring theatre suites or hospitals. A similar approach may be taken to analysing performance of a whole suite of theatres or hospitals. Table 2.3 and Figure 2.9 reproduce data from a study analysing

several thousand lists at two UK hospitals. The approach used reproduces that described by Pandit et al. (2012). Akin to the analysis in Table 2.2 and Figure 2.8, these hospitals have different ethos.

Whereas Hospital A has an ethos of completing all scheduled operations, almost regardless of how long they will take (note the considerable number of data points lying at almost twice the utilisation), Hospital B has the ethos of cancelling cases to avoid overrun (even if this means an underrun).

Dashboards and Statistical Process Control Charts

An alternative to the isograms plot is a 'dashboard'. In business, dashboards are visual displays of summary data that provide an 'at-a-glance' view of key

Table 2.3 Summary data for two UK hospitals (A and B) based on analysis of several thousand lists. Arbitrarily, a list was deemed to have finished early (or late) if it finished more than 10% outside the scheduled total list time.

	Cancellation rate (%)	Utilisation (%)	Proportion of lists finishing early	Proportion of lists finishing late	Efficiency ε (%)
Team A	1	105	2	32	83
Team B	10	83	39	5	81

Table 2.4 Summary data for a hypothetical team. Scheduled start time 08.00; end time 16.00; 480 min scheduled operating; always 8 patients scheduled

Day 1 Start 08.00; end 16.00; all 8 patients complete – ε = 100%

Day 2 Start 09.00; end 16.00; all 8 patients complete – ε = 88% (although all work has been done as on Day 1, 1 hour of theatre time was wasted through late start, so efficiency declines modestly)

Day 3 Start 09.00; end 18.00; all 8 patients complete – ε = 75% (the late start on Day 2 is now compounded by a late finish, so efficiency declines even further)

Day 4 Start 09.00; end 16.00; 6 patients complete – ε = 65% (the late finish on Day 3 is unsustainable, and patients are cancelled to end on time; efficiency falls dramatically)

Day 5 Start 08.00; end 16.00; 7 patients complete – ε = 88% (the team has resolved its start time issues and also achieves timely finishes, but can only really undertake 7 cases not 8 as originally thought; so it henceforth moves to booking just 7 patients; ε restored as a result)

Day 6 Start 09.00; end 16.00; all 7 patients complete – ε = 88% (this level of efficiency is sustainable and clearly relatively insensitive to start time)

Conclusion: With other issues resolved, from Day 6 the theatre manager needs to work with this team to identify the specific reasons for late starts. In the meantime efficiency is maintained by scheduling 7 not 8 cases. Later analysis shows the delay was due to a single blood test not being done in preoperative clinic, which then had to be done on day of surgery.

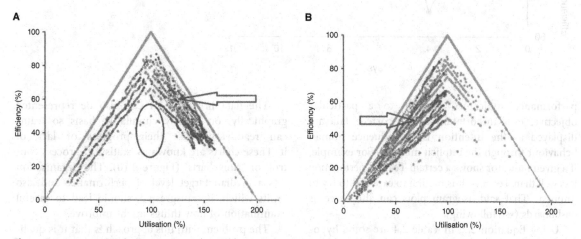

Figure 2.9 Isogram plots for the two hospitals in Table 2.3. Each point represents a single list. There is considerable overlap of data points (*n* > 3,500 in each panel). In the panel for Hospital A, the arrow shows where the concentration of data points lies, and the circle illustrates that relatively few data points lie within the 100% isogram triangle. In the panel for Hospital B, the arrow shows where the concentration of data points lies; well within the 100% isograms triangle and on its upslope. See also Figure 2.6 for interpretation of the scattergram plots.

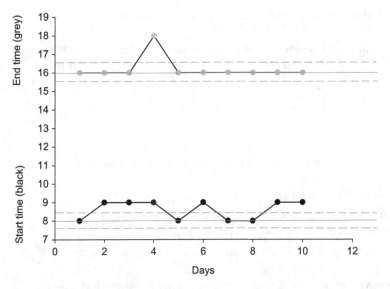

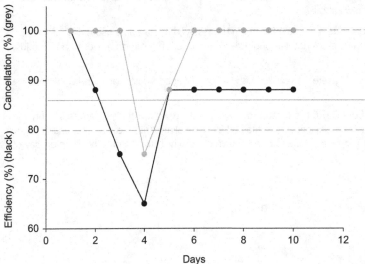

Figure 2.10 Statistical process control run charts of the data in Table 2.4. Days 7 onwards are when the hypothetical team reaches the sustainable and stable point. Top panels: start time (black) and end time (grey) are shown. The solid grey lines represent the median target value expected for the relative performance metric. The dashed lines are the limits of performance set by the organisation, exceeding which should trigger some investigation or analysis. Lower panel: efficiency (ε; in black) and cancellation rates (grey) for the days in question. There are several points to note. One is that end time does not correlate with start time (top panel); i.e., even when start time delayed, end time can be within schedule. Second, efficiency ε inexorably declines in the early days even though there is fluctuation in other metrics.

performance indicators relevant to a particular objective. It is important that the correct data are displayed as the intention is to influence human behaviour through the implicit message. For example, if a given indicator shows a certain Team B performing less well than Team A, it is natural to expect B to try to improve. That said, isogram plots can also serve as dashboards (see following).

Using Equation 2.2, in Table 2.4 are some hypothetical examples of a list over a period of several days, and how team behaviours might be influenced by the sequential results of ε (calculated using Equation 2.2).

The data in Table 2.4 can also be represented graphically, on a daily cumulative basis so teams can readily visualise their progress or lack of it. These charts are known as 'statistical process control' or 'run charts' (Figure 2.10). The organisation sets a median target level of performance and also limits which, if transgressed, should lead to careful examination of how things might improve.

The problem with this approach is that it is qualitative and not quantitative. Also, although it maps progress of a single team, it does not allow easily for direct comparison of data from different teams.

Applying ε Efficiency to Other Scenarios: A Typical US List

We now turn to another type of surgical list; the typical US list. Efficiency as described earlier using Equation 2.2 and ε is developed for list patterns resembling a 'typical UK NHS list'; that is, a block time for operating for 8, 10, 12 hours, etc., undertaken by a single surgical–anaesthetic–nursing team, the goal being to utilise the block time as fully as possible with no over-runs or cancellations. In a 'typical US list', there may be a block time assigned to a single OR, which is staffed by nursing and portering staff, and by a single anaesthesia team, but within this block time of 8, 10, 12 hours, etc., there may be several surgeons utilising portions of that time (and these portions varying day by day). In other words, for this typical US list, the understanding of 'block' differs according to perspective. From the perspective of the hospital or anaesthesiologist or OR team, the block is the whole time they are assigning to the OR time for the day. From the perspective of a surgeon, it is only the smaller block within this larger block that they are individually assigned.

It is possible and desirable to apply ε efficiency but with the modification that it must be viewed from these different perspectives. The ε efficiency from the perspective of the OR itself, the hospital, theatre staff or anaesthesia team (ε-OR) is essentially the same as in the case of a typical UK NHS hospital, and ε-OR relates to how well the OR block time is used as a whole. A small modification is needed for the calculation of ε-OR, which takes account of 'gaps' that may arise if, say, one surgeon utilises the OR for 1 hour in the morning, and then there is a gap of several hours until the next surgeon arrives for their case. The term 'fraction of scheduled time utilised' is therefore the fraction *after* taking into account any gaps like these within the day (see Excel spreadsheet – Efficiency Calculator-US at www.cambridge.org/9781316646830).

A second form of efficiency ε may also be estimated, as relating to the extent to which the individual surgeon is efficient in their own estimate of using their individual proportion of block time well (ε-surgeon). For example, a surgeon requests 4 hours of OR time but in fact uses only 2 hours on a given day. Then the quantity ε-surgeon can be calculated on the basis that this is a 2-hour underrun for that surgeon (ε-surgeon = 50% in this case). Equally, if the surgeon overruns by 2 hours having asked for 4 hours OR time, this is an overrun of 2 hours and therefore also

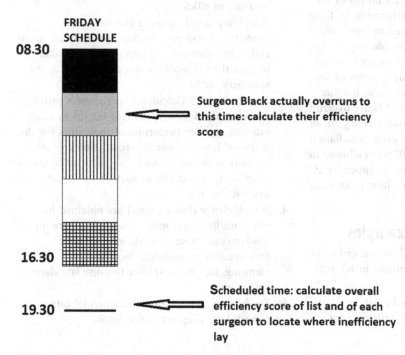

Figure 2.11 Example, in a 'typical US list' of how ε-surgeon (for each of the surgeons represented by shade) can be calculated as distinct from ε-OR for the list as a whole.

an ε-surgeon value of 50%. Cancellations can be factored in exactly the same way: a surgeon books four cases but on the day two are cancelled for a 50% cancellation rate and so on.

For clarity on this point, we will refer back to the surgeon panel in Figure 2.2 and reproduce it (Figure 2.11). In this example, Surgeon Black overruns; their efficiency ε-surgeon will be low as a result. The other surgeons (i.e., Grey, Striped, White and Hatched) all keep to their original stated times; their personal efficiency ε-surgeon scores will be high. However, the OR as a whole finishes early (at 16.30 hrs, instead of at its scheduled finish time as marked by arrow in Figure 2.11), so ε-OR is reduced. The theatre manager will be able to detect both the OR inefficiency and the surgeon-specific inefficiency and plan ways to tackle the problem, if recurrent. The theatre manager is also able to use this data to reassure the later surgeons, affected by the first surgeon's overrun: i.e., these later surgeons may wrongly perceive they themselves are inefficient because ε-OR is low, when in fact it is a surgical colleague who is inefficient.

In other words, whereas ε-OR is a means of estimating to the hospital how well a particular OR is used on any given day, ε-surgeon is a means of estimating how well the surgeon is performing by their own original estimates (and therefore how much unanticipated burden they may be placing on the system as a whole). The latter, ε-surgeon, clearly influences the former ε-OR. Placing a series of surgeons in the same OR consecutively who habitually underestimate the time they need, and hence overrun their potion of the list, will inevitably result in an overrun for the OR as a whole (or even cancellation for the later surgeon's cases if the OR is not allowed to overrun for other operational reasons). Appendix 2C outlines some practical scenarios of how to manage this situation.

Applying ε More Widely: Examples

Once ε is adopted, there are several ways it can enter the lexicon of surgical list management in advantageous ways:

Example: A hospital system or politician is challenged by the press about the 'efficiency' of

health service performance. There is concern about financial balance or cancellations or waiting for surgery. The hospital or politician can respond by citing in defence data of ε over time in its operating theatres; or, using ε constructively to identify specifically where the problems might lie (e.g., in underrunning or overrunning, or cancellation).

Example: Two theatre managers are competing for promotion; each can cite the aggregate ε for the theatre suites they respectively manage, in support of their applications.

Example: Two surgical–anaesthetic teams are under review; one of the metrics useful to compare their performance over time is ε.

Example: A team is concerned about the impact of a recent change in hospital policy on its performance; it can demonstrate whether this is the case using a run chart of ε.

Summary for the Theatre Manager

The main lessons of this chapter are these:

1. When assessing team performance or setting goals for surgical lists, use the composite quantitative measure of efficiency ε.

2. Avoid any single measure like utilisation, cancellation, overruns or start times; by all means collect this data (as it is necessary to calculate ε), but use the unbiased composite measure as the summary statistic.

3. Use the Excel ε Calculator spreadsheet provided (www.cambridge.org/9781316646830) to easily estimate the key performance indicators for the teams of interest over sustained times: present the data as means (SDs) in tables, or as isograms plots or as run charts as part of statistical process control.

4. If inefficiency (low ε values) are obtained for any team/list, investigate objectively where the fundamental cause of inefficiency may lie (preoperative assessment, poor list planning, factors conspiring to cause late starts or delays, etc.).

5. For how to address these fundamental causes, consult later chapters in this book.

Appendix 2A Using the ε Calculator Tool

Typical UK List: ε Calculator Tool

A simple tool (filename Efficiency E-calculator at www.cambridge.org/9781316646830) has been provided with this book to enable the reader to calculate efficiency ε using Equation 2.2. Open the tool, and there are several columns. These are, in turn:

Column A: manually enter the scheduled list duration. This is the agreed duration of the list, in minutes: if the list is scheduled to start at 08.30 and end at 16.30 this is 8 hours or 480 min, etc.

Columns B and C: here manually enter the scheduled start time and also the actual start times. The format has to be strictly 08:00 and not 0800 or 0900, etc (i.e., make sure to type in the colon). See Appendix 2B for further discussion on what is the 'scheduled start time', but generally this will be the locally agreed start. These two columns are used automatically to calculate column D.

Column D: a late start will be automatically entered, based on the data entered in the previous two columns. If there is an early start, a negative value will appear.

Columns E and F: here enter the scheduled time for the list to finish, and actual time the list finished (again, being careful to use the correct notation including use of colon).

Column G: in this column will automatically appear the actual minutes of surgery. This will be less than the scheduled list duration in column A if there are late starts, or early finishes. It will be greater than the value in column A if there are early starts or late finishes.

Column H: in this column will automatically appear the minutes of late finish (overrun). A negative value will appear for an early finish (underrun). These values are based in entries made in columns E and F.

Column I and J: in this column will automatically appear the % values for late start and late finish, respectively. There will be negative values for early start and early finish. These values are % of the scheduled list duration in column A.

Column K: in this column will automatically appear the list utilisation as a % value. This is calculated as the % of the actual minutes of surgery (from column G) and the scheduled list duration (column A).

Columns L and M: in this column will automatically appear the fractions (expressed as decimals) of scheduled time utilised and overrunning that are needed in Equation 2.2.

Columns N, O, P: into these columns should be manually entered, respectively, the number of cases scheduled, the cases completed and cases cancelled.

Column Q: in this column will automatically appear the cancellation rate as a %

Column R: in this column will automatically appear the fraction of scheduled cases completed, as a decimal, as is needed for Equation 2.2.

Column S: in this column will automatically appear the efficiency ε as calculated from Equation 2.2.

In this way, the ε Calculator Tool will generate almost all the key metrics needed to assess theatre performance. Each row can be used for a fresh list, if desired, and the columns should be 'dragged and extended' in the Excel function to complete the automatic calculations. Readers should practice using it, entering both real and hypothetical data, and explore it value and limitations. There are several points to note.

An early start per se will increase the total time spent operating (column G) and so will increase utilisation (to perhaps >100%) but will not of itself increase efficiency ε. That may seem surprising, but in fact, if at all, an early start required to complete all the cases is poor efficiency: it is exactly the same as a late finish. All the team has done is increase the list length to accommodate a presumably overbooked list. Then, an early start coupled with an early finish is neither penalised nor credited: if a list starts an hour early and finishes an hour early completing all its cases, ε is still 100%. The rationale for this is that this team has merely time-shifted its schedules, for whatever reason. There is no penalty (or reward) for doing so, and it is unlikely that this team will be required to undertake more cases at the end of the day from other theatres because it has 'finished early'. Note also that in this version of the ε Calculator Tool there is no explicit inclusion of the effect of long gaps within a list; these are assumed to be trivial. To include these, it is necessary to use the ε Calculator Tool-US.

Another point to note is that the data in Column A (scheduled list duration) should be consistent with the data in Columns B and E (scheduled start and end times respectively). If errors are made here, aberrant results may be obtained.

Typical US List: ε Calculator Tool-Gap

This calculator tool (filename Efficiency E Calculator-US Tool at: www.cambridge.org/9781316646830) is identical in every respect to the ε Calculator Tool described earlier, except that it factors in mid-list gaps. This the sum of the unproductive times within a list where no anaesthesia or surgery is conducted. An example would be from a typical US list, where an OR might be scheduled to accommodate one surgeon for an hour in the morning, then a long gap of many hours until the next surgeon for another hour's case. From the OR perspective, efficiency ε for this list is low, although it may be acceptable from each surgeon's perspective.

In this tool E Calculator-US Tool, if gap time is set to zero it functions identically to ε Calculator Tool. Note that the actual gap time needs to be measured directly by the theatre manager and entered into the program; it is not calculated automatically by the tool.

Appendix 2B Case Study: Managing Start Times of Surgical Lists – Should a Start Time Be Fixed as the Start of Surgery, or the Start of Anaesthesia?

The Problem

In a hypothetical hospital, start times for surgical lists have been historically defined as 08.30 each day, but it has never been clarified what this start refers to: start of anaesthesia, start of surgery or something else? A new national-level metric requires data to be returned to the health department, with flexibilities allowed for times to be locally defined, so long as hospitals are internally consistent so that their progress can be monitored.

It is self-evident that defining 08.30 to be the surgical start time would require anaesthetists to start earlier than this, which is acceptable to all in principle, but the question is then: how early? Equally, defining 08.30 to be the anaesthesia start time would then mean surgeons arriving later than this, which is also acceptable to all in principle, but then the question is: how much later?

What can the theatre manager do?

Data Collection

First, the important data set is: how long does anaesthesia take? Generally, anaesthesia techniques might be broken down by the type of anaesthesia the case needs. At the simplest level is a 'standard' anaesthetic, where the patient requires only intravenous induction plus a standard form of airway management (e.g., a supraglottic airway or tracheal tube). The most complex might consist of all this (and more; where tracheal intubation might involve advanced methods such as being fibreoptic-assisted), plus invasive monitoring lines, plus regional anaesthesia. The theatre manager might analyse by any number of categories of complexity in between, but we will take these two extremes for simplicity. The mean and standard deviation (SD) of the times is needed. For the simplest method of anaesthesia, a mean of 15 (5) min turns out to be needed; for the most complex it is 50 (15) min.

From these mean (SD) times, the normal distribution can yield the probabilities that for the simplest case, anaesthesia will be complete after 10 min, 15 min, 20 min and so on (these are: 16%, 50%, 84%). A probability distribution can be plotted for this case (Figure 2.12A). A similar plot can also be drawn for the most complex case, where the normal distribution means that the probability anaesthesia will be complete after 50 min will also be 50% (Figure 2.12B).

Conclusions

With these results, the theatre manager can offer the following observations:

1. Whether the hospital sets the start time of 08.30 to be the surgical start or anaesthesia start is technically irrelevant

2. However, the consequences of the choice can be defined, and depend on the mean (SD) anaesthesia times for the cases, which the theatre manager should publish

3. If 08.30 is regarded as the surgical start time, anaesthesia should start at a time before this, approximately equivalent to the mean published anaesthesia time for the case. Then both anaesthetist and surgeon will have a 50% of waiting for the other. That is, the anaesthetist may finish induction of anaesthesia before 08.30 on half the occasions and later than 08.30 on half the occasions. This seems fair to all.

4. If 08.30 is regarded as the anaesthesia start time, then the surgeon need not arrive in theatre until a time after this, approximately equivalent to the

A: Plot for short anaesthesia time

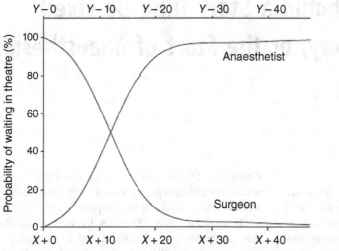

Time anaesthesia starts before surgical start time (Y) min

Time surgeon arrives in theatre after anaesthesia start (X) min

B: Plot for long anaesthesia time

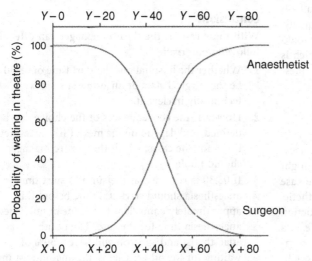

Time anaesthesia starts before surgical start time (Y) min

Time surgeon arrives in theatre after anaesthesia start (X) min

Figure 2.12 Panel A: Probability distributions for anaesthesia times for the simplest case, where total anaesthesia time is mean 15 (5) min. The plot is interpreted as follows. If the start time of 08.30 is regarded as when surgery should start (Y) and the anaesthetist starts 40 min before this (i.e., at 07.50) then there is a near-100% chance the anaesthetist will wait for the surgeon (who will only arrive at 08.30). The surgeon will not wait at all, as the patient will be ready. Conversely, if the start time of 08.30 is regarded as the anaesthesia start time, then this plot means that if the anaesthesia starts on time, the surgeon can be 0% confident (100% chance of waiting) of anaesthesia being complete if they arrive at 08.30, 50% confident of anaesthesia being complete at 08.45, 100% confident of anaesthesia being complete if they arrive at 09.00, and so on.

Panel B shows the same data for the longer case of mean 50 (15) min. The general shape of the curves are the same, although note the scales on the axes now differ. Again we see that if the anaesthetist starts very long before a fixed surgical start time, they will wait for the surgeon. If they start at a time approximately equivalent to the average anaesthesia time for this case, the chance of waiting for the surgeon (or surgeon waiting for anaesthesia to finish) is ~50%. Conversely, if the start time is defined as the start of anaesthesia, the surgeon should arrive at or after the average anaesthesia time for this case to be 50% or more confident that anaesthesia will be complete.

mean published anaesthesia time for the case. Then, the anaesthetist will have finished anaesthesia and be waiting on about half the occasions; anaesthesia will still be ongoing on half the occasions and the surgeon will have to wait. This seems fair to all.

5. Where necessary, individual performance can then be monitored by the degree to which they

adhere to their respective times, as dictated by the mean published anaesthesia time for the case. In other words, if start time is regarded as start of surgery at 08.30, how often does the surgeon arrive ready at 08.30, and on how many occasions does the anaesthetist start x min before this, where x is the mean anaesthesia time for the first case? If start time is regarded as start of anaesthesia at 08.30, how often does the anaesthetist start at 08.30, and on how many occasions does the surgeon arrive ready x min after this, where x is the mean anaesthesia time for the first case?

6. A question consequent to deciding start times is then to decide how many hours of surgery thereafter are to be scheduled, and how different contracts are arranged to achieve this. For example, if the start time is regarded as the start of surgery at 08.30, and it is agreed that there should be 8 hours of surgery thereafter, then clearly anaesthetists should be contracted for >8 hours

work because they will need to start sooner (as described earlier) to ensure this surgery start time. Conversely, if start time is regarded as the start of anaesthesia at 08.30, and it is agreed that there should be 8 hours of surgery thereafter, then clearly surgeons should be contracted for <8 hours work because they will need to start later than 08.30 (as described earlier). Or, surgeons' contracts should specify other tasks in this period after 08.30 and arrival.

7. All this is notwithstanding the need to perform the WHO premeet checklist where all staff need to attend a meeting before any anaesthesia or surgery starts. It is possible to fix the start time as being the time of the WHO meet, with anaesthesia starting immediately after this. If so, this is akin to regarding the WHO meet time as the start of anaesthesia, with the surgeon then leaving to return x minutes later, where x is the average time it takes for anaesthesia.

Appendix 2C Case Studies of Optimising Efficiency in a 'Typical US List'

We discussed how the measure of efficiency ε may be used within the context of a typical UK NHS list. We now discuss some practical problems faced by a theatre manager in the context of a typical US list.

Managing a Single Overrunning Surgeon and Follow-on Surgeons

The cardinal goals are (a) to maximise ε for each OR, (b) to maximise ε for each surgeon and (c) to maximise ε for the OR suite as a whole. In general, the first goal can be met by seeking to maximise the utilisation of each OR whilst preventing overrun of the OR. This will also automatically meet the third goal. Both goals can be met by managing the ε of the surgeon.

This can be demonstrated by a scenario where, if we consider two parallel ORs where one underruns (e.g., only 4 hours of 8 hours scheduled is used; ε 50%), while the other overruns (e.g., 2 hours over and above an 8 hour schedule; ε 25%). (No patients are cancelled.) The overall ε for this small OR suite is a meagre 37.5% (i.e., the average of 50% and 25%). One surgeon in the second OR overran their estimated time by 2 hours (when originally scheduled 4 hours; ε-surgeon 50%), while the first OR was simply underbooked.

This scenario can be avoided by detecting that an overrun is likely in the second OR, and responding promptly by moving the follow-on surgeons' cases to the first OR. Because these cases take 4 hours, then ε of the first OR will now be 100%, and that of the second OR 75% (6 hours of the OR utilised of 8 hours originally scheduled). The combined ε of the OR suite is now 87.5%. Note, however, that the ε of the overrunning surgeon remains low at 50% (ε-surgeon). This solution is depicted diagrammatically in Figure 2.13.

Several things are necessary for this to be possible:

1. There needs to be an active theatre manager, or separate 'floor manager' with real-time knowledge of events in each OR, with the power to make decisions to move cases

2. For multi-OR suites, ideally, a master dashboard is required, showing the real-time progress of each OR

3. The anaesthesiologist and OR team in OR1 need to have the correct skills to accommodate the follow-on cases from the OR2. Otherwise, clinical difficulties may be raised (e.g., it may not be possible to move specialised cases such as cardiac, or those requiring specialised equipment such as robotics).

More fundamentally, the sustained solution is to prevent the unanticipated overrun of the overrunning surgeon in the first place. Occasional overruns of this type are always going to happen, but where sustained over time such that ε-surgeon is consistently low for this surgeon, then data should be used better to schedule the list in the first place (see Chapter 4). In other words, if this is a consistent pattern, the overrunning surgeon should be allocated more scheduled time based on their known data, and the follow-on surgeons allocated to different ORs from the outset.

Managing Mid-List Gaps

Perhaps more challenging is how best to manage mid-list gaps, where Surgeon A has cases in the morning, but the follow-on Surgeon B has nothing until much later in the day. In this situation, the first surgeon's efficiency ε-surgeon has little tangible impact on the overall efficiency of the ε-OR. This is because this surgeon has the luxury of free space on the list; even if they overrun and their personal efficiency ε-surgeon is low, it does not influence ε-OR as a whole. Interestingly, personal efficiency ε-surgeon of Surgeon B could be much more influential, as if they overrun, then ε-OR as whole may be reduced.

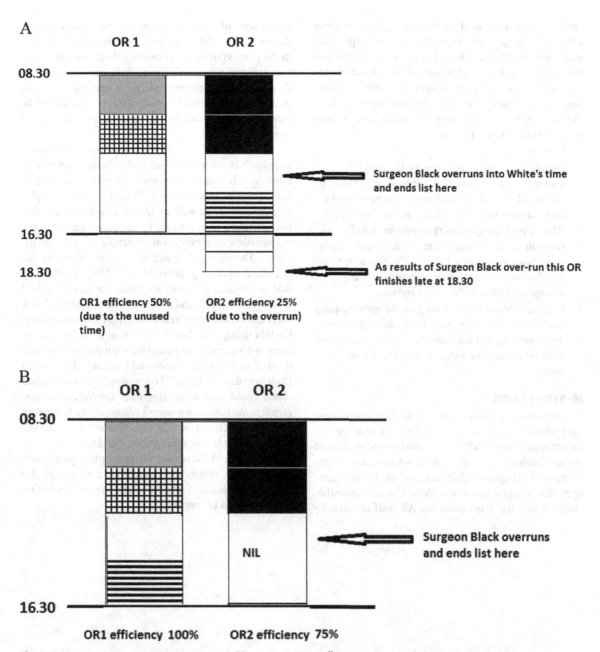

Figure 2.13 Managing one surgeon overrun in a 2-OR suite to maximise efficiency. A: Top panel, the problem. Each shade represents a different surgeon (the white block in OR1 represents unused time). In OR 1 there are two surgeons (Grey and Hatched). In OR2, Surgeon Black is scheduled for two blocks but overruns (arrow indicating the time they actually finish). As a result, Surgeons White and Striped finish late (bottom arrow). B: Bottom panel, solution. Surgeons White and Striped are moved to OR1.

However, it is still important to monitor the respective ε-surgeon data as this will generate useful data for consistency in list planning, especially if either of these surgeons at some other time has follow-on surgeons. In other words, if data shows

ε-surgeon to be consistently poor, then that will require analysis and adjustment.

However, the temptation for a theatre manager to fill the mid-list gap is fraught with risk and needs to be managed very carefully. In the sense that ε-OR could be very adverse, if by moving cases from other ORs to fill the gap, the original follow-on Surgeon B's start time is delayed. The list can then run late, and this can lead to staff frustration and loss of faith in the overall OR management system. Therefore, knowledge of ε-surgeon becomes very important: it is desirable only to move surgeons with very reliable ε-surgeon data to fill the gap.

In summary:

1. Mid-list gaps offer opportunity to collect ε-surgeon data on the first surgeon of the day, to use in other contexts (although overruns by the first surgeon will matter little on the day itself)

2. After a mid-list gap, overrunning by a follow-on surgeon can be damaging to ε-OR; hence, where there is a list with mid-list gap it is desirable to try to schedule only surgeons with very reliable ε-surgeon data as follow-on surgeons

3. It is desirable to fill mid-list gaps by moving cases from other ORs (especially from those that are overrunning), but then only cases from surgeons with very reliable ε-surgeon data should be moved.

Managing Teams

Whilst managing cases between ORs the theatre manager should not lose sight of how to manage the anaesthesia-theatre staff teams. If one anaesthesiologist always finishes late, while another always early, simply because of the optimisation tactics of the theatre manager, this will give rise to conflicts. The first anaesthesiologist will feel hard done by. All staff affected by movement of cases – surgeons, anaesthesiologists, theatre staff – should be made to feel equal partners in the process of decision making. This does not mean that they will necessarily have a veto, but any concerns they have about staying late on a particular day, or undertaking a particular case mix, etc., should all be listened to sympathetically and accommodated if possible.

One means of objectifying the debate is, of course, to publish in advance the general policies or principles upon which theatre management tactics are based. This involves education for all staff in the principles of efficiency ε, as well as in the understanding that maximising ε is important to maximise gains for the organisation as whole, and therefore for staff themselves. Therefore, it could be enshrined within the 'standard operating procedures' (SOPs) of theatres that movement of cases to maximise overall ε is a guiding principle – and so the philosophy of this book itself can be disseminated as an organisational policy. Certain things could even be written into contracts so there is no surprise or resentment on the part of staff, if asked to stay late, or given add-on cases transferred from another OR, etc. For example, a contractual clause could read something like: '*On the day of surgery it is the theatre manager's responsibility to manage cases within ORs such that the efficiency ε for the OR suite as a whole is maximised for the day*'.

The more objective are the principles upon which decisions are made, and the more transparent the reality that decisions will be made, the more satisfaction there will be overall.

Appendix 2D Case Study of Optimising Efficiency ε in a Typical UK Private Hospital

The flexibilities available to a theatre manager in this scenario are very limited. As described, the typical pattern of work superficially resembles the typical US hospital, with the very important proviso that anaesthetists are linked to individual surgeons, but they might also be covering other surgeons in the same OR for the whole day. This close anaesthetist–surgeon link constrains the ability of the theatre manager to move cases.

Thus, while it might be desirable from the private hospital's perspective to move cases from one OR to another (either to fill a mid-list gap, or to avoid an overrun in one OR), it may be impossible in practice if the anaesthetist also has to move, but cannot do so. In other words the commercial relationship between surgeon and anaesthetist is generally stronger and overrides the commercial relationship of these providers with the hospital. (Note that, as discussed, the hospital here is not an employer of these professionals).

Nevertheless, surgeon-specific ε-surgeon data are still very important, as these will help schedule series of surgeons to ORs in more optimal ways (e.g., surgeons with less-reliable ε-surgeon data should avoid having follow-on surgeons, whereas those with more reliable ε-surgeon data can be managed with more flexibility).

Appendix 2E Efficiency of the Emergency List

The method of calculating efficiency ε (Equation 2.2) cannot be used in context of an emergency list. Even an emergency list that is not used is serving an important function. To use a military analogy: what is the best measure of an efficient army in peacetime? Perhaps simply that there is peace. Many regulatory requirements correctly demand that there should be at least one emergency list, fully staffed and available 24 hours round the clock. There are exemptions for small hospitals that do not receive emergency cases, but even these hospitals have to make staffing provision for urgent cases that, say, need to come back to theatre for post-operative bleeding or other complications.

Therefore by definition 'utilisation' of an emergency list is an inappropriate measure of inefficiency. Also the notion of 'cases booked' is very fluid because these can change from minute to minute. At the extremes of utilisation some information is relevant. If the emergency list is so rarely used (e.g., one case per week) then consideration should be given to other ways of managing these rare cases. For example, flexibly using staff in recovery/PACU, and assigning perhaps a 'recovery/PACU anaesthetist' as the standby team. Or, seeking agreement that on any given day spare capacity on operating lists can be flexibly used for urgent cases. At the other extreme, if the emergency list is constantly full such that even urgent cases are waiting excessively, then perhaps more than one emergency list is needed.

More appropriate markers of the efficiency or performance of the emergency list are things like (a) the wait time between a decision to operate and actual surgery, (b) whether the actual diagnosis at operation confirms or not the urgency of the case (i.e., it would be undesirable if in fact a large number of non-urgent cases are being marked urgent) and (c) quality markers such as medium- to long-term patient outcomes like survival.

In some centres, a distinction needs to be made sometimes between an 'urgent bookable' list and a true 'emergency list'. Urgent cases are difficult to define and rely on individual surgical judgement, but where a case can be judged to wait 24–48 hours but no longer (e.g., a small abscess for drainage), a facility for booking the case onto a list in advance seems useful. This is distinct from a case that needs surgery immediately or at most within a few hours (e.g., an open limb fracture or testicular torsion). The point being that if the emergency list is full of the former cases, access to theatre for the latter may be delayed. Hence, some general principles are useful.

Because there is so little literature on managing an emergency list, the following rules are based on first principles, applicable to both urgent bookable and emergency lists:

1. It is useful to have a single 'floor manager' (usually an experienced consultant anaesthetist) who also acts primarily to manage the emergency list

2. However, the order of cases on the emergency list should be dictated by the surgeons, negotiating with each other their respective priorities. That said, sometimes order can be determined by resources, including availability of intensive or high-dependency care. For example, if one case needs an intensive care bed post-operatively but this will not be available till later, it may make sense to undertake a less urgent case first. Otherwise, the intensive care case will simply block the theatre or recovery/PACU while the team await the bed space in the intensive care unit

3. In this way, surgeons regulate themselves including any situations where cases are erroneously labelled urgent (e.g., for surgeon's own convenience). The floor manager may have a role to play in managing this.

4. If the emergency list is occupied, then where possible urgent cases should be accommodated onto space at the end of early-finishing elective lists (skill mix of staff permitting). The floor manager is in a position to identify those shorter urgent cases and use the Case Scheduling Algorithm CSA tool (see Chapter 4; and at: www.cambridge.org/9781316646830) to ensure cases can be reasonably accommodated. The need to avoid overrun of the elective list is greater in this scenario, so the CSA tool should be set to a very low probability of overrun if the add-on case is done.

Bibliography

Abouleish AE, Hensley SL, Zornow MH, Prough DS. 2003. Inclusion of turnover time does not influence identification of surgical services that over- and underutilize allocated block time. *Anesthesia and Analgesia* 96: 8138.

Association of Anaesthetists of Great Britain and Ireland. 2003. *Theatre Efficiency, Safety, Quality of Care and Optimal Use of Resources.* London: AAGBI.

Audit Commission. 2003. *Operating Theatres: Review of National Findings.* London: HMSO.

Audit Commission. 2004. *Payment by Results: Key Risks and Questions to Consider for Trust and PCT Managers and Non-Executives.* London: HMSO.

Berwick DM. 2005. Measuring NHS productivity: how much health for the pound, not how many events to the pound. *British Medical Journal* 330: 975–6.

Calvert N, Hind D, McWilliams R, Davidson A, Beverley CA, Thomas AM. 2004. Ultrasound for central venous cannulation: economic evaluation of cost-effectiveness. *Anaesthesia* 59: 1116–20.

Cegan PC. 2005. The easiest cut: managing elective surgery in the public sector. *Medical Journal of Australia* 182: 605–6.

Collantes E, Mauffrey C, Brewster M. 2008. A review of 1241 trauma cases: a study of efficiency in trauma theatres. *Injury: International Journal of the Care of the Injured* 39: 742–7.

Cutter RW, Carli N, O'Connor M. 2008. The modified staggered start. *Anesthesia and Analgesia* 106: S–72.

Dexter F, Abouleish AE, Epstein RH, Whitten CW, Lubarsky DA. 2003. Use of an operating room information system data to predict the impact of reducing turnover times on staffing costs. *Anesthesia and Analgesia* 97: 119–26.

Dexter F, Macario A. 1999. Application of information systems to operating room scheduling. *Anesthesiology* 91: 1501–8.

Dexter F, Wachtel RF. 2009. Influence of the operating room schedule on tardiness from scheduled start times. *Anesthesia and Analgesia* 108: 1889–901.

Durani P, Seagrave M, Neumann L. 2005. The use of theatre time in elective orthopaedic surgery. *Annals of the Royal College of Surgeons (Suppl.)* 87: 170–2.

Faiz O, Tekkis P, Mcguire A, Papagrigoriadis S, Renni J, Leather A. 2008. Is theatre utilization a valid performance indicator for NHS operating theatres? *BMC Health Services Research* 8: 28.

Foundation Trust Network. 2010. *FTN Benchmarking: Driving Performance Improvement in Operating Theatres.* London: NHS Confederation.

Gabel RA. 2003. Performance measurement. *American Society of Anesthesiologists Newsletter* 67: 5–6.

Gordon T, Paul S, Lyles A, Fountain J. 1988. Surgical unit time utilization review: resource utilization and management implications. *Journal of Medical Systems* 12: 169–79.

Gupta B, Agrawal P, D'souza N, Soni KD. 2011. Start time delays in operating room: different perspectives. *Saudi Journal of Anaesthesia* 5: 286–8.

Healey A, Undre S, Vincent CA. 2004. Developing observational measures of performance in surgical teams. *Quality and Safety in Health Care* 13 (Suppl. 1): i33–i40.

House of Commons Public Accounts Committee. 2006. *The Use of Operating Theatres in Northern Ireland.* Health and Personal Social Services, Seventh Report of Session 2005–6, London, HMSO.

Ivarson B, Kimbald PO, Sjöberg T, Larsson S. 2002. Patient reactions to cancelled or postponed heart operations. *Journal of Nursing Management* 10: 75–81.

Joshi GP. 2008. Efficiency in ambulatory center surgery. *Current Opinion in Anesthesiology* 21: 695–8.

Kelly MG, Eastham A, Bowling GS. 1985. Efficient OR scheduling: a study to reduce cancellations. *Association of Perioperative Registered Nurses (AORN) Journal* 41: 565–7.

Koenig T, Neumann C, Ocker T, Kramer S, Spies C, Schuster M. 2011. Estimating the time needed for induction of anaesthesia and its importance in balancing anaesthetists' and surgeons' waiting times around the start of surgery. *Anaesthesia* 66: 556–62.

Lawrentschuk N, Hewitt PM, Pritchard MG. 2003. Elective laparoscopic cholecystectomy: implications of prolonged waiting times for surgery. *Australian and New Zealand Journal of Surgery* 73: 890–3.

Macario A. 2006. Are your hospital operating rooms 'efficient'?: A scoring system with eight performance indicators. *Anesthesiology* 105: 237–40.

Macario A. 2011. The limitations of using operating room utilisation to allocate surgeons more or less surgical block time in the USA. *Anaesthesia* 65: 548–52.

Mangan JL, Walsh C, Kernohan WG, et al. 1992. Total joint replacement: implication of cancelled operations for hospital costs and waiting list management. *Quality in Health Care* 1: 34–7.

McIntosh C, Dexter F, Epstein RH. 2006. The impact of service specific staffing, case scheduling, turnovers, and first-case starts on anaesthesia group and operating room productivity: a tutorial using data from an Australian hospital. *Anesthesia and Analgesia* 103: 1499–516.

McWhinnie DL, Michaels JA, Collin J, Morris PJ. 1994. Resource implications of cancelled operations. *British Medical Journal* 398: 138–9.

Munoz E, Tortella B, Jaker M. 1994. Surgical resource consumption in an academic health consortium. *Surgery* 115: 411–6.

New South Wales Health Department. 2002. *Operating Theatre Management Report*. Sydney: Health Department.

Northern Ireland Audit Office. 2003. *The Use of Operating Theatres in the Northern Ireland Health and Personal Social Services*. Belfast: HMSO.

Office for National Statistics. 2004. *Public Service Productivity: Health, October 2004*. London: Office for National Statistics.

Overdyk FJ, Harvey SC, Fishman RL, Shippey F. 1996. Successful strategies for improving operating room efficiency at academic institutions. *Anesthesia and Analgesia* 85: 1232–4.

Pandit JJ, Abbott T, Pandit M, Kapila A, Abraham R. 2012. Is 'starting on time' useful (or useless) as a surrogate measure for 'surgical theatre efficiency'? *Anaesthesia* 67: 823–32.

Pandit JJ, Carey A. 2006. Estimating the duration of common elective operations: implications for operating list management. *Anaesthesia* 61: 768–76.

Pandit JJ, Westbury S, Pandit M. 2007. The concept of surgical operating list 'efficiency': a formula to describe the term. *Anaesthesia* 62: 895–903.

Pitches D, Burls A, Fry-Smith A. 2003. How to make a silk purse from a sow's ear – a comprehensive review of strategies to optimise data for corrupt managers and incompetent clinicians. *British Medical Journal* 327: 1436–9.

Queensland Health. 2005. *Policy Framework for Elective Surgery Services*. Queensland Government.

Rai M, Pandit JJ. 2003. Day of surgery cancellations after nurse-led preassessment in an elective surgical centre: the first 2 years. *Anaesthesia* 58: 692–9.

Ray N, Tung A, Glick DB. 2008. Who cares if I'm on time? *Anesthesia and Analgesia* 106: S-71.

Ray N, Tung A, Glick DB. 2008. Why rush? You won't get out any earlier!! *Anesthesia and Analgesia* 106: S-73. 43

De Riso B, Cantees K, Watkins WD. 1995. The operating room: cost center management in a managed care environment. *International Anesthesiology Clinics* 33: 133–50.

Saskatchewan Provincial Wait List Strategy Team. 2002. *Surgical Wait List Management: A Strategy for Saskatchewan*. Saskatchewan: Health Department of Saskatchewan.

Scottish Executive. 2006. *National Theatres Project: Final Report*. Edinburgh: HMSO.

Shafer S. 2006. Case scheduling for dummies. *Anesthesia and Analgesia* 103: 1351–2.

Sier D, Tobin P, McGurk C. 1997. Scheduling surgical procedures. *Journal of the Operational Research Society* 48: 884–91.

Silber JH, Rosenbaum PR, Zhang X, Even-Shoshan O. 2007. Influence of patient and hospital characteristics on anesthesia time in Medicare patients undergoing general and orthopedic surgery. *Anesthesiology* 106: 356–64.

Sokolovic E, Biro P, Wyss P, et al. 2002. Impact of the reduction of anaesthesia turnover time on operating room efficiency. *European Journal of Anaesthesiology* 19: 560–3.

Strum DP, Vargas LG, May JH, et al. 1997. Surgical suite utilization and capacity planning: a minimal cost analysis model. *Journal of Medical Systems* 21: 309–22.

Sury MR, Palmer JH, Cook TM, Pandit JJ. 2014. The state of UK anaesthesia: a survey of National Health Service activity in 2013. *British Journal of Anaesthesia* 113: 575–84.

Tait AR, Voepel-Lewis T, Munro HM, Gutstein HB, Reynolds PI. 1997. Cancellation of pediatric outpatient surgery: economic and emotional implications for patients and their families. *Journal of Clinical Anesthesia* 9: 213–9.

Tessler MJ, Kleiman SJ, Huberman MM. 1997. A 'zero tolerance' for overtime increases surgical per case costs. *Canadian Journal of Anaesthesia* 44: 1036–41.

Walsh U, Alfhaily F, Gupta R, Vinayagam D, Whitlow B. 2010. Theatre sending: how long does it take and what is the cost of late starts? *Gynecological Surgery* 7: 307–10.

Ward M, Sanders M. 2006. Section 13.4: Efficient Use of Planned Operating Lists. In Colvin JR (ed.). *Raising the Standard: a Compendium of Audit Recipes for Continuous Quality Improvement in Anaesthesia*, 2nd edn. London: RCOA.

Weinbroum AA, Ekstein P, Ezri T. 2003. Efficiency of the operating room suite. *American Journal of Surgery* 185: 244–50.

Widdison AL. 1995. Can we predict when an operating list will finish? *Annals of the Royal College*

of Surgeons (Suppl.) 77: 304–6.

Wright I, Kooperberg C, Bonar B, Bashein G. 1996. Statistical modeling to predict elective surgery time: a comparison with a computer scheduling system and surgeon-

provided estimates. *Anesthesiology* 85: 1235–45.

Wu R. 2005. Cancellation of operations on the day of surgery at a major Australian referral hospital. *Medical Journal of Australia* 183: 551.

Chapter

3

Defining 'Productivity'

Jaideep J. Pandit

Introduction

In this chapter, we discuss the concept of surgical list 'productivity' as distinct from 'efficiency', which we discussed in Chapter 2. In broad conceptual terms, efficiency rests on the notion of an input–output relationship. We put something in (e.g., effort or investment), and we get something out (e.g., use of time or resources or completed operations); efficiency is when we get the most out of what we put in. Productivity is, more simply, the crude or total amount we produce. This is rather like the gross domestic product (GDP) of a country, which can be very high, for larger, active economies, regardless of whether their economies are efficient or not at using investments.

As a word of warning, however, this chapter is not for the fainthearted. It is possible to skip this chapter without it affecting the reading of the remaining book. As our ideas of measuring theatre list performance develop, so too do our analyses become more sophisticated. As in the preceding paragraph, our definitions and distinctions become more subtle and therefore ever further removed from what we might regard as instinctive. Such is the case with 'productivity'.

Moreover, as we shall later discuss, it is not strictly necessary to measure productivity in every case faced by a theatre manager. We will see that a *sine qua non* for productivity is efficiency, and where there is a problem with a list or series of lists, it almost always lies with efficiency and rarely with productivity. So it is the content of the previous chapter that is really essential. It is rare in practise for a theatre manager to be challenged by a list that is already efficient.

Nevertheless, the ideas discussed in this chapter are important for a deeper understanding of how theatre lists work and how best to manage them. While it is entirely possible to skip this chapter without loss of continuity, the detail will certainly help those wishing to acquire the most advanced skills in theatre management. Again, most of the focus is for

the typical United Kingdom National Health Service (UK NHS) list, but a section deals with how the approach can apply to other scenarios.

Distinction between 'Efficiency' and 'Productivity'

In Chapter 2, we discussed the importance of achieving efficiency. We defined this as the ability to complete the planned caseload within the scheduled time, with no overruns and maximal utilisation of time. We showed how it was possible to quantify efficiency through the measure ε (Equation 2.2).

However, we also acknowledged there were some limitations of ε and that one of these was that it did not directly take account of midlist gaps – the times when no anaesthesia or surgery was conducted, but where staff were simply waiting for something else to happen before they could proceed. This might be a portering delay transporting the patient, or a tardy patient coming from home, or the cleaning of certain equipment, etc. That said, we did introduce a modified equation that was able to take this into account, especially for a typical US list or a private hospital list in the United Kingdom (see Excel E Calculator US Tool at: www.cambridge.org/9781316646830). We might wish in some circumstances to factor in these gap times more explicitly using another mathematical-analytic approach, different from that used for efficiency ε.

There are occasions, other than consideration of gaps, when the issue of 'productivity' – as a concept distinct from efficiency – may be important. Consider two orthopaedic lists in parallel theatres, each undertaking total knee replacements using similar surgical–anaesthetic techniques. Both start on time, both finish on time, there are no cancellations and negligible within-list gaps. Both these can be said therefore to have high or optimal efficiency ε. However, let us suppose that one team consistently performs five operations per day, whereas the other only performs three. We can immediately see that, even where maximal efficiency is achieved, there is a separate concept of how much work is actually delivered, through the notion of the knee replacements being akin to 'goods that are produced'. In this example, because there are no gaps or late starts or early finishes, the inescapable conclusion is that one team is working faster at the operations than the other. Intuitively, we feel that it is better that more operations are performed, and we say that one team is more 'productive' than the other (although they are equally 'efficient').

The words *efficiency* and *productivity* are sometimes used interchangeably in economics, and with different subtle senses. Appendix 3A outlines the different uses.

The Fallacy of 'Number of Operations Completed' as a Universal Measure of Productivity

The economist Harvey (1987) quotes a nice analogy to show how superficial measures of productivity like 'number of operations' are flawed. Worker A moves twice as many boxes as B in a given time; the intuitive conclusion is clearly that A is more productive than B. However, when the boxes are weighed, it turns out that B is moving twice as much weight as A; the real conclusion is quite different.

So there are several important prerequisites before we can simply count the 'number of operations'. First, efficiency must be adhered to. An orthopaedic list that completes five knee replacements versus three, but that finishes 2 hours later, is not necessarily 'better'. *Efficiency is therefore a prerequisite for any analysis of productivity*. This is a very important rule that should be remembered at all times; sacrificing productivity for efficiency is poor tactics.

Second, it is essential that *safety* is adhered to and that post-operative outcomes are the same. There is little point in undertaking five knee replacements if one was performed on the wrong leg and one resulted in fatal blood loss through errors. If so, the list that completes just one or two operations without complications is far more productive. Productivity should never entail working so fast or taking shortcuts as to endanger safety.

Third, following on from the safety notion, *quality outcomes* should be equivalent. The list that performs five knee replacements is not at all productive if none

of their patients can afterwards walk. There is a story from the old Soviet Union (where arbitrary targets were popular and enforced), where a ball-bearing factory was ordered to increase its tonnage of ball-bearings to an extent that was impossible (e.g., double production from 1,000 tonnes to 2,000 tonnes); that number of ball bearings could simply not be produced by the machines even working all day and all night. The chief manager solved this impossible dilemma by directing all efforts that year to producing a single giant (but useless) ball-bearing weighing 2,000 tonnes, which was much easier to do.

Fourth, in making any meaningful comparisons between teams, we need to appreciate differences between the modes of anaesthesia and surgery. It is readily appreciated that cardiac surgery is different from gynaecology. This does not preclude productivity comparisons of cardiac versus gynaecology teams (see later). However, the comparison is only meaningful if differences are appreciated. Moreover, even superficially similar specialties or teams can differ. An open cholecystectomy cannot be regarded as identical to a laparoscopic cholecystectomy. Nor can an anaesthetic that uses only a supraglottic airway be regarded as an identical intervention as one that involves tracheal intubation. It is self-evident that some anaesthetic or surgical techniques are always going to be quicker than others; this does not mean that those should be inherently preferable for reasons of productivity alone. Even where some interventions are due to the choice on the part of the practitioner (or patient), there should be no penalty for exercising that choice. Regional anaesthesia (a spinal, epidural or nerve blockade technique, with or without general anaesthesia) will generally take much longer than general anaesthesia alone, and it may even cause delays of discharge versus general anaesthesia. However, the practitioners that promote it will strongly argue that it yields better outcomes in terms of pain relief, reduced nausea and vomiting, less post-operative confusion, etc. (See the quality goal in the preceding paragraph.) In surgery, robotic prostatectomy takes much longer (and is more expensive) than conventional open surgery, yet again practitioners point to reduced blood loss, earlier discharge, etc. Often there is no science indicating which of the alternative techniques is preferable, and the issues are hotly debated in the literature. But until and unless there is professional consensus on a single technique, it is incorrect simply to credit the quicker methods with high 'productivity'.

Another related prerequisite for meaningful productivity comparisons is equal patient comorbidity, but this is something usually evened out over a sustained period of time over which data is collected. Operations in unhealthier patients can take longer, but an overall case mix of the healthy versus unhealthy should be broadly similar for teams undertaking the same operation.

So if all these prerequisites are met, then – and only then – is the 'number of operations' a simple and appropriate measure of productivity. Generally, this might apply to knee replacements or arthroscopies, hip replacements, vaginal hysterectomies, and so on – i.e., those operations that have generally accepted 'standard' techniques for surgery and anaesthesia underpinning them.

However, in real life these prerequisites are never met. There are always subtle differences that matter, and it is rare for a theatre manager ever to be able justify looking at crude 'number of operations' alone to performance-manage teams. The discussion will always boil down to details of technique, with the putatively underproductive team defending its practice by pointing to their better outcomes, patient satisfaction, etc. This is not a discussion that leads anywhere, and the theatre manager is advised against going down this route. Perhaps at best, the metric of 'number of operations' might be used to track productivity of a single team (which has always used the same methods) over time.

Moreover, the challenge is often not just to compare different lists performing broadly the same operation (e.g., knee replacements), but rather to compare teams undertaking a mix of operations (e.g., knee and hip replacements in different proportions). Or, to ask if one specialty's set of operations (e.g., knee replacements) is as productive as another (e.g., coronary bypass surgery). How is it possible, meaningfully, to compare productivity of teams performing *dissimilar* operations, or of *dissimilar* teams?

In the following sections we will answer this question using a method that can be applied universally, as well as discuss alternative methods that can be used for some specific situations.

Criteria That Need to Be Satisfied for a Universal Productivity Measure Φ

Based on the preceding considerations, we can define from first principles certain criteria to develop a universal productivity measure Φ:

(1) Φ should not be influenced by case mix. The type of operations conducted, or comorbidities in associated patient groups, should not influence whether a team is regarded as 'productive'. Intrinsic procedure duration should not be influential; i.e., Φ should not be influenced by short or long procedures, which should be viewed as equally potentially productive.

(2) Adoption of new techniques to achieve the same surgical aim should not be influential. For example, even after any 'learning curves', laparoscopic or robotic techniques (designed to improve outcomes, safety, pain scores or shortened post-operative stay), often take longer to perform, but Φ should not be adversely influenced by a move to inherently slower techniques. Thus, a team that previously completed, say, three open nephrectomies per list and that now completes just two laparoscopically has not suddenly become less productive (rather, it should be viewed as having started a new, different procedure).

(3) Φ should be in part determined by the *relative speed* of the given surgery. So long as conditions (1) and (2) are met, the faster a team operates, the more productive it is likely to be. Thus, a team consistently completing a hernia repair in 30 min should correctly be viewed as having a higher productive potential than a team that always takes 1 h undertaking exactly the same operation using the same techniques. A team wishing to be more productive should rationally try to operate more quickly – so long as this preserves quality of care. The professional challenge for the team, as always, is to increase its overall speed without compromising safety and outcomes. Therefore a suitable goal for any team is merely to be near to the median (or mean) of the operation time for the given operation – there can be no requirement or any expectation for any team to be faster than the median/mean.

(4) Φ should regard both anaesthesia contact time and surgical contact time with the patient as equivalent. This underlines that the 'speed' referred to in (3) is not just the speed of surgical 'cutting' but rather the speed of the team as a whole, from the point of induction of anaesthesia to the arrival of the patient after surgery in the recovery area. In other words, if a team is regarded as 'slow' for a certain operation, this could be

because of delays in opening surgical packs, or in positioning the patient; it does not necessarily indicate sluggish anaesthesia or surgical technique.

(5) As a consequence of point (4), maximising anaesthesia–surgical contact time means reducing the idle gap times between patients, when no anaesthesia or surgery is conducted. However, this reduction in gap time should only contribute to Φ if extra cases are accommodated into the saved time. Earlier finishes in themselves are not productive: they do not yield extra income (which accrues from cases) nor do they generally save staffing costs (if staff are employed for fixed base units of time). Unless, of course, this earlier finish avoids an overrun, which is otherwise expensive.

(6) Φ is only meaningful in the context of efficiency, ε. In other words, in any quantitative analysis it is ε that should have the biggest influence on Φ.

(7) As discussed earlier, measuring quantitative performance in terms of Φ is only meaningful where predefined quality or safety standards are met. A factory making more televisions than any other is unproductive if its televisions do not work, or frequently explode. This poses a challenge to the medical profession to define those quality and safety standards. An increasing number of specialties, most notably cardiac surgery, now do define minimum standards for risk-adjusted mortality rates, but this needs to extend to all aspects of anaesthetic–surgical care.

Development of a Formula Meeting the Specified Criteria

We describe here, in steps, how a universal formula can be developed based on the criteria defined earlier.

Productive Potential ρρ

First, it is necessary to define a 'productive potential' $\rho\rho$, for a surgical list as being:

$\rho\rho$ for a single operation = (relative operating speed, v) × (fraction of patient contact, τ)

Equation 3.1

Relative operating speed in Equation 3.1 is the team's speed expressed as an inverse proportion (decimal fraction) of the known mean or median speed for the operation. Thus if the reference, average speed for an inguinal hernia repair in a hospital is 50 min, and

the team's speed is 25 min, then the relative operating speed is 2.0 (twice as fast as the average). If team speed is 100 min then its relative speed is 0.5 (only half as fast as reference). The emphasis is on potential productivity because the factors detailed in other parts of the final equation will determine if this is translated into actual productivity. The reference for these speeds may be taken from published data, or from local analysis across several teams, or from the team itself (if assessing its progress over time).

Equation 3.1 applies only to a single operation. Because teams might undertake different specific operations on their lists, the relative speeds of all should be taken into account, and so in the final formula it is the 'team speed' that is relevant, not just the speed for any single operation:

$$\text{Speed, } v \text{ for the team} = \frac{(n_i x) + (n_2 \cdot y) + \ldots + (n_x \cdot z)}{n_1 + n_2 + \ldots + n_x}$$

Equation 3.2

where x, y, z, etc. are the type of operations (inguinal hernia, cholecystectomy, etc.), and n_1, n_2, n_3, etc. are the number of operations. Equation 3.2 encapsulates the notion that a team may be very fast at one operation (e.g., hernia) but slow at another (varicose veins). It can immediately be appreciated that calculating these speeds for all teams, for all their operations, can be quite labour intensive and laborious. It is often simpler to assume that the team operates at 'average' speed, with a value of 1.0.

Fraction of Patient Contact Time τ

This concept is based on the notion that a list is more productive the more patient contact time there is. Non–patient contact time includes waiting for patient arrival, cleaning theatres, etc. and does not progress surgery *per se*. Patient contact time is therefore the time actually spent conducting anaesthesia and surgery, expressed as a proportion of the total actual list time.

If a list started promptly at 09.00 and the last patient arrives in recovery at 17.00 the actual list duration has been 8 h. If six operations each of which lasted 1 h were completed, the patient contact is thus 6 / 8 = 0.75 (that is, 75% of the list time was spent with anaesthetist or surgeon in contact with the patient). In other words, patient contact time is the inverse of gap time, regardless of whether that gap arises at the start, middle or end of list:

$$Patient\ contact\ time,\ \tau = \frac{\sum(duration\ of\ operations\ conducted\ during\ scheduled\ list\ time)}{(time\ from\ scheduled\ start\ time\ to\ actual\ or\ scheduled\ end\ time\ of\ list^*)}$$

Equation 3.3

(*If the actual end time of list arises before the scheduled end time [i.e., underrun], then use actual end time. This way, the underrun gap is counted. If the actual end time of list is after the scheduled end time of list, use the scheduled end time.)

Let us imagine a list whose scheduled list start time is 08.00 and end time at 16.00. It starts late at 09.00 and ends late at 17.00. The denominator in Equation 3.3 is 8 hours. If the sum of the duration of operations (during the scheduled list time) is 6 hours (i.e., the total of gaps within the list is 1 hour), then the numerator is 6. Thus τ becomes 6/8, or 0.75 (75%). If this list finished early at, say, 15.00 instead of late at 17.00, then the denominator becomes 7. Thus τ becomes 6/7, or 0.86 (86%).

Patient contact time τ can be increased by reducing gaps, including reducing late starts. In turn, this could be achieved in theory by the following:

(a) Booking more, rather than fewer, cases on a list (with the aim of increasing utilisation; notwithstanding the risk of overrun or cancellation).

(b) Parallel processing of anaesthesia. This scenario is possible in the UK NHS, where there are generally 'anaesthetic rooms' adjoining the main OR. If there are two anaesthetists (e.g., consultant and trainee) or anaesthetic teams, the next patient can be induced and prepared in the anaesthetic room while the previous patient is being awoken and extubated in the OR. The turnover/gap time between cases is therefore minimal or zero.

(c) Operating more slowly increases τ: this is a perverse way of maximising contact time, and it also adversely influences the 'speed' in Equations 3.1 and 3.2, so the overall gain of this tactic is nil.

Putting the Formula Together

Equations 3.1–3.3 together with Equation 2.2 can be combined to yield an empirical formula that fulfils the criteria we specified for a universal understanding of productivity:

$$\Phi = 111 \times \left[\varepsilon - 10^{(0-\rho\rho)}\right]$$

Equation 3.4

Or, to use all terms of the equations:

$$\Phi = 111 \times \left[\varepsilon - 10^{(0-[\nu \cdot \tau])}\right]$$

Equation 3.5

This formula suggests that productivity ϕ is a function of efficiency ε and productive potential $\rho\rho$ (itself a function of operating speed ν and patient contact time τ). When this equation is plotted graphically, it is seen that the relationship is, however, an asymptotic one: it tends to a maximum of ~100% value for ϕ as the variables increase, in a curvilinear manner.

An oddity of the equation is that where efficiency ε is 1.0 and operating speed ν is 1.0 (the average) and patient contact time τ also 1.0, $\phi = 111\%$. This suggests it is possible to have a 'higher than perfect' productivity, but in practice perfect efficiency ε is never achievable, and some shortcomings always occur. Realistic maximum values might be more like: $\varepsilon = 0.9$, $\nu = 1.0$ (the average) and patient contact time $\tau = 0.9$, which yields $\phi = 97\%$. So Equations 3.4 and 3.5 are designed to deliver ϕ of near 100% for maximal values of the variables. ϕ can exceed 100% only in exceptional circumstances of extremely high efficiency, speed and patient contact.

We have already regarded surgical operating lists not as a factory or conveyor belt as is so often an analogy mistakenly used, but as analogous to antique clock restoration, i.e., a series of skilled, non-repetitive task. In an antique clock restoration firm, high productivity results when the company estimates its workload accurately, for example by accepting enough clocks for repair to fill its time, but not too many that it needs to cancel or postpone orders or pay staff overtime. This is akin to sensible booking of patients onto operating lists to achieve efficiency ε. Staff should spend as much of their time working on the clocks, rather than in idle gaps or break time (a notion akin to maximising patient contact, τ). Finally, for any given clock, staff should ideally take no longer than the average time in repair for the complexity of the task. This is akin to our notion of speed, ν.

Graphical Analysis of Productivity Index ϕ

Plotting Equation 3.5 results in a family of curves. As team speed ν and patient contact τ increase (their product being productive potential, ρρ; see Equation 3.1), this increases ϕ but in a non-linear manner. As productive potential ρρ increases, the marginal gains made become less and less pronounced. In other words, if a team is already working at average speeds, or slightly above, or already minimising gaps to appropriate levels, further increases in speed or squeezing gaps to elimination gain relatively little extra productivity ϕ – this is the 'law of diminishing returns'. However, doing these things is very influential for a team that is extremely slow or suffering very long gaps.

The plot also shows that efficiency ε sets an envelope for productivity ϕ. In other words, the effect of increasing team speed ν and/or patient contact τ depends on the prevailing efficiency ε. Productivity ϕ gains are modest if ε low. This is an important result: a team that is fundamentally inefficient cannot compensate for this by working fast or eliminating all gaps.

Figure 3.1 can be usefully divided into quadrants, based on arbitrary thresholds. We can assume that efficiency ε > 85% is high, and that a productive potential ρρ > 90% is high. Then, we can see where teams that are efficient but unproductive versus productive and inefficient might lie (Figure 3.2, upper panel). For teams that are both inefficient and unproductive, Figure 3.2 helps show that the first step should be to become more efficient, that is, to move up to the next efficiency ε curve – and only then seek to improve operating speed or reducing gaps (arrow

marked 'Step 1', Figure 3.2, lower panel). Attempts simply to work faster and eliminate gaps will (because of the intrinsic shape of the curves) only make modest gains and leave the team potentially productive, but inefficient (arrow marked 'limited gains', Figure 3.2, lower panel).

Using Φ in Practice: Rules of Thumb

It would be unusual to use Φ routinely. The reason is that most surgical lists face the fundamental problem of inefficiency (i.e., under- or overrunning or cancellation). Because efficiency is a prerequisite for productivity, there is no point in expending the greater effort of measuring productivity in an inefficient system. The lists that are efficient are few and far between, in whom we might address their productivity as an end in itself. Appendix 3A outlines the steps of calculation involved.

Nevertheless, a theatre manager may be faced with some challenges that require productivity Φ to be calculated separately. One is, of course, a demand from more senior managers who might wish to know the true capability of the organisation, were it able to run efficiently at all times (e.g., for forward planning). A second might be in settling disputes between different teams or when they compete for resources. For example, an operating room (OR) expansion may be planned, and it is decided to offer this to the 'most productive' specialty as a reward. How, then, to compare, say, cardiac surgery performance versus orthopaedic versus gynaecology? Who is best placed to make the best use of this additional investment? Appendix 3B outlines the comparison of several teams.

If it is necessary or desirable to track Φ on a daily or regular basis, then the theatre manager can reduce the calculation requirements by making certain assumptions (which evidence suggests are not far from reality). One is to assume that most teams, on average over a range of cases, work at median speeds (i.e., ν is ~1.0). It is common to find some teams fast at some things, but very rare to find teams fast at everything. A second is that gap time is ~10–15% (i.e., that patient contact time τ is ~0.9). Unless there is strong evidence to the contrary – and then a sample of observations of the team might be taken – these are safe assumptions. Figure 3.3 repeats an analysis performed by Pandit et al. (2012) from a large number of lists in two

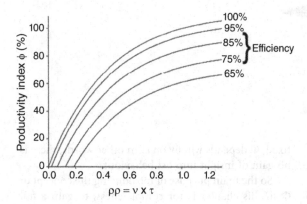

Figure 3.1 Plot of productivity index ϕ against productive potential ρρ, for efficiency values 65%–100%.

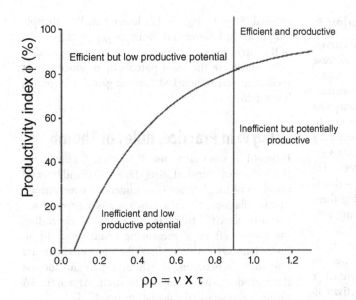

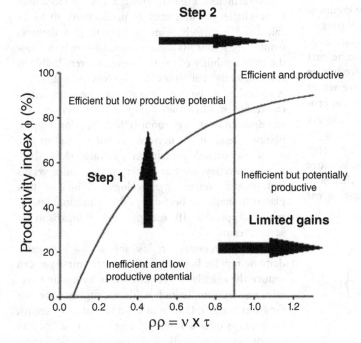

Figure 3.2 Top panel: Dividing Figure 3.1 into quadrants by efficiency and productivity. Bottom panel: If a team is inefficient and unproductive, the first recommended step is to seek efficiency and move from one efficiency curve to a higher curve (Step 1); then as a second step, seek to improve operating speed and eliminating gaps, whilst on the higher efficiency curve (Step 2). The goal of simply working faster whilst remaining on lower efficiency curve will yield only modest gains for the effort (arrow marked 'limited gains').

hospitals (>14,000 lists) showing gap time is ~10–15% of total list time.

If these assumptions are made, then this makes the calculation of Φ much easier. However, making these assumptions does not add anything to the concept of efficiency, ε, as then it means that with ν and τ fixed, Φ depends wholly on ε! In other words, there is no gain of insight into list behaviour.

So the main purpose of introducing the concept of Φ in this chapter is for completeness, to gain a full understanding of the core principles underlying the measurement of list performance.

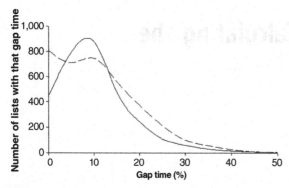

Figure 3.3 Histogram of the distribution of gap times from two UK NHS hospitals.

Applying φ to a Typical US List or UK Private List

Although the preceding discussion has been presented with a typical UK NHS list in mind, the approaches are readily adaptable to other situations. The broad principles are already described in Chapter 2.

For a typical US list, as for efficiency ε, φ could be assessed separately for the OR itself (or a suite of ORs), or for each surgeon who operates within a single OR. The same holds true, as already discussed in Chapter 2, for a typical UK private list. In essence, in the same way as each surgeon's efficiency ε can be assessed for their scheduled time slot within an OR, so too can their individual φ be estimated.

There is a case to be made that in these circumstances individual surgeons or anaesthetists should themselves keep their own tally of ε or φ for their own lists. They are in the best position to calculate, for example, their own timings for operations (i.e., team speed, ν) and could use this as evidence of audit in their personal portfolios. These records could then be compared with standards held by the hospitals for specialties as a whole.

Appendix 3A. Case Study: Calculating the Parameters of φ

Table 3.1 shows the timings for a typical (urology) list. Following it are the calculated parameters (Figure 3.4).

There is no doubt, however, that calculating the parameters is laborious, especially if it is to be repeated over several lists. The especially time-consuming step is the calculation of team speed, for which there is no ready algorithm. This may change in future with (a) accurate coding of each operation and (b) linking that coding to data on duration of procedure.

Table 3.1 A typical surgical list showing the timings for each episode. Following is listed the results of calculating the key parameters. The reference time for the operations can be taken (as in this case) from the team's own past performance (e.g., average of its last 10, 20, 30 procedures), or from published data or national reference norms (of such exist). Data in columns 3,4,5 in minutes.

Time	Operation	Team operation time	Gaps	Reference time for operation(s)	Relative speed
09.00			5		
09.05	Start of cystoscopy	25		33	1.32
09.30	End				
	Gap		5		
09.35	Start of cystoscopy	34		33	0.97
10.09	End				
	Gap		1		
10.10	Start of cystoscopy	45		33	0.73
10.55	End				
	Gap		10		
11.05	Start of cystoscopy	30		33	1.10
11.35	End				
	Gap		5		
11.40	Start of cystoscopy	25		33	1.32
12.05	End		5		

Table 3.1 (*cont.*)

Time	Operation	Team operation time	Gaps	Reference time for operation(s)	Relative speed
12.10	Start of cystoscopy	40		33	0.83
12.50	End				

Summary data

Scheduled time for list = 09.00 – 13.00	240 min
Number of patients scheduled/cancelled	6/0
Late start	5 min
Underrun	10 min
Gap time (% or fraction of list)	13%
Patient contact index, τ (% or fraction; from Equation 3.3)	87%
Weighted mean speed, v (from Equation 3.2)	1.05 (105%)
Efficiency, ε	**95.8%**
Productivity index, φ	**0.93 (93%)**

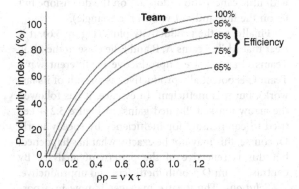

Figure 3.4 The data in Table 3.1 plotted on the productivity plot. Note the x-axis position of 0.87 x 1.05 = 0.91, the point lies on the ε curve of 96%, and the y-axis position of φ is 93%.

Appendix 3B. Case Study: Comparing Teams' Productivity Φ

A theatre manager is asked by supervisors to produce data on the performance of five teams, A–E, who undertake completely different types of surgery. Table 3.2 shows the data extracted. Some things are immediately clear. First, overall start times are not too problematic – late starts are a trivial feature here. Second, there is a wide range of utilisation. Team C underutilises while Team D overruns. Team C appears to try to compensate for this (either volitionally or subliminally), as its speed is quite high. However, this does not work: cancellation rates are unacceptably high, and consequently, its efficiency ε is very low. Cancellations on this team may in fact be the cause of the underruns (e.g., perhaps problems with preassessment are the root cause).

Team D, in contrast, has an ethos of overrunning to complete the cases booked (hence cancellation rates are low), but Team D also appears slower than average. Because of the extreme overruns, Team D's efficiency ε is comparable to Team C's. They also have similar productivity index Φ. Teams A, B and E seem overall reasonable, and the manager can probably discount them from further analysis.

The manager can also now perform graphical analysis. Figure 3.5 shows the efficiency ε isograms

for the teams. Figure 2.6 in Chapter 2 discussed how to interpret these plots. This confirms that Team C underruns with cancellations (dots lie on the upslope and within the triangle) and that Team D overruns with little cancellation (dots are on the downslope but lie on the line and not within the triangle).

Finally, on the productivity plots (Figure 3.6), it is clear that while Teams A, B and E lie close to the ideal, Teams C and D are unproductive in different ways. Team C is potentially productive (as a result of its fast work), but it is inefficient. In essence, it has followed the arrow marked 'limited gains' in Figure 3.2 – i.e., tried to compensate for inefficiency by speedy work. Of course, this may not be exactly what has happened, but this is reflective of the pattern of analysis. By contrast, Team D is both inefficient and unproductive.

Solutions. The theatre manager is now in a position to offer solutions. Team C needs to (a) prevent cancellations and (b) work more slowly – less rushed – at least in the first instance. It may seem paradoxical to suggest that Team C should 'work slowly'; better phraseology is that Team C should be shown that working as fast as it does is achieving neither efficiency nor productivity. If the team speed is its natural rhythm, then all well and good. If, however, the

Table 3.2 Comparison of team performance. Data are median values or number (proportion), for $n = 20$ lists.

Team	Start time (min)	Utilisation (%)	Efficiency ε (%)	Team speed (%)	Patient contact time (%)	Cases completed/ cases booked (cancellation rate, %)	Productivity index φ (%)
A	–3	91	84	117	96	36/39 (7.6)	84
B	9	91	89	111	92	41/42 (2.4)	88
C	–8	88	69	120	23	66/84 (21.4)	68
D	–8	120	75	78	94	43/46 (6.5)	63
E	0	92	85	88	98	19/21 (9.5)	79

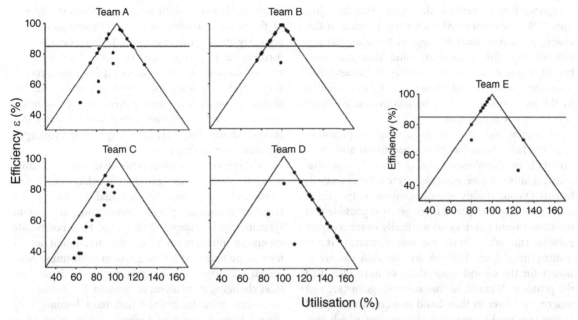

Figure 3.5 Data in Table 3.2 plotted on efficiency isograms. There is an overlay of points, but the patterns reflect the data in the table.

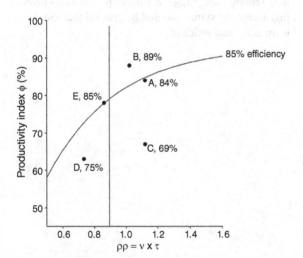

Figure 3.6 Data for the teams in Table 3.2 plotted on productivity plots. The graph is divided by the vertical line into quadrants as shown in Figure 3.2. The numbers by each team refer to their efficiency (Table 3.2).

team speed is compensatory or a reflection of a rushed culture, then in fact, gains can be made by slowing down. Root causes for cancellation may lie in poor preassessment of patients, or indeed overbooking of the list such that remaining cases are cancelled

(i.e., the team prefers an underrun versus overrun at the end of the day).

The solutions for Team D are completely different. This team needs to book fewer cases, to avoid the overruns, or it needs to work to different scheduled times for the list (e.g., be assigned a 10- or 12-hour list rather than an 8-hour list; see Chapter 5 for how this can be done). Because it works unusually slowly, it would benefit from at least average working speeds, but this apparently slow speed may be a result of organisational chaos as a result of the overbooking of cases.

In this way, the theatre manager has provided targeted solutions by careful analysis and also – equally importantly – excluded several teams from further investigation and so saved much time.

The Problem of Intractably Low Productivity

The preceding example is a constructive analysis of teams' performance where some clear solutions present themselves through analysis. Let us now consider a case where analysis seems fruitless.

There are two orthopaedic teams in parallel theatres specialising only in knee replacements. They both start and finish on time, with an equal number of few or no cancellations. Their efficiency ε score is consequently high. However, one team routinely completes five operations; the other completes just three. (We have discussed such a team earlier in this chapter). Further analysis suggests there are no significant gaps for either team, and they are using broadly the same method for surgery and anaesthesia. Thus their patient contact time, τ, is equivalent. It is in the team speed, ν, that the less-productive team falls short – it is just slower.

Assuming that there is not a simple explanation (e.g., the faster team has more anaesthesia and nursing staff, or the slower team is the only one that teaches), this is a rare example where a fuller analysis by patient comorbidity or individual specialty-specific times may help the theatre manager. It is possible that the slower team operates on medically more complex patients (though unlikely for this scenario). If the 'cutting time' from knife-to-skin to skin closure is slower for the second team, then we have identified the problem. It could be that some surgeons are just inherently slower in their hand movements or spend longer in careful haemostasis at each step, which may be a choice rather than necessity. If the anaesthesia induction time is slow, then that also locates the problem. Unfortunately, naturally slow paces are difficult or impossible to resolve. One anaesthetist might draw up all their anaesthetic agents shortly in advance of the patient arriving in the anaesthetic room and regularly inserts the canula while the nurse is performing basic preoperative checks (name, number, etc.) so that the patient is distracted from this procedure. Another anaesthetist might habitually only do things in strict sequence: patient arrives – nurse checks – canula – preparing drugs, etc. Clearly this is much slower, but there is no way that this colleague can now change that rhythm.

If there are no causes other than inherent slowness, the theatre manager therefore has only a few choices. One is to provide additional staffing support (e.g., to encourage parallel processing, assist with speeding up key steps). This would be a potentially expensive intervention where the investment would have to be balanced by the gains in performing additional surgeries. A less-expensive option is to consider changing team members around. For example, if the teams have been fixed and have become very closely knit, gravitating towards the pace of their slowest member, then exchanging team members may reinvigorate things. A final option is to do nothing, accept the status quo and be grateful that the slow team is at least efficient.

Appendix 3C. Squeezing Productivity from a Surgical List; or Squeezing Too Hard?

The problem discussed in Appendix 3B highlights the dual role of a theatre manager in both managing the data and managing people.

Imagine a surgical list whose main operation is a single, long procedure (e.g., hemicolectomy or radical cystoprostatectomy, or radical pelvic debulking surgery for ovarian cancer). The team is scheduled 8 hours for their weekly list. They work well and invariably complete the main operation but also schedule two short cases such that they rarely if ever overrun. Thus, anaesthesia starts at the scheduled start time of 08.30, and the surgeon habitually arrives at 09.30 when anaesthesia is complete (involving as it does several invasive lines). But late starts for anaesthesia or late arrival of the surgeon are very rare. The main operation concludes at ~15.00. The two short cases that follow are usually complete by ~16.00 and rarely later than 16.30, which is the scheduled finish time of the list. There are few cancellations on any given day (and therefore underruns), as preassessment is diligent. There are few overruns. Both the ε score and ϕ score for this team appear high: the team is highly efficient and also acceptably productive.

There is then an organisational drive for increased 'productivity' as a result of which the surgeon is requested to add a local anaesthesia (LA) case to the start of the list, to be performed during the hour that the anaesthetist is inducing the major case and inserting invasive lines, etc. The idea is that, because the anaesthetist is not needed for an LA case (flexible cystoscopy, or removal of minor lump/stitches, etc.), the surgeon and scrub team can do this alone, in the OR. This assumes that there is a separate anaesthesia or induction room for anaesthesia to occur, and itself is a form of parallel processing, mentioned earlier.

Whether this proposal is wise or not is open to debate. First, the real gains are undoubtedly small. Even if the LA waiting list is very long, this is not an important solution to that other problem: performing one patient per week will hardly dent a large waiting list. A different consideration is whether the proposal is disruptive to a team that clearly has an efficient rhythm and works well. Will the surgeon be distracted or tired by the addition of another case, however small? Might it then slow down the speed of the major case, leading to overrun (and hence be counterproductive)? The scrub team may already spend the hour of anaesthesia opening and checking packs and equipment for the major case – if they now have to service the LA case, will this now delay entry of the major case into the OR? That all said, it could be that the team welcomes this idea and is easily able to accommodate an extra small LA case in this way.

The point of this example is to demonstrate that, although the proposal to squeeze one more case undoubtedly leads to increase ϕ in an analytical sense, the theatre manager is not there to increase ϕ as an end in itself. The theatre manager is there to use data such as ϕ or ε to inform discussions and decision making around theatre management.

Appendix 3D. Justifying the Productivity Index Φ

The word *productivity* has various meanings, whether used in economics, engineering or administration. The Organisation for Economic Co-operation and Development (OECD) has suggested over twenty definitions, encompassing both *productivity* and *efficiency* as sometimes used interchangeably. The OECD emphasises that each industry should develop its own agreed-on measures. In other words, there does not seem to be a universal definition of *productivity* versus *efficiency*, and the literature in theatre management is also confusing.

While we do not intend to consider in detail how our notion of productivity Φ might map onto the various formal economic measures, there are some parallels. The economist Sumanth (1984) has written extensively about the concept of productivity. His view (consistent with notions in this chapter) is that efficiency is a necessary but not sufficient condition for productivity; i.e., a *sine qua non*. The two can be distinguished, and the economist quotes a medical analogy. A surgeon amputates a leg in half the time as before and claims that efficiency has doubled: this is true. However, it was the wrong leg, so productivity has drastically declined.

Many other aspects of our discussion in Chapters 2 and 3 are supported by several results from the literature. Although late starts are often blamed for inefficiencies, few objective studies suggest they are influential – Lebowitz (2003), Ray et al. (2008) and Cutter et al. (2008) all affirm that starts as late as by 15 min have no discernible impact on performance, and Macario (2006) makes explicit that delays of <45 min rarely matter. In essence, it is difficult to show objectively that late starts have a detrimental impact on performance, when in reality there exist more influential adverse factors such as overrunning or cancellation.

In this chapter we have been rather dismissive of the need to analyse in detail the gaps between cases and have modelled them as having only a modest effect on performance. Gaps are subjectively felt to be important, but objective analysis suggests that gap (turnover) times are in practice modest. Mathias (2000), Abouleish et al. (2003) and Dexter et al. (2003) have all shown that even eliminating gaps has little overall effect – such that Brenn et al. (2003) even go so far as describing analysis of turnover (gap) times as 'meaningless', implying that the effort is rarely worth the expense.

Ultimately this is the point. Overanalysis is all very well, but the ultimate issue is whether the investment in the factor identified as responsible for poor performance is worth the investment of a solution. If the only thing that starting on time or eliminating small gaps can achieve is a few minutes earlier finish to the list, then what exactly has been gained? Tangible gains occur only if extra cases can be realistically added to fill the time saved, or where long overruns are prevented.

Recently, the productivity index has been justified by analogy with cricket scores, as both represent a form of analysing the best use of resources (Tavare and Pandit, 2018).

In the next appendix we consider an alternative approach to analysing productivity.

Appendix 3E. Data Envelopment Analysis

Data envelopment analysis (DEA), also termed 'frontier analysis', is a performance measurement technique that measures the *relative efficiency* of *decision-making units* (*DMUs*) in organisations. A DMU is a distinct unit within an organisation that has some, but not complete, flexibility with respect to decision making. We can regard a DMU in the DEA theory as a surgical-anaesthetic team, whose performance we are seeking to examine or compare with others.

Consider four teams, undertaking the same type of surgery in the same way (e.g., knee replacements) for which we have a single performance measure (number of operations completed) and a single input measure (number of staff). In this example, 'number of operations' is valid because the same techniques are being used.

Table 3.3 shows the data. Clearly both the number of operations and the number of lists available to each team varied; hence, the fourth column shows the ratio per list. The fifth column shows the normalised ratio, taking Team A arbitrarily to be the norm.

This data might be used to set targets for Teams B–D against the performance of Team A (e.g., for each team to increase its normalised operations/list by 10% per month or per year until it reaches Team A's performance).

However, as we have already discussed, rarely do such teams exist undertaking only one type of surgery – they will more commonly undertake each to a mix of, say, knee and hip replacements. Table 3.4 highlights the problem we discussed, that different teams might compare differently, depending on the focus of the enquiry. So, Team A does the most knees; Team C does the most hips. Which is the higher performer? And how poor, if at all, are the others? Or are they not poor at all – perhaps they are just focussing on the correct balance rather than any single output?

In this chapter, we addressed this problem by disregarding 'number of patients'. Thus the data in Tables 3.3 and 3.4 is irrelevant to our universal measure ϕ, focussing on average speed ν, contact time τ and efficiency ε. Another approach – and this introduces the DEA method – is to plot the different ratios (Figure 3.7). Then after plotting the points (from the last two columns in Table 3.4), lines are drawn from the maximum points, connecting them and the axes so as to create a boundary or frontier.

The positions on the graph represented by Teams A and C represent the performance superior to the other teams. The resulting limit created by the lines is called the *efficient frontier* and represents the performance that the teams B and D could aspire to. It is important to stress in this approach that any teams lying on these boundary lines are all equivalently

Table 3.3 Hypothetical data for four teams conducting a certain number of operations (same type of surgery) on assigned lists.

Team	No. of operations	No. of lists	Operations/ list	Normalised operations/ list
A	125	18	6.94	1.00
B	44	16	2.75	0.40
C	80	17	4.71	0.68
D	23	11	2.09	0.30

Table 3.4 Hypothetical data for where a combination of operations are undertaken.

Team	No. of knees	No. of hips	No. of lists	Knees/ list	Hips/ list
A	125	50	18	6.94	2.78
B	44	20	16	2.75	1.25
C	80	55	17	4.71	3.23
D	23	12	11	2.09	1.09

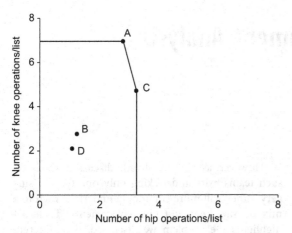

Figure 3.7 Data from Tables 3.3 and 3.4 plotted, with lines joining the 'highest-performing' teams.

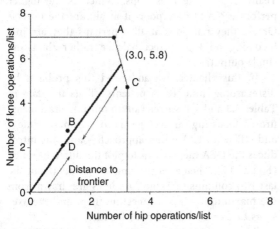

Figure 3.8 Calculating the (in)efficiency of Team D.

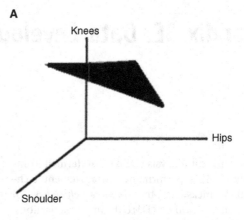

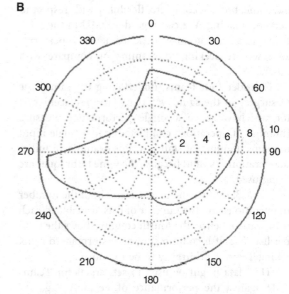

Figure 3.9 A: Hypothetical three-dimensional DEA plot. The floating shape is the efficient frontier. B: polar plot. Here the efficient frontier is conceptualised as the edges of the shape formed, with the dials being the various measures of performance, and the distance from the centre being the degree of performance by measure.

efficient – the boundary represents the line of '100% efficiency' (efficient, that is, in the sense of DEA). Note, however, that this is only a relative efficiency as based on the data available. Teams A and C might increase their numbers of knees and/or hips such that the boundary shifts to the right and higher.

If Teams A and C are to be regarded as 100% efficient, how inefficient are Teams B and D? This can be estimated by drawing a straight line, from the origin, through the team's point (D is shown in Figure 3.8) until it intersects the efficient frontier (here, at the intersection the number is 3 hips/list and 5.8 knees/list). These numbers represent the mix of cases that Team D could achieve as based on its current state, working as efficiently as possible.

The distance the team lies along this line towards the efficient frontier represents the current efficiency of Team D. This can be easily calculated (from the slope of the line) as ~36%.

The further problem – which we have already discussed – is that teams will conduct more than even just two operations. Two operations lends itself well to simple graphical display as shown; we can imagine that with three operations, a three-dimensional graph becomes necessary (and this is still interpretable; Figure 3.9A). Where more than three measures are of interest, one graphical method is the polar plot (Figure 3.9B). The quality measures of efficiency suggested by Macario (2006) could be plotted in this way. However, these plots become more difficult to immediately grasp the results for any one team.

It is still possible to undertake the same analysis as described for the two-operation example, but using mathematics rather than graphs. In other words, DEA requires the inputs (e.g., number of lists available) and outputs (types of operations) for each team to be specified and then defines efficiency for each team as a weighted sum of outputs divided by a weighted sum of inputs (e.g., the ratio columns in Tables 3.3

and 3.4). The result is a series of linear equations that can be solved by linear programming, producing a numerical output (of efficiency) for each team of interest.

Although complex DEA analysis of this sort has been applied in the context of operating theatres as a research or educational tool, there is sparse evidence that it has been used to inform practical decision making. The two-operation example given earlier works well, but like the consideration of productivity ϕ, it is presented in this chapter to enable a wider understanding of approaches, rather than to suggest it is an essential tool to solve many day-to-day problems.

Bibliography

Abouleish AE, Hensley SL, Zornow MH, Prough DS. 2003. Inclusion of turnover time does not influence identification of surgical services that over- and underutilize allocated block time. *Anesthesia and Analgesia* 96: 813–8.

Abouleish A. 2008. Increasing operating room throughput: just buzzwords for this decade? *Anesthesiology* 109: 3–4.

Basson MD, Butler T. 2006. Evaluation of operating suite efficiency in the Veterans Health Administration system by using data-envelopment analysis. *American Journal of Surgery* 192: 649–56.

Brenn BR, Reilly JS, Deutsch ES, Hettrick MH, Cook SC. 2003. Analysis of efficiency of common otolaryngology operations: comparison of operating room vs. short procedure room in a pediatric tertiary hospital. *Archives of Otolaryngology, Head and Neck Surgery* 129: 435–7.

Bridgewater B. 2005. Mortality data in adult cardiac surgery for named surgeons: retrospective examination of prospectively collected data on coronary artery surgery and aortic valve replacement. *British Medical Journal* 330: 506–10.

Cutter RW, Carli N, O'Connor M. 2008. The modified staggered start. *Anesthesia and Analgesia* 106: S–72.

Dexter F, Abouleish AE, Epstein RH, Whitten CW, Lubarsky DA. 2003. Use of operating room information system data to predict the impact of reducing turnover times on staffing costs. *Anesthesia and Analgesia* 97: 1119–26.

Dexter F, O'Neill L. 2004. Data envelopment analysis to determine by how much hospitals can increase elective inpatient surgical workload for each specialty. *Anesthesia and Analgesia* 99: 1492–500.

Harvey J. 1987. Measuring productivity in professional services. *Public Productivity Review* 11: 29–38.

Lebowitz P. 2003. Why can't my procedures start on time? *AORN Journal* 77: 594–7.

Lehtonen J-M, Kukala J, Kouri J, Hippelainen M. 2007. Cardiac surgery productivity and throughput improvements. *International Journal of Health Care Quality Assurance* 20: 30–52.

Macario A. 2006. Are your operating rooms 'efficient?': a scoring system with eight performance indicators. *Anesthesiology* 105: 237–40.

Mathias JM. 2000. Operating room efficiency: benchmarking operating room turnover times. *Operating Room Manager* 16: 1–4.

Office for National Statistics. 2006. *Public Service Productivity: Health*. London: Office for National Statistics.

www.statistics.gov.uk/articles/ nojournal/ PublicServiceProductivity Health(27_2_06).pdf.

Organisation for Economic Co-operation and Development. 2001. *Measuring Productivity. OECD Manual: Measurement of Aggregate and Industry-Level Productivity Growth*. Paris: OECD Publications.

Pandit JJ, Abbott T, Pandit M, Kapila A, Abraham R. 2012. Is 'starting on time' useful (or useless) as a surrogate measure for 'surgical theatre efficiency'? *Anaesthesia* 67: 823–32.

Pandit JJ, Stubbs D, Pandit M. 2009. Measuring the quantitative performance of surgical operating lists: theoretical modelling of 'productive potential' and 'efficiency'. *Anaesthesia* 64: 473–86.

Ray N, Tung A, Glick DB. 2008. Who cares if I'm on time? *Anesthesia and Analgesia* 106: S–71.

Royal Statistical Society Working Party on Performance Monitoring in the Public Service. (2004). 2005. Performance indicators: good, bad and ugly. *Journal of the Royal Statistical Society A* 168: 1–27.

Schmenner RW. 2004. Service business and productivity. *Decision Sciences* 35: 333–47.

Schreyer P. 2005. Measures of productivity. Proceedings of the

Conference on Next Steps for the Japanese System of National Accounts. www.esri.go.jp/en/workshop/050325/0503325main-e.html.

Scott S. 1987. *Productivity Management: Planning, Measurement and Evaluation, Control and Improvement.* New York: John Wiley and Sons.

Seim AR, Dahl DM, Sandberg WS. 2007. Small changes in operative time can yield discrete increases in operating room throughput. *Journal of Endourology* 7: 703–8.

Smith MP, Sandberg WS, Foss J, et al. 2008. High-throughput operating room system for joint arthroplasties durably outperforms routine processes. *Anesthesiology* 109: 25–35.

Strum DP, Sampson AR, May JH, Vargas LG. 2000. Surgeon and type of anesthesia predict variability in surgical procedure times. *Anesthesiology* 92: 1454–66.

Sumanth DJ. 1984. *Productivity Engineering and Management.* New York: McGraw-Hill.

Tavare A, Pandit JJ. 2018. When rain stops play: a 'Duckworth-Lewis method' for surgical operating list productivity? *Anaesthesia* 73: 248–51.

Zbinden AM. 2002. Introducing a balanced scorecard management system in a university anesthesiology department. *Anesthesia and Analgesia* 95: 1731–8.

Chapter 4

Case Scheduling

Jaideep J. Pandit

Introduction

All that has been discussed in the preceding chapters – achieving efficiency ε (Chapter 2), and productivity φ (Chapter 3) – requires that the surgical list is well planned in the first place. This is the important topic of 'case scheduling'. In the next chapter we will discuss the separate but related topic of 'list scheduling' (i.e., the number of lists to assign to each team and the optimum duration of those lists: this is 'capacity' for the team and is discussed in Chapter 5).

The reason why good case scheduling is important is readily apparent. If in a typical United Kingdom National Health Service (UK NHS) list a team is assigned 8 hours of time on its list, but schedules cases on its list that clearly will take longer than this, then overrun or cancellation will result. If a pseudorandom method of scheduling results in just one or two small cases being listed, then the list will greatly underrun, and resources are wasted. Similar chaos can result in a typical US list. A US surgeon regularly demands the full 8 hours of the operating room (OR) time that is staffed, but habitually only uses 4 hours – simply because the sum of duration of cases scheduled is never going to last anywhere near 8 hours. Or conversely, the surgeon habitually uses 10 hours; in both cases resources are wasted or mis-used.

In this chapter, we will discuss how to schedule cases onto a list such that as much time as possible is utilised, with low chance of overrun or cancellation as a result. We will focus on the planning around a typical UK NHS list, but will discuss how the principles are readily applicable to other scenarios.

Fallacies Surrounding Case Scheduling

First, we will discuss certain fallacies commonly associated with case scheduling, including: the fallacy that case durations are unpredictable, that mean (or median) case times are all that matter, and that

surgical (cutting) time – or anaesthesia controlled time – should always be measured separately.

The Fallacy That Case Durations Are Unpredictable

One of the commonest fallacies heard in ORs, theatre coffee rooms, surgeons' changing rooms or committees is that 'the duration of an operation is unpredictable'. This fallacy rests on the idea that any task – especially a surgical operation – is a complex series of steps, the duration of the one step dependent on how easy or difficult was the preceding step. Consequently, the duration of the whole procedure is deemed 'unpredictable'.

If this were true, then the duration of everything in life would be unpredictable. We would not know how long it would take to have a shower, to drive to work, or to schedule for evening dinner. We would be constantly surprised by the time and be unable to plan anything. In clinical practice, nobody of any seniority would ever be able to guess if a toenail removal would take more or less time than a combined heart–lung transplant. We would all end up commiserating with each other: 'how long is a piece of string?'; 'anything could happen!', etc.

Clearly even on first principles these imagined scenarios are silly. Surgical operations (and the anaesthetic interventions that underpin them) fall into discrete categories, characterised by aliquots of time that, while not identical for all elements within a category, are broadly similar within any category (i.e., there is a median and a variance of the times). Thus a toenail removal is on average very much shorter than the average heart–lung transplant (although there may have once, sometime, somewhere, been an unusual toenail removal that lasted longer than an unusually quick heart–lung transplant). So it follows that surgical operation times are *predictable*, at least by their groups.

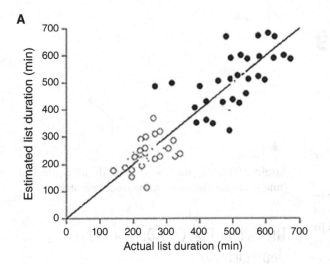

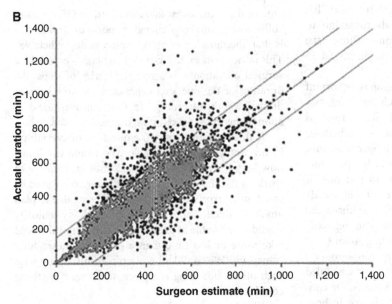

Figure 4.1 A: Previously unpublished estimates by surgeons of published surgical lists for 4- to 6-hour lists (white circles) and 8- to 10-hour lists (dark circles), for a large number of lists. There is data overlay of points. The line represents the line of identity. In a previous study, similarly good predictions were obtained by asking different staff groups such as anaesthetists, anaesthetic assistants and theatre staff (Pandit and Carey, 2006). B: Previously unpublished data from two hospitals (black and grey circles) for > 8,000 lists showing the good predictive ability of surgeon to actual duration (significant data overlay). The three straight lines represent the line of identity (middle) and the 95% confidence interval for the predictions.

Moreover, much research has confirmed that experienced staff groups can predict the duration of surgical operations extremely well. Figure 4.1 repeats methodology from previously published studies, showing the estimated duration of lists by surgeons matches very well the actual durations that occurred.

There is one caveat to operations (and therefore duration of surgical lists) being predictable: that is the 'open-and-shut' case. Particularly in cancer surgery, some operations can be predictably very long, with much careful dissection being necessary. However, even with the best preoperative planning and imaging

of the tumours, sometimes it is found only soon after the operation starts that the patient is inoperable because the tumour has spread. Therefore, these operations can either be very long or very short, and this may be unpredictable. However, this is an exception, and how to handle it is discussed later.

The Fallacy That Mean (or Median) Operation Times Are All That Matter

In Figure 4.1 the mean operation times have been estimated by the staff group (similar results arise if medians are used), and these match the actual means (or medians) that occurred. This result should not lead to the fallacy that all that is required for good list planning is knowledge of the means (or medians), and that all it takes to plan a list is to sum the means/ medians case times.

The fallacy can best be presented by the following example. A surgical list is scheduled to last 4 hours. The team specialises in, say, hernia repair, which is an operation known on average to last 1 hour. The fallacy is that if four cases are booked onto this list, it can be expected to finish within time. It will not; it will commonly overrun.

The reason for this is that means or medians alone do not take account of *variation*. Variation is best represented for our purposes by standard deviation (SD), or range or interquartile range. So, each hernia in reality lasts one hour ± ~20 minutes. This means that, given 100 hernias, 95 of them will take between 20 minutes and 120 minutes, 68 of them will take between 40 and 80 minutes, and so on (assuming the distribution is normal or Gaussian). To express this differently, the reasonable best-case scenario is that each of the four hernias will take 40 minutes (total 160 minutes); the worst-case scenario is that each will take 80 minutes (320 minutes). So from this data, all we can say is that this list of four hernias will only run to time on half the occasions.

The means/medians alone have therefore not really helped us schedule the cases very well; the missing data is the variance (SD). Readers will commonly come across commercial theatre scheduling software models that use only the means or medians of the operation times. They should beware, because purchasing such software or adopting such models will lead to operational chaos.

We discuss later how the data of SDs can be used to develop a method of probabilistic scheduling.

Fallacy of the Importance of Measuring 'Surgical Cutting Time' Separately from 'Anaesthesia Controlled Time')

One of the paradoxes of working in the operating theatre environment is this. Ask a surgeon how long a particular operation in which they are specialised will take, and they will likely respond with a surprisingly low estimate. An example is a dynamic hip screw (DHS); most responses to this question yield answers approximating 20 minutes. Yet, ask the same surgeon how long a list of DHS cases will take, and they will provide (as shown by Pandit and Carey, 2006) an estimate that is surprisingly accurate – and in this more accurate estimate, each DHS will have the more realistic duration of ~90 minutes. How is this possible, for the surgeon to be both correct and incorrect in answer to fundamentally the same question?

A very dramatic example of this scenario happened recently, when I approached an extremely experienced and skilled surgeon colleague who had the previous day undertaken a very complex tumour removal, deep inside the abdomen, near the pancreas and kidneys. The case had been postponed from days before because of lack of remaining OR time. When I asked him how long it had taken, he honestly and seriously replied it has taken him exactly 15 minutes. Surprised, I checked the theatre computer to find that in fact, the case had lasted almost 4 hours, as expected. Was my colleague deluded? Cleary not; but what was the explanation?

In fact, this scenario is perfectly understandable and helps highlight the fallacy of 'specialty-specific times'. Surgeons will, quite understandably, focus or recall only those times within the operation that matter to them, and perhaps by which they judge their own or each others' performance. For a DHS operation, the time that matters to a surgeon is that from the first incision to completing the insertion of the dynamic hip screw. To many surgeons, the positioning of the patient, the preparation and cleaning of skin, the closure of tissue layers (and certainly the anaesthetic time) do not matter at all. For the tumour in question in the preceding story, the only time that mattered was that from when the tumour was exposed to when it was removed from the body, which was indeed ~15 minutes. The entire process of the hours of dissecting down to free the tumour and careful closure was – for the purposes of the question asked – completely irrelevant to the surgeon. I clearly recall another surgical colleague – a senior professor – once holding aloft a piece of liver, dripping with blood and shouting proudly, 'The operation is over'; when in fact there were clearly several hours of surgery still to complete.

Yet, when asked the subtly different question about list durations, surgeons quite correctly estimate very well because then they automatically take into account all the other times that really make up the case duration.

This is not a critique of surgeons. The important message is that if asked a question about a task upon which one is entirely focussed, it is natural to answer the question only in relation to that task. It is notable that the patient pathway within the theatre suite is a series of several steps, with different professionals leading each step (Figure 4.2). The question is: does this mean that in order to understand the process as a whole, we must deconstruct it into each of its component times?

On one level or in certain circumstances this may be necessary. For example, it may be important to know how long the patient is spending in recovery/post-anaesthesia care unit (PACU). Or, how many days on the ward post-operatively – in order to reduce these respective stays. Yet on another level, the danger of excessive deconstruction is demonstrated by the following *reductio ad adsurdum*. Even if we promote the idea of 'surgical cutting time', why stop there? Why not then deconstruct things further to measure 'incision time', 'closure time', etc.? And deconstruct

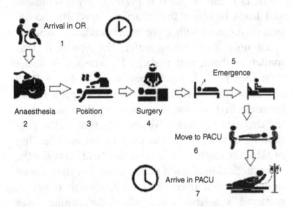

Figure 4.2 Patient pathway in theatre. The total case duration starts with the arrival of the patient in the OR or anaesthesia room. At this point, the patient is checked, regulatory paperwork completed, monitors applied. Then, anaesthesia begins (e.g., with intravenous induction or regional blockade). After entry of the patient into the OR (or after completion of anaesthesia in the OR), the patient is positioned, skin prepared. Then, surgery can begin (after the WHO timeout), and surgery is complete after the last skin suture. Anaesthesia reversal or emergence may begin in OR (e.g., by using reversal of neuromuscular blockade) and at some suitable point, the anaesthetist will judge that it is safe to transport the patient to recovery/PACU area (e.g., in some centres this may be with the patient still to some extent anaesthetised, breathing via a supraglottic airway). The case ends with arrival of the patient in PACU with suitable handover of care. While the anaesthetist is in PACU, the anaesthesia assistant is cleaning and preparing the OR/anaesthesia room for the next patient. The time from this event to the arrival/start of anaesthesia in the next patient is the gap or turnover time. The total case duration is the time from step 1 to step 7.

anaesthesia into 'canula insertion time' or 'intubation time', etc.

Then, we also encounter a paradox in trying to measure specialty-specific times. Even if we accept that 'surgical cutting time' is easily identified, what might be regarded as the time in control of the anaesthetist? This is referred to sometimes in the literature as the 'anaesthesia control time' (ACT). In part, this is the induction, step 2 (Figure 4.2). But the anaesthetist is present throughout until step 7. Should not the whole of steps 2–7 be the ACT? Yet, while it can be argued that emergence (step 5), ending with extubation, is 'under control' of the anaesthetist, the pharmacology of emergence is in fact almost entirely a passive process, not under control of anyone. Some patients inherently take longer to wake, regardless of anaesthetic technique or interventions because of their innate biology.

The real question for an organisation is: what is the value of the effort expended in identifying specialty-specific times? As will become clear in this chapter, any gains are modest. For list planning what is really important to measure is the total case time – the time for all the steps from 1 to 7. It is *team* performance being primarily measured, and all other deconstructed measures are secondary.

Probabilistic Case Scheduling

We introduced earlier the notion of variation (SD) in timings as being important. Here we show how these variations can be used to adopt a method of case scheduling that relies on probabilities, rather than certainties. Although a mathematical concept, there is also a linguistic consequence. Rather than saying, 'This list of cases will (or will not) be finished within the scheduled time for the list' (i.e., linguistic certainty), we will now say, 'This list of cases has a certain probability $x\%$ of being finished within the scheduled time for the list' (probabilistic language). We can then have a separate discussion of what value x has, or what value it should have.

Mathematics: Developing the Formula

A list is composed of several operations. The mean estimated list duration is the sum of the operations (Mx) listed and the 'gap time' (Gt), which can be expressed as a proportion of the scheduled duration of the operating list (St). Literature suggests (as we discussed in Chapter 3) that Gt averages ~10%.

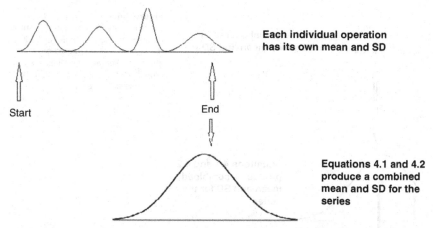

Each individual operation
has its own mean and SD

Start   End

Equations 4.1 and 4.2
produce a combined
mean and SD for the
series

Figure 4.3 Understanding Equations 4.1 and 4.2 pictorially. In these plots, the x-axis is time and the y-axis can be considered to be a histogram of the operation finish times. The surgical list has a defined start time and end time (arrows). Each operation (four are shown here) has its own mean and SD, shown as four Gaussian curves. The total may (as shown) or may not overlap/exceed the end time for the list. Equations 4.1 and 4.2 convert these four separate Gaussian curves into one combined curve (lower panel), whose mean (peak of the curve) is the sum of mean (peak of curve) times of each of the four operations, and whose SD is the pooled SD, which may (as shown) or may not overlap/exceed the end time for the list. Given the list has a known duration (e.g., 480 minutes) then the combined mean and SD (e.g., 480 ± 60 minutes) can be compared to assess the probability of the series of operations overrunning or not this duration.

Equation 4.1 gives the mean duration from the start of arrival of the first patient on the list in the anaesthesia room (or OR) for induction of anaesthesia, to the arrival of the last patient on the list in the recovery/PACU area.

Estimated mean duration of list =

$$(M_1 + M_2 + \ldots M_x) + (G_T \cdot S_T) \qquad \text{Equation 4.1}$$

Each operation has its own variance (SD). There are two ways to calculate a pooled SD for the series of operations listed. One is a pooled SD for an estimated mean (i.e., which is akin to the standard error of the mean):

Pooled SD for the mean time of the series of operations

$$= \frac{\sqrt{SD_1^2 + SD_2^2 + \ldots SD_X^2}}{x} \qquad \text{Equation 4.2}$$

An alternative is the pooled SD for the sum of a series of discrete times:

Pooled SD for the sum of a series of times

$$= \sqrt{SD_1^2 + SD_2^2 + \ldots SD_X^2} \qquad \text{Equation 4.3}$$

In these equations, x is the number of operations and SD_x is their individual SD. For example, a hypothetical list of two inguinal hernia repairs (mean time

63 min ± SD 11 min) and one mastectomy (mean time 101 min ± SD 12 min) scheduled into a 240-min operating list yields an estimated time (including 24 min representing the 10% gap time) of 63 + 63 + 101 + 24 min = 251 min ± pooled SD of 11.3 min.

The actual difference between these two quantities is very small, and the literature suggests that Equation 4.2 works somewhat better in practice (Proudlove et al., 2013).

Thus Equations 4.1 and 4.2 yield a simple formula that, for any series of operations, will produce a mean ± SD of the time of the list as a whole. The next step is to compare this result statistically with the desired finish time of the list. Pictorially the process can be understood by considering Figure 4.3.

The process has been made easy through a Case Scheduling Algorithm (CSA tool), which is a simple Excel-based program (filename CSA Scheduler Tool at: www.cambridge.org/9781316646830). Indeed, it is not only the list duration that can be compared with the combined mean and SD; any chosen time point can be used, and two are especially relevant.

A theatre manager will, of course, wish a surgical list to be completed as near to its scheduled time as possible. However given there is uncertainty and variation, the theatre manager will have in mind two other time points. One is the minimum amount of

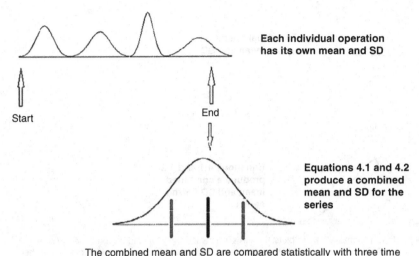

Each individual operation has its own mean and SD

Start

End

Figure 4.4 How Equations 4.1 and 4.2 can be used to generate statistical comparisons against three relevant time points. The combined mean and SD (lower plot) indicates the probability the list is ongoing at the three relevant time points.

Equations 4.1 and 4.2 produce a combined mean and SD for the series

The combined mean and SD are compared statistically with three time points: scheduled end of list (black line); minimum utilisation time and maximum utilisation time (grey lines)

list time that should ideally be used (i.e., the minimum utilisation of the list). If any less is used, this is regarded by the organisation as underrunning. The time point is arbitrary but, say, for a 480 minute list the organisation might like at least 420 minutes to be used. The second is the maximum time the list can overrun before it is regarded as unacceptable. Again, this is arbitrary, but could also be by 60 minutes (i.e., total list time 540 minutes). Or, each of these could be 30 minutes or whatever. The importance of Equations 4.1 and 4.2 is that the combined times generated can be used to compare against each of the three time points: the scheduled end time for the list, the minimum time the list should be utilised and the maximum overrun allowed. Figure 4.4 illustrates this.

The next section describes the use of the CSA tool.

Using the CSA Tool

Figure 4.5 shows an output from the CSA tool using the example we used earlier in the text, of four hernia repairs each of duration 60 min (SD 20 min). What is striking is that even where the sum of means of the operations are close to 240 min (the sum is a little more to take account of gap time, embedded in the CSA tool), there is only a very low (12%) probability that this published list will finish on time: i.e., an 88% chance it will overrun. This underlines the fallacy of using means to schedule cases onto a list – the SDs must also be taken into account.

Note also the ability to set the outer limits for time. The published list will of course utilise the minimum time desired (100% probability), but in fact, it is so overbooked that there is still a 38% chance it will overrun 270 minutes.

What is to be done? The theatre manager should not allow this list to go ahead as published. Instead, one of the 60 min cases should be replaced with a shorter 30 min case. Let us see in Figure 4.6 the result of doing this. There is a remarkable transformation in fortunes, with a 69% chance of finishing on time (i.e., more likely than not) and just a 2% chance of overrunning the outer limit of time. Interestingly there is now a small chance (12%) that the list may not exceed the minimum time. If this is a concern (although there is no reason it should be), further list adjustments can be made.

A Case Scheduling Heuristic for Theatre Managers

What we have shown here is a heuristic – a rule of thumb, or protocol – that theatre managers can follow to optimise their case scheduling. We will list the steps of the heuristic:

(1) Obtain mean and SD times for the operations in question.
(2) Enter the data for each operation into the CSA tool, along with the scheduled time of the list and the agreed minimum and maximum times.

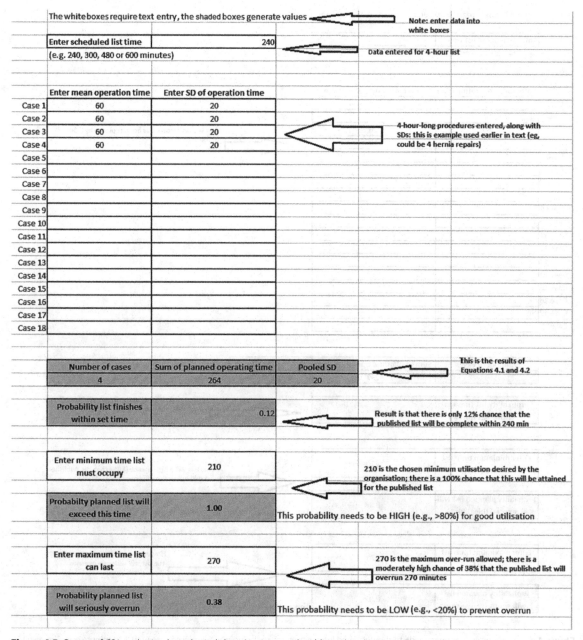

The white boxes require text entry, the shaded boxes generate values → Note: enter data into white boxes

| Enter scheduled list time | 240 |
| (e.g. 240, 300, 480 or 600 minutes) | |

← Data entered for 4-hour list

	Enter mean operation time	Enter SD of operation time
Case 1	60	20
Case 2	60	20
Case 3	60	20
Case 4	60	20
Case 5		
Case 6		
Case 7		
Case 8		
Case 9		
Case 10		
Case 11		
Case 12		
Case 13		
Case 14		
Case 15		
Case 16		
Case 17		
Case 18		

← 4-hour-long procedures entered, along with SDs: this is example used earlier in text (eg, could be 4 hernia repairs)

Number of cases	Sum of planned operating time	Pooled SD
4	264	20

← This is the results of Equations 4.1 and 4.2

Probability list finishes within set time	0.12

← Result is that there is only 12% chance that the published list will be complete within 240 min

Enter minimum time list must occupy	210

← 210 is the chosen minimum utilisation desired by the organisation; there is a 100% chance that this will be attained for the published list

Probabilty planned list will exceed this time	1.00

This probability needs to be HIGH (e.g., >80%) for good utilisation

Enter maximum time list can last	270

← 270 is the maximum over-run allowed; there is a moderately high chance of 38% that the published list will overrun 270 minutes

Probability planned list will seriously overrun	0.38

This probability needs to be LOW (e.g., <20%) to prevent overrun

Figure 4.5 Output of CSA tool using hypothetical data. Arrows provide additional explanation of the results.

(3) Ensure that (i) there is a high probability (>80%) that the provisionally published list will finish within time whilst (ii) have high probability (>80%) of utilising the minimum time and (iii) a low probability (<20%) of exceeding the maximum time.

(4) If not, then either add or replace cases by time accordingly to achieve the goal set out in (3).

The heuristic relies, of course, on certain requirements: *Knowledge of the mean and SD times*. This is essential for the process to work. However, it is also

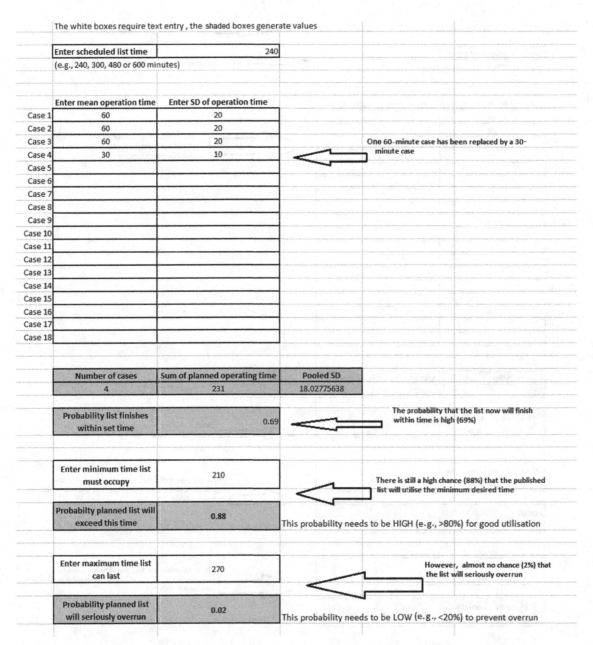

The white boxes require text entry , the shaded boxes generate values

Enter scheduled list time	240

(e.g., 240, 300, 480 or 600 minutes)

	Enter mean operation time	Enter SD of operation time
Case 1	60	20
Case 2	60	20
Case 3	60	20
Case 4	30	10
Case 5		
Case 6		
Case 7		
Case 8		
Case 9		
Case 10		
Case 11		
Case 12		
Case 13		
Case 14		
Case 15		
Case 16		
Case 17		
Case 18		

One 60-minute case has been replaced by a 30-minute case

Number of cases	Sum of planned operating time	Pooled SD
4	231	18.02775638

Probability list finishes within set time	0.69

The probability that the list now will finish within time is high (69%)

Enter minimum time list must occupy	210

There is still a high chance (88%) that the published list will utilise the minimum desired time

Probabilty planned list will exceed this time	0.88

This probability needs to be HIGH (e.g., >80%) for good utilisation

Enter maximum time list can last	270

However, almost no chance (2%) that the list will seriously overrun

Probability planned list will seriously overrun	0.02

This probability needs to be LOW (e.g., <20%) to prevent overrun

Figure 4.6 An adjustment has been made to the published list in Figure 4.5, replacing one 60-minute case with a 30-minute one. The result is a remarkable transformation of the predictions.

essential knowledge for hospitals to function. We emphasised in this book that 'time' is the relevant currency for efficient operating theatre management. Without knowledge of time, then no planning is possible. It is rather like trying to run a supermarket without knowing the preferences of the customers, or running any business without having core knowledge of expenditure and income. It just is impossible. Any theatre manager asked to optimise theatre efficiency but not provided with access to operation timings with SDs (or working in a system that cannot easily produce such data) should probably resign, as their task is impossible. Such a hospital will be doomed to financial and organisational failure.

We discuss later the separate limitation of the situation where there is no data for a specific operation, or where the times are too variable, and we describe how to manage this. But this is quite different from not having access to *any* timing data.

Agreeing minimum times to be utilised and maximum times not to be exceeded. This is purely arbitrary and achieved by local agreement. It will be part of a manager's skills to have a mature conversation with staff and with more senior management to agree on what these limits should be. Senior management cannot insist on a list *never* finishing 'early'; staff cannot insist on a list *never* finishing 'late'. The real questions are, for example: how early are senior managers prepared to let staff go home early? How late are staff prepared to stay late, if perchance the list finishes late? The answers to these set the 'tolerance levels' of the formula.

The narrower these tolerance limits, the more difficult it will be to match the published list to the agreed times. For example, if a 240-min list can only be scheduled to finish between 235 and 245 min, the opportunity for adjusting the list to this degree of accuracy is limited. In other words, these are not meaningful limits. Yet the wider these tolerance limits, the more pointless becomes the activity of case scheduling in the first place. For example, if a 240-min list could acceptably be scheduled to finish anywhere between 5 min and 480 min, then clearly it is possible to book anything (or nothing) at all, and for things still to be acceptable. The whole point of the CSA tool is lost.

Adjusting cases. Cases on the list can only be adjusted if two preconditions are met. First, that there are enough cases on the waiting list to replace the provisionally booked cases. This is certainly the case in the UK NHS, where there is a large pool of patients waiting. However, it may less so in a typical US surgical list, or a UK private hospital list. Clearly then, the theatre manager is constrained by what flexibilities are available.

Second, the wider surgical–anaesthetic team should find it acceptable that in essence their individual control over list composition is taken over by what is after all a computer algorithm, the CSA tool. They may feel disempowerment by loss of clinical freedoms. By way of reassurance, it must always be emphasised that clinical skill mix, or other factors

unknown to the CSA tool, must supervene in any final decision on scheduling.

Limitations of the CSA Tool and How to Manage Them

Clearly no intervention is perfect, and the CSA tool has its limitations.

Probabilistic Language

Perhaps the biggest strength of the CSA tool is also its main limitation. The CSA tool output is phrased in terms of probability, not certainty: i.e., that a provisionally booked list has x% chance of finishing by the scheduled time. The wider theatre team should be comfortable with this sort of language and also at ease with, on different days, interpreting how to respond to the specific value of x.

For example, let us suppose on one day the team is faced with a CSA tool-booked list that estimates there is a 75% chance of finishing on time, with a 35% chance of overrunning an hour beyond time. On another day it is faced with a CSA tool estimate that the list has an 80% chance of finishing on time, but a 40% chance of finishing an hour beyond time. Are these lists equally acceptable? This is an unanswerable question, and teams themselves need to develop familiarity with probabilistic thinking and language to make the best sense of the CSA tool outputs. It is hoped that a combination of practice and training will produce the necessary familiarity with the new language.

Absence of Data

For some operations, there will never be any timing data. One example is a completely new procedure. For procedures that have nationally or internationally published timing data, but that are new to the team, it may be unwise simply to translate that other data to the local situation (as there will always be a learning curve to perform the surgery). Sometimes, a robust *mean* value may be available (e.g., just three or four procedures have been performed), but too few cases have been undertaken to produce a meaningful SD. Data can also be 'absent' where multiple procedures are performed in the same patient at one sitting. The total duration of the operation is then going to be somewhat less than the simple sum of the individual procedures, but hard data may not be available.

Solution: Where the mean is known or estimable, use an estimated SD that is approximately one-third the value of the mean (e.g., mean 60 min, SD 20 min). For multiple procedures in one operation, the sum of means for each procedure might be used as an estimate (perhaps with 10% subtracted) and then SD assumed to be one-third of this. Where the mean is unknown, use the *β distribution* (see later) to yield a mean and SD for the CSA tool.

Wide Variation of Data

Another problem, touched upon earlier, is when the procedure has extremely wide variation (SD). An example of this is the open-and-shut case (often in cancer surgery). Such cases can yield a mean procedure time, but will have huge SD variation. The mean is then not an appropriate reflection of the true operation duration. The wide SD values simply make the process of prediction ever more uncertain. Figure 4.7 shows an example similar to that in Figure 4.5 (same scheduled list duration; four cases of an hour each), but where each case has a huge SD. The result is uncertainty of when this list will finish: the probability that it will finish to time is almost the same as that it will overrun. This makes it difficult or impossible for the team to know what will happen on the day.

Solution: There is no perfect technical solution to this problem. Certainly, the CSA tool can assist in selecting cases to optimise the predictive probabilities, but ultimately the solution will lie in engaging with staff affected, perhaps through contracts (see Chapters 6 and 7). A 'swings and roundabouts' approach may need to adopted wherein it is agreed that the casemix is fundamentally variable, and so staff will sometimes be released very early (swings), but at other times have to stay very late (roundabouts). Another pragmatic solution is to agree with other patients (who have relatively short operations scheduled) that they are on 'short call': if the putatively long case does not go ahead, they are willing to be ready and waiting, fasting on the day of surgery, to come in at short notice as replacement cases.

No Replacement Cases and Single-Case Lists

The heuristic based on the CSA tool requires there to be suitable replacement cases on the waiting list. If the replacement cases have similar means/SDs as the originally booked cases, then the list scheduling cannot be improved, and there will need to be different discussions with staff and other managers as to whether to over- or underrun the list.

The CSA tool works best, the more diverse cases there are on a waiting list to schedule. If a list consists of only one case, then there is only one mean and SD to consider. You have what you have and cannot conjure up cases. The CSA tool can still be used: it will still generate a probability of finishing to time, and the probabilities of finishing *x* hours late, etc. But then it needs to be used in a different way. Rather than being used to adjust casemix (which is impossible because the given case has to be done, sooner or later), the CSA tool is used to estimate the list duration and adjust it accordingly.

Let us suppose a list is normally scheduled for 8 hours. The surgeon has to do a single case of mean duration 8 hours (SD 60 min). The locally agreed policy is for lists to be scheduled with 80% probability of finishing on time and 20% or less probability of finishing late. As it stands, this case has only a 21% chance of finishing on time and a 42% chance of running beyond an hour over time. What we then do is adjust not the casemix, but instead the scheduled time for the list. We find that at 600 min (10 hours) the probability of finishing on time is now 88% and the probability of running beyond 660 min (11 hours) very low, just 1% (Figure 4.8). Thus, staff can be informed of the changed list length – suitable arrangements can be made, by staffing with those who can stay late, and also extra payment arrangements made as per contract, all well in advance.

Non-Gaussian Data: Using the β Distribution

This discussion also touches upon whether the operation timing data are Gaussian or non-Gaussian (Figure 4.9). Non-Gaussian distributions for operation times can be relatively easily detected by having large differences between the mean and the median and also having very wide SDs (e.g., SD > 50% of the mean value).

If Gaussian statistics are applied to non-Gaussian data, there will arise an error in the estimates that is broadly proportional to how large is the disparity between assuming Gaussian distributions for non-Gaussian data. Often, that disparity is in practice small, and the assumption does not matter (or at least, the assumption is better than using no quantitative method at all and relying only on guesswork).

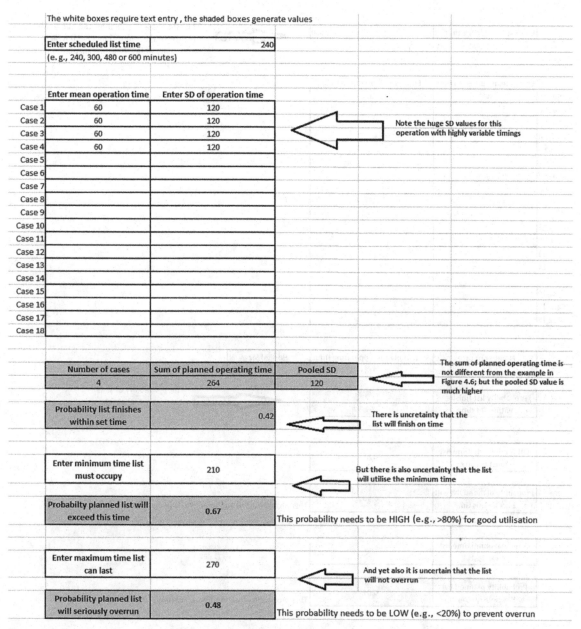

The white boxes require text entry , the shaded boxes generate values

Enter scheduled list time	240

(e.g., 240, 300, 480 or 600 minutes)

	Enter mean operation time	Enter SD of operation time
Case 1	60	120
Case 2	60	120
Case 3	60	120
Case 4	60	120
Case 5		
Case 6		
Case 7		
Case 8		
Case 9		
Case 10		
Case 11		
Case 12		
Case 13		
Case 14		
Case 15		
Case 16		
Case 17		
Case 18		

Note the huge SD values for this operation with highly variable timings

Number of cases	Sum of planned operating time	Pooled SD
4	264	120

The sum of planned operating time is not different from the example in Figure 4.6; but the pooled SD value is much higher

Probability list finishes within set time	0.42

There is uncrertainty that the list will finish on time

Enter minimum time list must occupy	210

But there is also uncertainty that the list will utilise the minimum time

Probabilty planned list will exceed this time	0.67

This probability needs to be HIGH (e.g., >80%) for good utilisation

Enter maximum time list can last	270

And yet also it is uncertain that the list will not overrun

Probability planned list will seriously overrun	0.48

This probability needs to be LOW (e.g., <20%) to prevent overrun

Figure 4.7 Example data for a list consisting of hugely variable cases using the CSA tool.

Complete solutions are not easy. The mathematics of non-Gaussian distributions can become very complicated, and there are no ready-to-access algorithms that make calculation easy.

Solution A: Median and Interquartile Range. A solution can be used if the mean and median for an operation time are very different. This difference indicates that the data are likely non-Gaussian. Then, the CSA scheduling tool can still be used, but instead of the mean, the median time can be used. Instead of the SD, the interquartile range (IQR) for the time can be used. The dataset for the durations can be divided into four quartiles, and the IQR is the values between the middle two quartiles (i.e., 25%–75% range of the

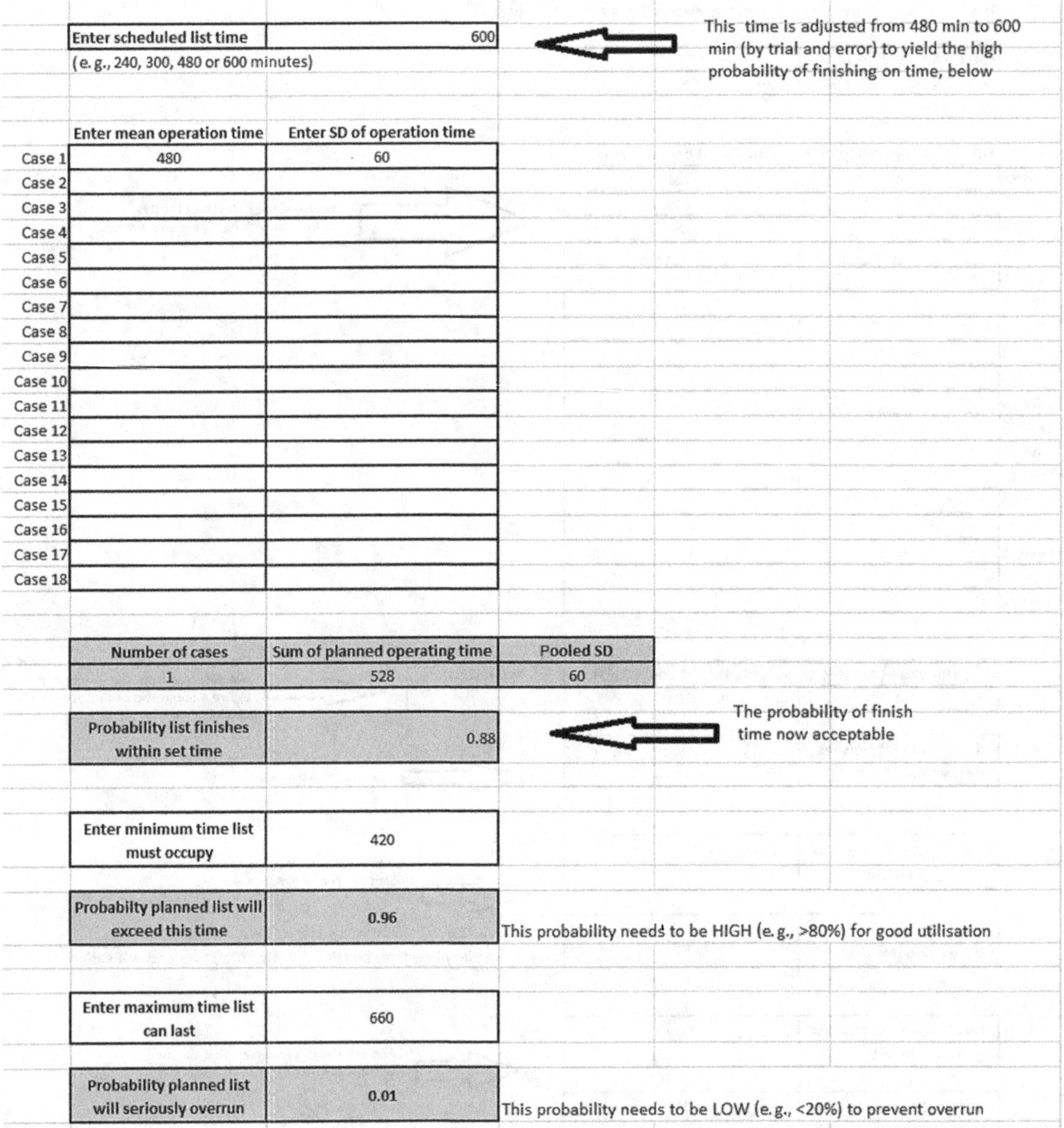

Enter scheduled list time	600
(e. g., 240, 300, 480 or 600 minutes)	

This time is adjusted from 480 min to 600 min (by trial and error) to yield the high probability of finishing on time, below

	Enter mean operation time	Enter SD of operation time
Case 1	480	60
Case 2		
Case 3		
Case 4		
Case 5		
Case 6		
Case 7		
Case 8		
Case 9		
Case 10		
Case 11		
Case 12		
Case 13		
Case 14		
Case 15		
Case 16		
Case 17		
Case 18		

Number of cases	Sum of planned operating time	Pooled SD
1	528	60

Probability list finishes within set time	0.88

The probability of finish time now acceptable

Enter minimum time list must occupy	420

Probabilty planned list will exceed this time	0.96

This probability needs to be HIGH (e. g., >80%) for good utilisation

Enter maximum time list can last	660

Probability planned list will seriously overrun	0.01

This probability needs to be LOW (e. g., <20%) to prevent overrun

Figure 4.8 For when there is a single case, adjusting the list duration to achieve high probability of finishing on time.

data). For example, a hypothetical operation may have a mean time of, say, 90 minutes with an SD of 120 minutes. The very wide SD indicates likely non-Gaussian distribution. The corresponding median for this operation might be 60 minutes (again, the large difference between mean and median indicating non-Gaussian data). The interquartile range might be 40–85 minutes; that is, 50% of the data lies within these values. We could use the value 45 minutes (i.e., the range of the IQR) instead of the SD.

Solution B: The β Distribution. The β distribution or three-point method can be useful in these circumstances. The method works as follows. For any operation with unknown or non-Gaussian time

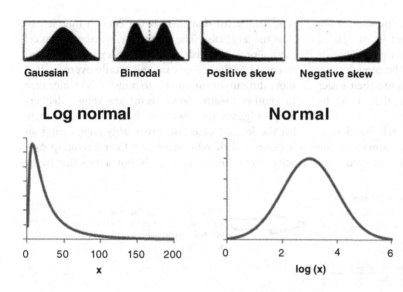

Figure 4.9 Examples of different distributions. In each panel, the x-axis is the operation time in minutes, and the y-axis the number of operations with those times, for a large number of operations for a single procedure. The shapes are, in turn, Gaussian (normal); bimodal (e.g., where one group of patients with the condition takes a short time; another group takes a longer time); positively skewed (where most operations take a short time, but some take much longer); or negatively skewed (where most operations take a long time, but some can be short – perhaps in open-and-close surgeries). Lower panels: if a positive skew (left bottom) is plotted on a logarithmic x-axis (right bottom), it will appear normal.

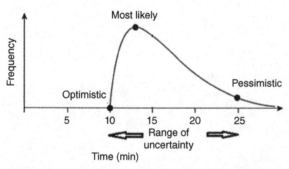

Figure 4.10 The shape of the β distribution and how it works to estimate a mean and SD. For the example shown (where $o = 10$, $m = 13$ and $p = 25$), $\mu = 14.5$ and SD = 2.5.

distributions, estimate the *optimistic time* (o) and the *pessimistic time* (p), and the most likely time (l). The mean time (μ) is given by:

$$\mu = \frac{[o + 4l + p]}{6} \qquad \text{Equation 4.4}$$

and the standard deviation is given by:

$$\text{Variance} = \frac{(p - o)^2}{36} \qquad \text{Equation 4.5}$$

With SD being the square root of this variance value (i.e., $(p - o)/6$). In this way, the mean μ and SD for each of these unknown timed operations can be entered into the CSA tool and the probabilities estimated. Figure 4.10 shows the principles of how this

method operates. A beta-distribution calculator tool is provided at: www.cambridge.org/9781316646830.

Ordering Individual Cases on a List

The CSA tool helps in selecting the correct cases, by their individual case durations, that could be scheduled onto a list. What it does not do is determine the order in which these cases should best be done. Where all cases are of the same or similar duration and SD, then it hardly matters what the order is. However, where these are different, the order may matter.

One commonsense factor that will be influential is the timing of the availability of equipment. Another factor may be urgency: it is always advisable to perform the most urgent case earlier. Patient comorbidities may also be influential; e.g., diabetic patients or those with latex allergy should be scheduled before other cases, where possible. Other more tactically related factors include the length of the case and the variation (SD) of the case.

Duration of Case Time. An analogy can be made with packing a suitcase. Generally it is wisest to pack the largest items first and then fit the smaller items around these. If there is no longer much space, then some smaller items may be left behind or transferred to another bag. It is generally the case that the larger items are deemed more important to take. Similarly in surgery if the longer cases are scheduled first there is a higher chance of their completion before the scheduled end time of the list. There is, of course, then a risk that some of the smaller cases overrun or are cancelled, if there turns out not to be enough time. Ideally these remaining smaller cases are then easier to transfer to neighbouring lists that may be finishing early.

If instead, the smaller cases are scheduled first, then the team may be faced with a dilemma with the last case. The smaller cases may have utilised such time on the list that there is not enough time left to start the large case. The dilemma is whether to cancel the major case, finish early and underrun, or instead to complete the major case and greatly overrun. It is more difficult or impossible to transfer the major case to another theatre. Some teams are known deliberately to 'game' the system such that they knowingly list the longest case last, predictably engineering an overrun and thereby increasing their operating capacity, week on week. This is not a practice to be

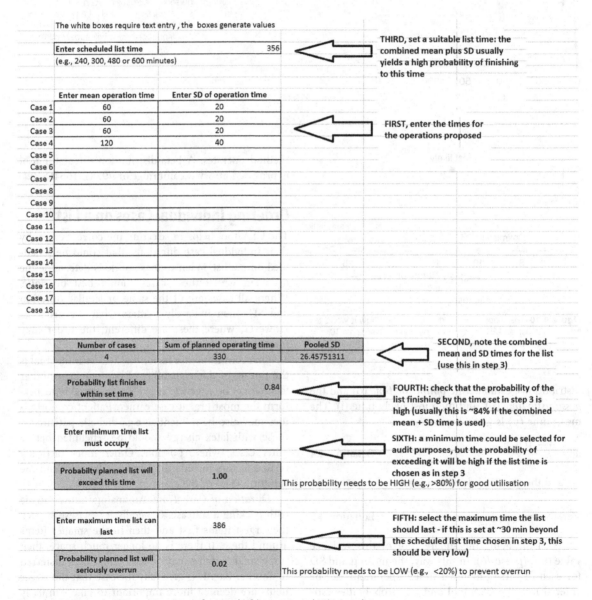

Figure 4.11 Using the CSA tool in context of a typical US list or a typical UK private list.

encouraged (for reasons of cost and operational chaos), as already discussed.

Variation of Case Time. Similarly, if cases with the widest variation (SDs) are scheduled first, then it is easier to make on-the-day decisions about the other more reliable cases later during the list. If highly variable cases are left to the end of the list, then it is difficult to make reliable decisions based on data. Happily, it is mathematically the case that the longer cases also generally have the wider variation in duration, at least by absolute times, so again it is the more variable cases that should be scheduled first.

Using the CSA Tool for a Typical US List or a Typical UK Private List

Much of the preceding discussion has applied to scheduling cases on a typical UK NHS list where the goal is to fill a block of time from a very large pool of cases from the waiting list. In a typical US list or a typical UK private list, the surgeon is seeking variable time on a list on any given day. The host organisation, however, will still need to know how long the surgeon

will likely take for the cases to be scheduled. The CSA tool is still valid, if used in a slightly different way from that described earlier.

First, no block time is entered for the list, nor are any minimum or maximum times entered. Instead, the case times to be scheduled are simply listed. This will yield the combined mean and pooled SD time for the proposed list. Adding the pooled SD to the combined mean generally provides a good estimate of the suitable time for the list (i.e., a time by which the list will have a high chance, >80%, of being complete). An upper limit of time can also be set, as being, say, 30 min more than this mean + combined SD time (the exact figure being up to each organisation). A lower limit can also be set, for purposes of audit. Figure 4.11 shows the steps to take.

The difference of this procedure and the typical UK NHS scenario is that the scheduled list time is therefore not one set in stone from the outset, as a block time, but rather highly responsive to what the surgeon is booking. The accuracy of actual performance can then be compared – using the methods described in previous chapters – against this time.

Appendix 4A: Ideal Scheduling Pathways

Ideal Scheduling Pathway for a Typical UK NHS List, Where Data Is Known

The following steps can be used to schedule a list:

(1) The surgeon decides surgery is necessary in clinic and books the patient for surgery on the waiting list.

(2) The system or bookings team wait-lists the patient by operation type, or code, which is associated with a case duration time (either automatic, or using lookup tables; these times being obtained either from the team's own averages or from agreed-on norms).

(3) Well ahead of the actual day of surgery, a provisional list of cases is constructed from those on the waiting list using the CSA tool. The aim is to have >80% probability of finishing before the scheduled list duration, but <20% chance of overrunning by the locally agreed maximum duration.

(4) This provisional list is sent to both surgeon and anaesthetist for the list (and ideally the theatre nursing staff lead), so there is universal buy-in to the list construct. That way, all specialists are given opportunity to adjust the list based on clinical and other information that may not be known simply by the timings used in CSA tool. For example, a patient may be more complex than indicated by the average times, or may in fact be planned for local rather than general anaesthesia, or need special equipment, etc. This step of buy-in is important so that if on the day of surgery there is an overrun there is less staff resentment.

(5) A final list is published at a suitable time before day of surgery (e.g., a week before).

(6) The theatre manager will then know the cases for each list in each theatre on the day of surgery and also their probable finish times. The manager can then create provisional backup plans in the event of overrunning, underrunning, etc., such as to identify theatres where cases might be moved, if needed.

(7) After the day of surgery, the actual times for each case are used by the system to update the team's average times for that case (i.e., later informing step (2), above).

Ideal Scheduling Pathway for a Typical UK NHS List, Where Data Is Not Known

Slightly different from where times are known, the following steps can be used to schedule a list:

(1) The surgeon decides surgery is necessary in clinic and books the patient for surgery on the waiting list, listing the patient case descriptor along with the time the case will take. This will ideally be the total case time or, by local agreement, the β distribution method can be used and the surgeon asked to estimate optimistic, pessimistic and mean times.

(2) Weeks ahead of the actual list, the bookings team draws up a provisional list of cases constructed from those on the waiting list using the CSA tool. The estimated total case times is used, with SDs approximating ~30% of this time. The aim is to have >80% probability of finishing before the scheduled list duration, but <20% chance of overrunning by the locally agreed-on maximum duration.

(3) This provisional list is sent to both the surgeon and the anaesthetist for the list (and ideally the theatre nursing staff lead), so there is universal buy-in to the list construct. If different staff have different estimates for total case time, the three times (surgeon, anaesthetist, staff) can be used in two possible ways to recalculate the list using the CSA tool: (i) take the average of the three times, assuming SD is ~30% of each mean; (ii) use the β distribution method, as described earlier. The method will have to be agreed locally.

(4) A final list is published at a suitable time before day of surgery.

(5) After the day of surgery, the actual times for each case are used by the theatre manager or bookings team to create a database of the team's actual average times for that case (i.e., later informing steps (1), (2) and (3)).

Ideal Scheduling Pathway for a Typical US List, or UK Private List

The additional challenge for the theatre manager here is to know in advance the duration of each surgeon's cases to plan the staffing for the theatre suite as a whole.

(1) The surgeon decides surgery is necessary in clinic and books the patient for surgery on the waiting list. The surgeon lists the patient case descriptor along with their estimate of the total case time for the case (if accurate times are not known, the β distribution method may also be used), or the case is associated automatically with the mean total case time from a database by the system or bookings team.

(2) As far ahead of actual list as is locally agreed, the bookings team draws up a provisional list of cases constructed from those on the waiting list using the CSA tool, assigning the surgeon an OR duration. The aim is to have >80% probability of finishing the booked cases before this scheduled list duration, but <20% chance of overrunning by the locally agreed maximum duration.

(3) This list is sent to the theatre manager, who will have similar information for the day from all surgeons using the ORs. The theatre manager will be able to decide from this which surgeons might follow on which others, or which surgeons need an OR to themselves for the full day and for how long.

(4) A final set of lists for the OR suite is published no later than the agreed time, say, a week before surgery.

(5) After the day of surgery, the actual times for each case are used by the system or bookings team to create a database of the surgeon's actual average times for that case (i.e., later informing steps (1) and (2)).

Bibliography

Broka SM, Jamart J, Louagie YAG. 2003. Scheduling of elective surgical cases within allocated block-times: can the future be drawn from the experience of the past? *Acta Chirurgica Belgica* 103: 90–94.

Denton B, Viapiano J, Vogl A. 2007. Optimization of surgery sequencing and scheduling decisions under uncertainty. *Healthcare Management Science* 10: 13–24.

Dexter F, Macario A, Qian F, Traub RD. 1999. Forecasting surgical groups' total hours of elective cases for allocation of block time: application of time series analysis to operating room management. *Anesthesiology* 91: 1501–8.

Dexter F, Traub RD. 2002. How to schedule elective surgical cases into specific operating rooms to maximize the efficiency of use of operating room time. *Anesthesia and Analgesia* 94: 933–42.

Dexter F, Traub RD, Macario A, Lubarsky DA. 2003. Operating room utilization alone is not an accurate metric for the allocation of operating room block time to individual surgeons with low caseloads. *Anesthesiology* 98: 1243–49.

Dexter F, Traub RD, Qian F. 1999. Comparison of statistical methods to predict the time to complete a series of surgical cases. *Journal of Clinical Monitoring* 15: 45–51.

Eijkemans MJC, van Houdenhoven M, Nguyen T, et al. 2010. Predicting the unpredictable: a new prediction model for operating room times using individual characteristics and the surgeon's estimate. *Anesthesiology* 112: 41–49.

Jones JW, McCullough LB. 2007. Ethics of over-scheduling: when enough becomes too much. *Journal of Vascular Surgery* 45: 635–6.

Lacqua MJ, Evans JT. 1994. Cancelled elective surgery: an evaluation. *American Surgeon* 60: 809–11.

Macario A, Dexter F. 1999. Estimating the duration of a case when the surgeon has not recently performed the procedure at the surgical suite. *Anesthesia and Analgesia* 89: 1241–5.

Macario A. 2009. Truth in scheduling: is it possible to accurately predict how long a surgical case will accurately last? *Anesthesiology* 108: 681–5.

Pandit JJ, Carey A. 2006. Estimating the duration of common elective operations: implications for operating list management. *Anaesthesia* 61: 768–76.

Pandit JJ, Tavare A. 2011. Using mean duration and variation of procedure times to plan a list of surgical operations to fit into the scheduled list time. *European Journal of Anaesthesiology* 28: 493–501.

Proudlove N, Hine A, Tavare A, Pandit JJ. 2013. Improvements and corrections to estimating probabilities in the formula for planning a list of operations to fit into a scheduled time. *European Journal of Anaesthesiology* 30: 633–5.

Schofield WN, Rubin G, Piza M, et al. 2005. Cancellation of operations on the day of intended surgery at a major Australian referral hospital. *Medical Journal of Australia* 182: 612–5.

Stepaniak PS, Heij C, Mannaerts GHH, et al. 2009. Modeling procedure and surgical times for current procedural terminology-anesthesia-surgeon combinations and evaluation in terms of case-duration prediction and operating room efficiency: a multicenter study. *Anesthesia and Analgesia* 109: 1232–45.

Strum DP, May JH, Vargas LG. 2000. Modeling the uncertainty of surgical procedure times: comparison of the log-normal and normal models. *Anesthesiology* 92: 1160–67.

Testi A, Tanfani E, Torre G. 2007. A three-phase approach for operating theatre schedules. *Healthcare Management Science* 10: 163–72.

Wachtel RE, Dexter F. 2004. Differentiating among hospitals performing physiologically complex operative procedures in the elderly. *Anesthesiology* 100: 1552–61.

Capacity Planning

Jaideep J. Pandit

Introduction

Common questions facing a theatre manager include: how many operating room (OR) sessions does one specialty need versus another? How many ORs in total do we actually need to staff? These are all questions of *theatre capacity*, in essence the time available for surgery.

In reality the answers to these questions about theatre capacity are often dictated by historical norms. For example, a vascular team has always operated Mondays and Tuesdays; the two surgeons retire, and their successors will also be allocated Mondays and Tuesdays, and so on. Rarely in practice – at least in the United Kingdom (UK) – is the situation reassessed to ask if these two OR slots are sufficient, insufficient or just right. This chapter introduces a method to estimate how much capacity is needed. The main focus is for a typical UK NHS list, and later we will see how the methods can be adapted for other list types.

Understanding Demand to Understand Capacity

The first step in understanding 'capacity' is to understand 'demand' – what it is and how it is best measured. It is essential to measure demand and capacity in the same units of measurement. The most appropriate and accurate measure is *time*. It is readily understood that theatre capacity is the minutes or hours available (per week or on any given day) to a surgical team, to a surgeon or to the specialty or hospital as a whole. Therefore, it follows that demand is correspondingly the minutes of surgery booked from surgical clinic. As we shall see, this makes it possible to match the two at least in a probabilistic way.

As ever, we will first discuss and discard erroneous ways of measuring demand.

Fallacies in Demand Measurement

Incorrect measures of demand include: number of surgical clinics, number of patients seen in clinic or booked from clinic for surgery, size of waiting list by number of patients waiting or population demographics. Yet all these measures are far more commonly used than is the estimated time required for the surgery of the patients booked from clinic.

It is self-evident that the number of surgical clinics undertaken by the surgical team is irrelevant. A team may undertake many clinics for historical reasons, or book a low proportion of patients for surgery even if they undertake a large number of clinics. Likewise, the fallacy of considering the number of patients is readily seen when we consider that the operations for which they are booked may have very variable durations (e.g., an eye clinic will book many more cataracts per clinic than a cardiac clinic books heart valve replacement surgery, but the time demands of the sum of operations booked may be similar).

The size of the waiting list may appear an attractive measure for assessing demand. If, say, vascular surgery has many more patients waiting for longer than 6 months than does urology, it is tempting to conclude that vascular surgery needs more surgical capacity. Again, it is not the number of patients waiting that matters, but the sum of times that their listed operations will take that should determine capacity. If the vascular patients are all perchance varicose vein operations, but the urology patients are all radical cystoprostatectomies or ureteric reimplantations, then urology demand may in fact be much higher.

Population demographics might help at a strategic level in that the proportion of elderly patients, the prevailing socioeconomic conditions and the prevalent diseases may help in planning hospital service across a region. However, it is less helpful at a tactical level where theatre capacity across specialties needs to

75

be planned over time cycles of months or a few years at a time. Rarely is it the case that analyses of entire populations generate such accurate demand data to help a theatre manager plan surgical ORs.

Relationship between Demand, Capacity and the Waiting List

This section will show how these three quantities are intimately linked, and it will demonstrate some of the quantitative relationships between them. At all times henceforth, demand, capacity and the waiting list are all described in units of time (minutes of surgery/anaesthesia needed or available), regardless of how many patients are waiting, or booked for surgery.

Let us imagine a hypothetical surgical team that (for purposes of illustration) remarkably and reliably over several years books patients from its outpatient clinics for elective surgery whose operations always need a total of exactly 3,000 min/week of operating time. How much theatre capacity should this team be allocated? Figure 5.1 shows that if the surgical capacity is set at exactly 3,000 min/week (capacity option 1), this always matches the demand precisely. No waiting list results. If, alternatively, the capacity is instead fixed at any value greater than 3000 min/week, then there will always be spare (excess) capacity (capacity option 2; Figure 5.1). Theatre time might be wasted or need to be assigned regularly to another team. If, however, capacity is for some reason fixed at any value less than 3000 min/week, then there is an inevitable shortfall in capacity (capacity option 3). A cumulative backlog of patients will result.

The rate at which this backlog develops can be readily calculated. It is proportional to the disparity between the capacity and the demand: the lower the

capacity option 3 is set at, the faster will be the rate of accumulation of the waiting list. Thus for this hypothetical example, if the capacity is set at a low 2,400 min/week, the backlog (waiting list) develops at a rate of 600 min/week (600 being the difference between 3,000 and 2,400). If capacity option 2 is set at just 1,000 min/week, then the waiting list accumulates at 2,000 min/week, and so on (Figure 5.2).

In this hypothetical scenario, capacity setting is very easy. Unfortunately, real life is not so straightforward. It is certainly possible for the capacity offered to be near-constant over many years, and this is in large part a theatre manager's role. For example, a surgical list may always be staffed by contractual cross-cover arrangements or locum staff. However, it is the demand that will vary from week to week: it will not be constant as suggested in Figure 5.1.

There are, of course, several self-evident reasons for this. Referral rates from primary care to surgical clinic may themselves vary, and at staggered times. The nature of patients' problems (casemix) will vary: even for, say, an orthopaedic team not every patient will need the same knee replacement. Some may need an arthroscopy, others a hip replacement and so on. Even for the same planned operation the surgical time required may vary due to patient comorbidity. Some patients may be amenable only to certain types of surgery such as laparoscopic or robotic methods, which themselves may have inherently greater variation than other techniques.

Selecting Capacity Where Demand Is Variable

Figure 5.3 shows the more common scenario where demand varies from week to week. In this plot, the

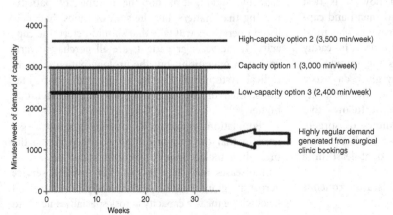

High-capacity option 2 (3,500 min/week)

Capacity option 1 (3,000 min/week)

Low-capacity option 3 (2,400 min/week)

Highly regular demand generated from surgical clinic bookings

Figure 5.1 Elective demand in terms of bookings for surgery from a hypothetical outpatient clinic generating demand for surgery with remarkable consistency (bars, min/week). Also shown (horizontal lines) are three options to set capacity for this team: option 1 (matching the demand); option 2 (exceeding the demand); or option 3 (less than the demand).

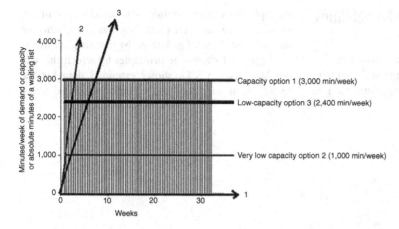

Figure 5.2 Illustrating the rate of growth of a waiting list (in minutes; lines with arrows). The slope of this rate of growth is proportional to the disparity between the capacity set and the demand generated. Thus, if capacity set very low (horizontal line option 2) the growth rate is high; somewhat less for when it is set moderately low (horizontal line option 3); but not at all when capacity matches demand (horizontal line option 1).

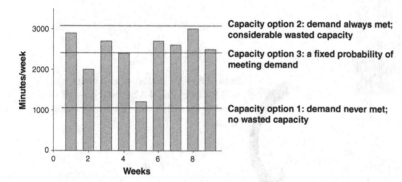

Figure 5.3. Similar to Figure 5.2 for a more realistic surgical team with variable weekly bookings. The capacity options 1–3 are discussed in text.

mean demand is still 2,400 min/week – the same as the very regular hypothetical team in Figure 5.1. What capacity should we allocate this team?

This problem in setting the correct capacity is much more difficult. The problem in large part arises because 'spare' or excess capacity in one week cannot be carried forward to the next week: 'time' is not a quantity that can be saved up for use sometime in the future. As we noted in the Introduction (Chapter 1), in this way and many others, hospitals are not like factories where manufactured products can be stored up for release into the market later, or the conveyor belt can be sped up to make up for lost time. In other words, the problem is that the weeks when demand outstrips capacity always contribute to a backlog, but the times where capacity outstrips demand cannot always compensate, and capacity is wasted - that time cannot be carried forward. Later we do explore ways in which this excess capacity could be used to tackle a waiting list.

The problem in Figure 5.3 can be stated in terms of probabilities. One certainty within Figure 5.3 is that if we set the capacity below any of the weekly

demands generated (option 1) then for sure – with 100% probability – we will never absorb the demand. There will be an inevitable waiting list generated. Of course, one advantage is that we will also be more certain of utilising the capacity we are allocating (notwithstanding problems of efficiency, ε, within any given list; see Chapter 2).

Another certainty is that if we set the capacity to exceed all weekly demands generated (option 2), then we can be sure – with 100% probability – of always absorbing demand. There will be no waiting list, but that will be at the cost of much wasted, unutilised capacity (regardless of its intrinsic efficiency ε; a team will simply not have enough work to fill all the time it has been allocated).

For any capacity we allocate between these limits of certainty (option 3), there is a fixed probability or meeting or not the weekly demand generated (Figure 5.3). We have in this manner illustrated the broad relationship between demand, capacity and the waiting list. We will now turn to discussing how to quantify the impact of the capacity we allocate.

Converting Capacity Options to Probabilities of Meeting Demand

It would be desirable and important to know how any one of the capacities we select in Figure 5.3 can be converted into a probability of meeting demand. For example, for capacity option 3 it would be important to be able to say: 'This capacity has x% chance of meeting the demand generated by this surgical team'.

Figure 5.4 shows the principles by which this can be done. Figure 5.4A shows extended data for the hypothetical surgical team's clinic bookings, along

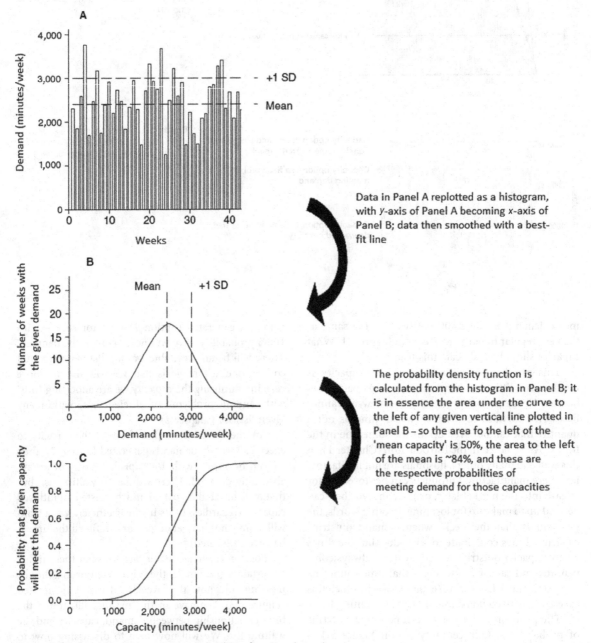

Data in Panel A replotted as a histogram, with y-axis of Panel A becoming x-axis of Panel B; data then smoothed with a best-fit line

The probability density function is calculated from the histogram in Panel B; it is in essence the area under the curve to the left of any given vertical line plotted in Panel B – so the area fo the left of the 'mean capacity' is 50%, the area to the left of the mean is ~84%, and these are the respective probabilities of meeting demand for those capacities

Figure 5.4 Converting capacity options to probabilities of meeting demand.

with the mean and SD time for these cases. Figure 5.4B shows this same data as a simple histogram. The smoothed line is the best fit for the distribution of times, and in this case follows a near-normal or Gaussian distribution. Figure 5.4C is what is called the 'cumulative probability density function' derived from Figure 5.4B.

So we now have a very simple method of converting our capacity options to probabilities. For the data in Figure 5.4, if the team is allocated a weekly capacity of ~2,500 minutes/week, it will have only a ~50% chance of meeting its demand week on week; i.e., half of its caseload in the long run will be diverted to generating a waiting list. If allocated ~3,000 minutes/week, then it will have ~84% chance of meeting it demand, and just ~16% of its caseload in the long run will be diverted to generating a waiting list. And so on.

What Level to Set Capacity? – The Problem of Waste

The question for the theatre manager, working together with the team and the organisation as a whole, is then: 'What probability of meeting demand is acceptable?' A politically driven agenda might insist that there should be no waiting list at all. Under such conditions a capacity of 3,000 minutes/week is unacceptable, and capacities of at least 3,500 minutes/week or more are necessary.

However, the price of such a simplistic political agenda is 'waste'. Recall that the amount of surgical theatre time wasted is simply the inverse of that utilised. Let us look again at the data in Figure 5.4 and replot this as the maximum percentage of time that could be utilised or wasted, if a certain capacity is allocated to this team. If this team is awarded 3,000 minutes/week of theatre time, we know from Figure 5.4 that this will ensure their weekly demand from clinic is met ~84% of the time. However, this does not mean that in 84% of weeks the lists will be guaranteed to be full of cases. In fact, it means that for most of these lists the capacity greatly outstrips the demand: note that the mean + SD line in Figure 5.4 is much higher than any of the blocks, for most of the weeks. It can be readily calculated that at a capacity of 3,000 minutes/week, for the demand shown in Figure 5.4, only 20% of this overall capacity (600 min) will be utilised (at a maximum) week on week; 2,400 minutes/week could be wasted. The waste is negligible if only 2,000 minutes of capacity are

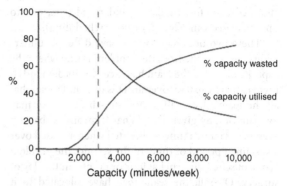

Figure 5.5 The inverse relationship between waste and utilisation for the data in Figure 5.4.

allocated (Figure 5.5) but then we know that this will also mean that for half the weeks, this capacity will be inadequate to meet demand.

In other words, a second parallel question to be answered is: 'How much waste of the capacity can we tolerate?' To summarise, here are the sensible questions, based on the data that a theatre manager could reasonably ask, to assess what level of capacity should be allocated to a team:

1. What probability of meeting weekly demand should we accept?
2. What proportion of wasted capacity should we accept?
3. If we allocate capacity with a high probability of meeting weekly demand, how should we best manage the likely wasted OR time that will result?
4. If we allocated capacity with low probability of meeting weekly demand, how should we best manage the likely waiting list that will result?

It is readily seen that points 3 and 4 are mutually exclusive, but that both involve more qualitative approaches, as are discussed in the following examples.

Clarifying the Meaning of 'Waste'

In the preceding discussion, the term *waste* is used in the specific sense of theatre time that is allocated to a team, which the team cannot fill because for that week or time period, it does not have sufficient cases booked from its clinics. This is a somewhat different sense in which we used *waste* in Chapter 2 on theatre efficiency. In that chapter, the wasted time referred to unused time within a list. In the case of utilisation of a single theatre list, underrunning is a form of waste where the allocated time for the day is underused (e.g., due to unanticipated cancellation or poor scheduling).

These two notions of waste have different underlying causes. In the first, the problem is one where the capacity allocated the team has exceeded its demands – there is spare capacity overall. This does not mean that all the team's lists will underrun – indeed they may overrun on any given day. What it means is that, on average, too much time is allocated when assessed over a sustained period of time. In the second, the problem is one of scheduling, behaviour or events on the day of surgery. Overall, the team may have allocated to it excess capacity or inadequate capacity – this is irrelevant. What is happening here is that, on the day, one or more factors have caused the list to underrun.

In summary, wasted time due to overallocation of capacity is quite different from wasted time due to underrunning on the day of surgery.

Finally, there is an important sense in which waste is important and necessary as clearly demonstrated in the tone of this current chapter. Without any waste we have by definition allocated less time than a team needs overall. Therefore, a politician who at once demands that 'there must be no waiting list' and that

'there must be no waste' is talking nonsense. As we have shown earlier, the two are locked in an inverse relationship – more waste means excess capacity and no waiting list; less waste can only arise with inadequate capacity and a waiting list.

A Note on Non-Gaussian Distributions

For simplicity and better to illustrate the principles, strictly Gaussian distributions have been used in the preceding examples. Non-Gaussian distributions are also possible for demand data and arguably more likely than Gaussian, but in fact the cumulative probability distributions are quite similar. Figure 5.6 shows that for a wide variety of non-Gaussian distributions, the probability density function are similar to the extent that capacities set at ~80% of the range of variation in demand (vertical dotted lines) always capture ~80% of the proportion of weeks of demand (horizontal dotted lines).

Further to emphasise this point, Figure 5.7 shows a large dataset from a real surgical team; again setting capacity at ~80% of the range captures ~80% of the weekly demands.

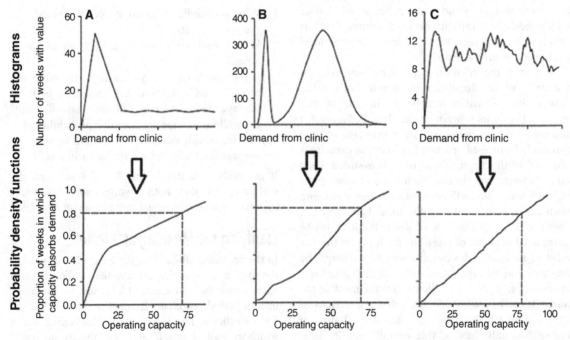

Figure 5.6 Cumulative probability density functions for three non-Gaussian distributions. A: skewed; B: bimodal; C: pseudouniform. The top three panels are the histograms of the demand from hypothetical clinics (arbitrary units), corresponding to Figure 5.4B. The lower three panels are the corresponding cumulative probability density functions derived from these, corresponding to Figure 5.4C. For each (dotted lines) 80% of the range of distribution meets 80% of demand.

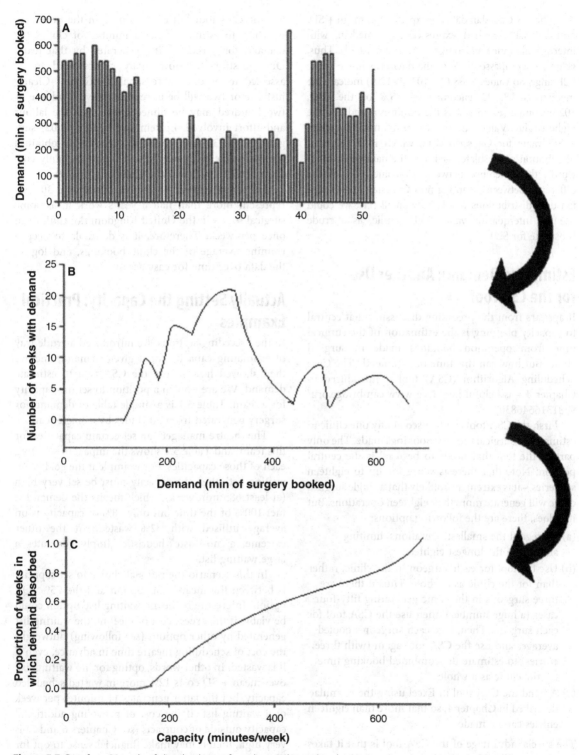

Figure 5.7 Data from 56 weeks of clinic bookings of a real surgical team (one lead surgeon), presented in the same panel types as in Figure 5.4).

Whereas Gaussian data are expressed as mean + SD, non-Gaussian are best expressed as a median, with interquartile range and range (e.g., a (b–c [d–e]). Thus, value c encompasses 75% of the dataset, while e is the full range. So values of 88 (22–102 [1–120]) indicate the median is 88, 22 encompasses 25% of the data, 102 encompasses 75%, 1 is the minimum and 120 the highest value. Value c therefore approximates the mean + SD value for Gaussian data, which in a Gaussian distribution encapsulates ~84% of the dataset. In other words, the difference between 75% and 84% as the difference between assuming non-Gaussian and Gaussian data distributions is relatively small (i.e., we could use the interquartile value, 75th centile, as a crude substitute for SD).

Estimating Demand: Another Use for the CSA Tool

It appears from the preceding discussion that central to capacity planning is the estimation of the surgical time from operation bookings made in surgical clinic. But how can this time be estimated? The Case Scheduling Algorithm (CSA) tool – introduced in Chapter 4 – is helpful here (see www.cambridge.org/9781316646830).

First, the CSA tool can be used at any one clinic to estimate the surgical time for bookings made. The only part of the tool that needs to be used is the central portion. Note that there is space for up to eighteen surgeries – it is extremely unlikely that a single surgical clinic will generate more than eighteen operations. But if it does, there are the following options:

(a) Disregard the smallest operations, limiting analysis to the longest eighteen
(b) Use the tool for each surgeon in the clinic, rather than for the clinic as a whole. Thus if there are three surgeons in the clinic generating fifty-four cases (a huge number), then use the CSA tool for each surgeon. Then, take each surgeon's pooled averages and use the CSA tool again (with three entries) to estimate the combined booking time for the clinic as a whole
(c) Amend the CSA tool in Excel using the formulae described in Chapter 4, so that more than eighteen entries can be made

The special advantage of the CSA tool is that it takes into account the likely gap times as well. Figure 5.8 shows one example clinic.

The CSA tool can then be used in the next step, which is to estimate from a number of clinics the demand for surgery being generated by that team. One question is: How many clinics need to be assessed to produce a reasonable estimate? Clearly just one or two will be unrepresentative. And one or two hundred may be unnecessary given the labour and effort involved. Epstein and Dexter (2002) suggest at least 30 data points is necessary to obtain a representative estimate. This is almost certainly correct in strict mathematical terms (Figure 5.9).

However, context is always important: 30 lists represent more than half a year's work if, as some surgical teams in the United Kingdom do, clinics run once per week. Therefore, it is desirable to keep a running average of the clinic bookings, and log all the data over time for easy access.

Actually Setting the Capacity: Practical Examples

In the preceding sections, we introduced a crude way of estimating capacity for a given demand, and we then showed how to use the CSA tool to estimate demand. We are now in a position to set the capacity for a team. Table 5.1 is a simple table of demand for surgery generated from 30 clinics by a single team.

The theatre manager can set certain capacities for this team, and Table 5.2 shows the impact of selecting each of those capacities. For example if the goal is 'no waiting list', then the capacity must be set very high (at least 685 min/week), which means the demand is met 100% of the time but only 68% of capacity is on average utilised with 32% wasted. At the other extreme, a 'no-waste' heuristic simply generates a large waiting list.

In this scenario the rational choice to set capacity is between the mean + SD option and the 75% IQR option. Interestingly the 'no waiting list' option could be viable if the excess cost of meeting the waiting list generated by other options (see following) outweighs the cost of scheduling theatre time in advance, even if it is wasted. In other words, opting for 'no waiting list' over mean + SD costs 12% more in wasted scheduled capacity, but the latter generates 11 minutes per week of a waiting list. If the cost of providing additional capacity outside of contracts (see Chapters 6 and 7) is very high, then it may make financial sense to opt for 'no waiting list'. The excess capacity could be used in other ways (see following section).

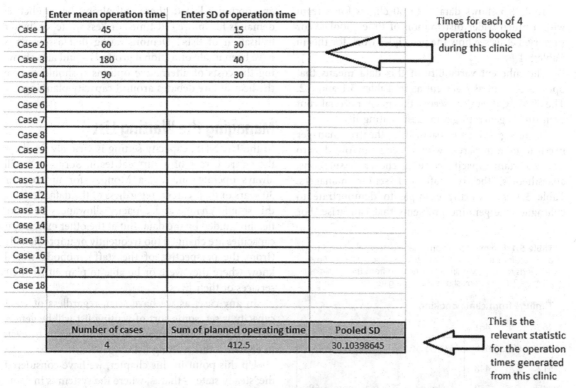

	Enter mean operation time	Enter SD of operation time
Case 1	45	15
Case 2	60	30
Case 3	180	40
Case 4	90	30
Case 5		
Case 6		
Case 7		
Case 8		
Case 9		
Case 10		
Case 11		
Case 12		
Case 13		
Case 14		
Case 15		
Case 16		
Case 17		
Case 18		

Times for each of 4 operations booked during this clinic

Number of cases	Sum of planned operating time	Pooled SD
4	412.5	30.10398645

This is the relevant statistic for the operation times generated from this clinic

Figure 5.8 Example output from using the CSA tool as applied to a single clinic. In this hypothetical clinic, four bookings for surgery were made. Using lookup tables, or locally available software, the operation times associated with each of these procedures are readily entered, along with the SDs for each operation. The combined mean and pooled SD represents the demand for surgical theatre time generated by this clinic.

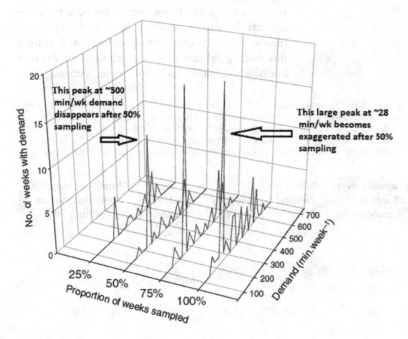

This peak at ~500 min/wk demand disappears after 50% sampling

This large peak at ~28 min/wk becomes exaggerated after 50% sampling

Figure 5.9 Three-dimensional histogram from the data in Figure 5.7 for the 56 urology clinics. If the first 25% of the clinics (14) are sampled to generate the estimated demand, there is a clear peak at ~500 minutes/week. This largely disappears as more lists are sampled. Instead, a larger peak emerges at ~280 min/week from when ~50% (28) clinics are sampled.

Table 5.3 shows data from 30 clinics for a team with a much wider distribution of times booked for surgery. Let us see how the principles work for this in Table 5.4.

The inherent variability of this data means that options are not as clear cut as in Tables 5.1 and 5.2. The 75% IQR option seems the most rational, but even this is generating a modest waiting list.

In using this approach, the theatre manager needs to be transparent with all teams involved as to why a certain capacity is being chosen – surgeons, anaesthetists, theatre staff and senior managers. Table 5.4 is a worthy example to demonstrate to colleagues the genuine problems that can arise. For

any option selected, there will always be conflicting demands for 'more OR time', or 'less waste' or 'better utilisation of lists'. Demonstrating that assessments have been made on rational grounds – and also showing the costs of alternative options – should reduce the heat of any debates around capacity planning.

Managing the Waiting List

In the UK NHS, capacity setting is virtually fixed for the entire career of a surgical team. Surgeon X will always operate on, say, a Monday for up to over 30 years of their career, regardless of the data. Perhaps this should change and capacity allowances be more flexibly guided by the data. But at the other extreme, if capacities are changed too frequently or unpredictably (from the perspective of the staff), nobody would know where they were or be able to plan either their services or their lives.

In any case, as we have seen, regardless of what capacity is set, some sort of waiting list will be generated. This section illustrates how to manage – or even to exploit – this waiting list.

Up this point in this chapter, we have considered the 'steady state' – that is, where the system is in some artificial equilibrium condition. We have not yet taken account of the influence of time itself within the process. Figure 5.10 illustrates what is really happening. A surgeon undertakes a clinic, during which certain patients are booked for surgery. These patients do not immediately head to the operating theatre but are booked onto a waiting list. It is from this waiting list that cases are extracted for the next available surgical list. So some patients may

Table 5.1 Summary data from one hypothetical surgical team over 30 clinics (each cell represents one clinic). Data are time demands for surgery (minutes) generated from the 30 clinics as a whole. The inset box shows the aggregate data.

Timings from clinic bookings		
463	386	461
405	605	415
512	526	448
445	596	259
322	671	336
517	348	513
383	489	399
451	407	578
685	410	345
374	605	561

Mean = 463 SD = 106

Maximum = 259; maximum = 685

Median = 449 (IQR 385–525)

Table 5.2 Setting capacity (column 2) by four different heuristics (column 1) for the data in Table 5.1. The total capacity over 30 weeks (column 3) is dictated by the heuristic. The percentage of weeks in which demand is captured (column 4) is simply the number of weeks in Table 5.1 where the demand generated is below the capacity being set. The percentage of capacity being utilised (column 5) is the minutes of the captured weeks from column 4, divided by the total capacity in column 3. The percentage of capacity wasted is the inverse of column 5. The waiting list generated in the last column is the sum of the clinic times not captured by the capacity set. IQR is the interquartile range (at the 75th decile).

Heuristic to set capacity	Capacity set (min/ week)	Total capacity over 30 weeks (minutes)	% weeks demand met	% capacity utilised	% capacity wasted	Minutes of surgery/ week diverted to waiting list
No waiting list	685	20,550	100%	68%	32%	0
Mean + SD	569	17,070	77%	80%	20%	11
75% IQR	525	15,750	73%	84%	16%	21
No waste	258	7740	0	100%	0	206

theoretically wait only days, or perhaps to the next week. Others may wait longer. Factors such as urgency or the need to deal with the longest waiting patients are also influential.

It can readily be seen how the demand-for-surgery calculations in the preceding sections help estimate the capacity needed. If the match of the capacity on the surgical list matches the demand generated perfectly, the size of the waiting list will be static. If capacity is less than the demand, the waiting list will grow at the rate described in Figure 5.2.

It can be seen that in some ways, a modest waiting list helps plan and utilise capacity. Indeed, waiting a little can bring benefits if there is a chance that underlying conditions improve such that surgery is no longer needed, or patients change their mind about surgeries that are not strictly necessary. This can bring its own problems if these decisions are made after the list is compiled and there is a

cancellation on the day of the procedure. However, great care should be taken, as during prolonged waits conditions can worsen, patients can suffer in pain or at worst, die. So fundamental to waiting list management is the need to prioritise patients most in need.

Managing Excessively Large Waiting Lists

We have seen that, regardless of the capacity selected, some waiting lists will accrue over time. Limits should be set as to how long patients should wait and also how large the waiting list should be at any given time. The following options are generally available:

1. Increase the regular capacity allocated to the team; either by lengthening the duration of each surgical list or by increasing the total number of regular surgical lists allocated to that team.
2. Create *ad hoc* lists temporarily, known as 'waiting list initiatives'.
3. Use a 'standby' list of waiting patients who are able and willing to be called at short notice on the day of surgery, as soon as it becomes clear that there is space on a given day's list.
4. Use capacity at other hospitals, by transferring care. This can be done by high-level strategic agreements across regions or nationally. It is easier where hospitals are closer so that travel times for patients are small, but more difficult where long distances are involved. The third-party hospitals might be private providers rather than the NHS (such transfers being generally easier within the NHS as there is no real transfer of funding).

Which of these is the optimal solution depends on local circumstances. Generally, options 3 and 4 require high levels of patient cooperation. In option 4, patients will be operated on by a different surgical team from

Table 5.3 Summary data from one hypothetical surgical team over 30 clinics (each cell represents one clinic). Data are time demands for surgery (minutes) generated from the 30 clinics as a whole The inset box shows the aggregate data.

Timings from 30 clinic bookings				
0	77	395		
297	78	404	Mean = 295 SD = 242	
271	81	428		
0	151	456	Maximum = 0; maximum = 841	
155	233	545		
44	258	609	Median = 284 (IQR 76–428)	
34	320	718		
26	323	731		
58	370	841		

Table 5.4 Setting capacity (column 2) by different heuristics (column 1) for the data in Table 5.3. Layout as in Table 5.2.

Heuristic to set capacity	Capacity set (min/ week)	Total capacity over 30 weeks (min)	% weeks demand met	% capacity utilised	% capacity wasted	Minutes of surgery/ week diverted to waiting list
No waiting list	841	25,230	100	35	65	0
Mean + SD	537	16,110	77	50	50	28
75% IQR	428	12,840	73	67	43	51
No waste	13	390	0	93	7	283

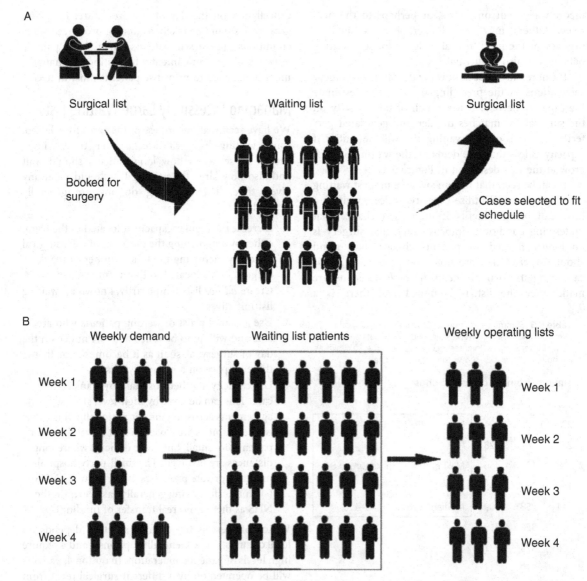

Figure 5.10 Panel A: Sequential illustration of how patients booked in clinic first enter a waiting list, and it is from this waiting list that cases can be selected for the surgical list, days, weeks or months in advance. Panel B: Week-on-week illustration of patient flow into and out of the waiting list, ideally filling the list capacity through optimal scheduling.

the one they have consulted in clinic. Option 1 requires changes to staff contracts (discussed in Chapters 6 and 7). Option 2 is potentially expensive, as the additional lists are generally regarded as extracontractual services. Option 4 is also potentially expensive, if transfers are made to the private sector. If made within the NHS, then very good planning and scheduling of cases is required across hospitals, so information technology coordination may be a fundamental requirement if

this option is to work well. Figure 5.11 is an adaptation of the top panel of Figure 5.10 to show the options.

Demand and Capacity Matching at Every Step in the Patient Pathway?

Figures 5.10–5.11 highlight the fact that we should ideally consider the demand-capacity step at each stage of the patient pathway. The figure is expanded

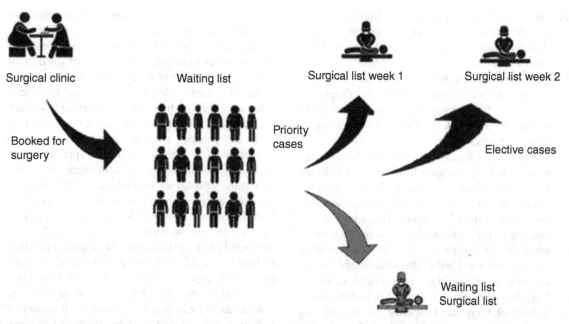

Figure 5.11 The bigger picture. As in Figure 5.10, patients enter a waiting list but from this are prioritised certain cases (e.g., due to clinical need, or being the longest waiters or those who can be accommodated best into the following week's list). Other patients are scheduled later (elective cases). There is an overflow arrangement, as described in text, for managing the waiting list (grey) which can be a combination of additional regular list-time, or *ad hoc* waiting list initiatives, or transfer to another hospital.

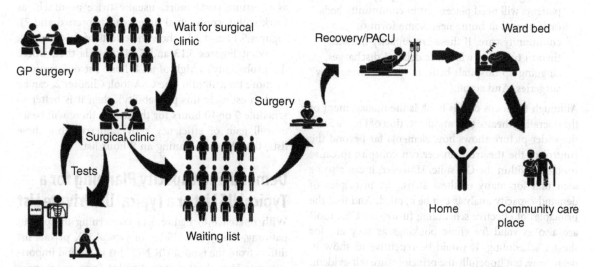

Figure 5.12 The patient pathway into and out of surgery. GP = general practitioner; PACU = post-anaesthesia care unit.

to show this (Figure 5.12). We can identify necessary demand-capacity calculations at each step in this path:

1. Access to the general practitioner (GP) or community physician. These will have a limited number of clinic slots, so there may be access delays or bottlenecks here.

2. Access to the surgeon: surgical clinics need scheduling in the same manner as surgical lists (see Chapter 4). They can also overrun or underrun in the same way as surgical lists and also need demand-capacity analysis (i.e., analysis of the time needed to see the GP referrals).

3. Even before booking for surgery, there may be need for further tests (X-ray and exercise testing is shown in Figure 5.12), and each of these may be capacity-limited.

4. We have discussed the wait for surgery and management of the surgical list in this chapter, but also on day of surgery there can be bottlenecks in recovery area/PACU, which can cause delays within the surgical list.

5. The pathway critically relies on ward beds (even for day cases, day surgery beds may be a limiting factor). Ward beds can cause backward-delays to discharges from recovery/PACU and/or can be a bottleneck to the whole system (i.e., a patient needing an inpatient ward bed cannot even be scheduled for surgery if there is no bed available). The relevant ward bed in this sense might also be an intensive care or high-dependency bed, which being fewer are also constrained as bottlenecks.

6. In hospital, there may be specific care needed with its own limited capacity (e.g., physiotherapy, or further treatment such as radio- or chemotherapy), but hopefully the patient is dischargeable home. However, a proportion of patients will need placement in community beds – or if nursed at home need some form of community care. If these are capacity-limited, then in turn this will cause delayed discharges, clogging up hospitals beds, in turn delaying new surgeries. And so on.

Although the focus of this book is the management of the operating theatre (the middle section of Figure 5.12) the wider picture shows how elements far beyond the control of the theatre manager can conspire to cause problems within the OR suite. However, it can also be seen that for many of these steps, the principles of demand-capacity analysis can be applied. And that the principles of effective scheduling (using the CSA tool) are also as valid for clinic bookings as they are for theatre scheduling. It would be repetitive to show in detail how, but hopefully the principles are self-evident.

Planning Capacity of a Single List

Hitherto, we have considered the question of how to allocate capacity over the week – i.e., over a sustained period of time – to a surgical team.

Now we ask the separate question: How do we schedule the list time, to avoid under- or overrun for a single surgical team? We might, for example, use the

preceding analysis to determine correctly that one team needs a weekly capacity of 18 hours per week, but is that best allocated as two 9-hour lists, or as one 10-hour list and one 8-hour list? In other words, how is the optimal length of a single list calculated?

Let us consider a hypothetical surgical team, currently assigned an 8-hour (480 min) list for cases each Monday, from 9:00 am to 5:00 pm. However, the time of the last patient's exit from theatre and arrival in recovery/PACU is always reliably ~6:15 pm. The mean of the actual hours of surgery is therefore 9 h 15 min (555 min; with an as-yet-undefined SD). There is therefore always a ~75 min overrun. If, however, 9 hours (540 min) were allocated, there would be a smaller ~15 min overrun. If 10 hours are allocated, there would be a ~45 underrun. The question is, which of these is optimal? And how does the data, especially the SD, help estimate what the optimal list length is?

The efficiency concept ε can assist us here (see Chapter 2). We can first assume that each minute of overrun is as inefficient as each minute of underrun. We can then insert a different assumption that each minute of overrun is twice as inefficient as each minute of underrun (this assumption can be justified as overtime costs more, usually twice as much, as work within contractual time; see Chapters 6 and 7). Figures 5.13 and 5.14 show the effects of this analysis.

What Figures 5.13 and 5.14 show is that, where the probability is high of an 8-hour list overrunning by more than 40 min (the CSA tool, Chapter 2, can be used to estimate this probability), then it is better to schedule 9 or 10 hours for the list, as there will be an overall gain of efficiency ε by underrunning these lists, than by overrunning an 8-hour list.

Demand and Capacity Planning for a Typical US List or a Typical UK Private List

With reference to Figure 5.11 concerning the patient pathway, the typical US list or typical UK private list differs from the typical UK NHS list in several important ways. First, there is no waiting list. Surgeons manage their own time and schedules, so as soon as a patient is ready and booked for surgery, the expectation is that the patient will be scheduled for surgery. The surgeon will, of course, generate a variable demand for surgery from clinics, but is not constrained to fit this demand into a fixed block time so Figure 5.10B rarely applies.

The question of assessing the 'demand for surgery' generated from clinics is, however, exactly the same as

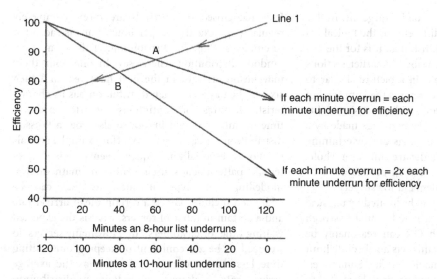

Figure 5.13 The *y*-axis is efficiency ε, calculated using principles in Chapter 2. The two single-arrow lines are read from the first *x*-axis, representing the decline in ε with minutes of overrun for a list scheduled at 8 hours; the steeper-declining arrow is if the inefficiency of overrun is twice that of underrun. The double-arrow line (line 1) shows the decline in inefficiency if this same hypothetical list is scheduled at 10 hours (to be read from the lower *x*-axis). Thus (in)efficiencies are equal for the two lines, at points A and B, respectively. At point A, efficiency ε is ~90% if an 8-hour list overruns by ~60 min and also if a 10-hour list underruns by ~60 min. At point B, where it is assumed inefficiency is greater with over- than underrun, (inefficiency) is ~85% if an 8-hour list overruns by ~40 min and if a 10-hour list underruns by ~80 min.

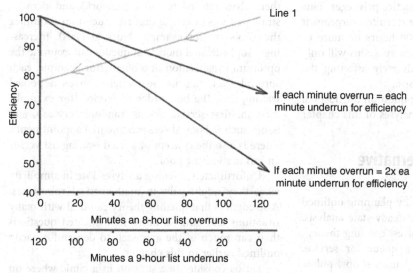

Figure 5.14 Similar plot to Figure 5.13, with the double-arrow line showing data for a 9-hour list underrunning (read from lower *x*-axis).

the question of optimising the scheduled list time for that surgeon, week on week, as was discussed in detail in Chapter 4. The CSA tool is used to estimate the time the surgeon needs on any given day, given the bookings made from an earlier clinic. In other words, the surgeon is working to a variable capacity, related to the demand. If in one week 100 hours of surgery

are booked from clinic, the surgeon will expect 100 hours of theatre time the following week for this demand. If the next week it is just 50 hours, then the surgeon will expect 50 hours (all estimated using the CSA tool; see Chapter 2). And so on.

However, it is the hospital that faces the challenge of deciding how much overall capacity it needs to accommodate the demands of *all* its surgeons. In this way, the problem is subtly different for the typical US list or the typical UK private list, than it is for the UK NHS list. The modelling described in earlier sections still applies, but, for example, in a picture similar to Figure 5.3, the bars would represents the sum total of bookings made by all surgeons with practising rights at that hospital, and not just the bookings made by a single surgeon. The total bookings are determining the capacity of the hospital's theatre suite as a whole. The hospital's calculations are then probability estimates of meeting the total demand for surgery.

Sometimes this capacity will be limited by physical constraints. Let us suppose a new hospital has been built with ten ORs. If each OR can reasonably be staffed for 10 hours per day; this sets an absolute limit of 100 hours of surgery available per day. Sometimes, physical capacity is available but needs to be staffed to provide actual capacity. If the new hospital cannot recruit staff (poor contracts, unpopular geographical location, etc.) then its functional (true) capacity will be much lower than its physical (theoretical) capacity. These considerations are important in questions like how many surgeons to grant practice privileges. This new hospital might already have recruited surgeons it knows are likely to generate 100 hours or more of surgery each week; recruiting new surgeons will only create scheduling problems, adversely affecting the experience of its existing surgeons.

Nevertheless, in each case or question the hospital can use the demand-capacity analyses of this chapter to solve most problems.

Queuing Theory: An Alternative Approach

The approach to demand-capacity planning outlined earlier might be described as a steady-state analysis. A more dynamic analysis involves 'queuing theory', which perceives 'demand' as a queue for service. Queues are seen every day in banks, shops, public transport, etc., and can be described as a system where a customer arrives for service at a counter or point. It does not matter for mathematical analysis whether the service is a surgery clinic, surgery OR, shop or bank. The process is defined by its key elements, which are

1. How frequently 'customers' arrive
2. The rate at which they are 'served' (i.e., the time it takes to serve them)
3. The number of 'servers' available

It is recognised that arrivals are rarely completely regular (e.g., exactly ten per hour) but instead often resemble a Poisson distribution. This is a near-random distribution where, say, in one hour there may be no arrivals, in the next hour ten, and then six, etc. Just as a Gaussian distribution has its characteristic features for continuous data (for example, time in min or weight in kg), so also does a Poisson distribution for categorical data (for example, arrivals per hour), especially infrequent events. This characteristic pattern lends itself readily to mathematical modelling. The type of questions that can be addressed include: 'Given a certain mean arrival rate and a certain number of servers, what is the expected waiting time for customers?' or 'How many servers do we need to be x% confident of keeping our waiting time less than y minutes?' As long as the average arrival rate is known and Poisson distribution assumed, robust conclusions can be drawn using the models.

The simplest queue is one where there is a single arrival point and a single server; in reality many queues can coexist and involve multiple servers (often themselves interrelated in a network) and demonstrate patterns of arrival that are much more complex than Poisson (for example, block arrivals). Increasingly sophisticated models of queues can examine the optimum organisation of a queue (for example, each surgical team has its own queue versus a pooled waiting list), the best order of service (for example, 'first in, first served' versus 'random service'), and issues such as booked versus sequential appointments. There is also the concept of a fixed waiting list versus an infinite waiting pool.

Unfortunately queuing analyses lose in simplicity what they might gain in mathematical robustness. A strength is that queuing theory can deal with many situations and address more sophisticated questions than can much of the approach to demand-capacity outlined earlier in this chapter.

Let us consider one surgeon in a clinic where on average four patients arrive per hour, with a mean consultation time of 10 min each. With an average of just 40 min each hour in total taken in consultations (i.e., 20-min free time in the clinic), intuition might suggest that there is unlikely to be any waiting time. Yet queuing theory predicts (accurately) that patients will wait in clinic for a mean of 20 min, which seems surprisingly long. To reduce this wait, a second surgeon is employed. Having doubled the capacity, we might expect the waiting time to halve to 10 min (double the servers, halve the capacity, surely?). In fact, and as predicted by the theory, waiting time declines dramatically to just over 1 min. If, then, managers are tempted to increase bookings because of this second surgeon's presence, such that patients' attendances double from four to eight per hour, the expectation might be that waiting time will simply double to a modest (and acceptable) 2 min. Unfortunately, the increase is much more marked to (a possibly unacceptable) 8 min.

Some user-friendly applets are readily available online, but none are specific for problems faced by theatre managers every day. Because there are no simple rules or 'off the peg' analyses tools available to solve the problems, we do not expand on queuing theory in this chapter.

However, one important result from queuing theory, consistent with the approach of this chapter, is that the size of the queue and wait time are inversely related to the utilisation of the system (Figure 5.15),

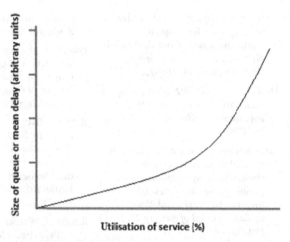

Figure 5.15 Queuing theory predicts that as utilisation of the service increases, especially > 80%, the size of queue (waiting list) or delay (waiting time) increase.

with the size of the queue or delay in service markedly increasing if utilisation exceeds ~80%.

Bibliography

Bailey NTJ. 1952. A study of queues and appointments systems in outpatient departments with special reference to waiting times. *Journal of the Royal Statistical Society Series B* 14: 185–99.

Bailey NTJ. 1954. Queuing for medical care. *Applied Statistics* 3: 137–45.

Bellan L. 2008. Changes in waiting lists over time. *Canadian Journal of Ophthalmology* 43: 547–50.

Buhaug H. 2002. Long waiting lists in hospitals. *British Medical Journal* 324: 252–3.

Carter GM, Cooper RB. 1972. Queues with service in random order. *Operations Research* 20: 389–405.

Castille K, Gowland B, Walley P. 2002. Variability must be managed to reduce waiting times and improve care. *British Medical Journal* 324: 1336.

Cayirli T, Veral E. 2003. Outpatient scheduling in health care: a review of literature. *Production and Operations Management* 12: 519–49.

Chalice R. 2008. *Improving Healthcare Using Toyota Lean Production Methods*, 2nd edn. Milwaukee: Quality Press.

Dexter F, Epstein RD, Traub RD, Xiao Y. 2004. Making management decisions on the day of surgery based on operating room efficiency and patient waiting times. *Anesthesiology* 101: 1444–53.

Dexter F, Macario A, Qian F, Traub RD. 1999. Forecasting surgical groups' total hours of elective cases for allocation of block time: application of time series analysis to operating room management. *Anesthesiology* 91: 1501–8.

Dexter F, Macario A, Traub RD, Hopwood M, Lubarsky DA. 1999. An operating room scheduling strategy to maximize the use of operating room block time: computer simulation of patient scheduling and survey of patients' preferences for surgical waiting time. *Anesthesia and Analgesia* 89: 7–20.

Doig A. 1957. A bibliography on the theory of queues. *Biometrika* 44: 490.

Epstein RH, Dexter F. 2002. Statistical power analysis to estimate how many months of data are required to identify operating room staffing solutions to reduce labor costs and increase productivity. *Anesthesia and Analgesia* 94: 640–3.

Gallivan S, Utley M, Treasure T, Valencia O. 2002. Booked inpatient admissions and hospital capacity: mathematical modeling study. *British Medical Journal* 324: 280–2.

Gans N, Koole G, Mandelbaum A. 2003. Telephone call centers: tutorial, review and research prospects. *Manufacturing and Service Operations Management* 5: 79–141.

Gauld R, Derrett S. 2000. Solving the surgical waiting list problem? New Zealand's "booking system". *International Journal of Health Planning and Management* 15: 259–72.

Gorunescu F, McClean SI, Millard PH. 2002. Using a queuing model to help plan bed allocation in a department of geriatric medicine. *Healthcare Management Science* 5: 307–12.

Harrison A, Appleby J. 2009. Reducing waiting times for hospital treatment: lessons from the English NHS. *Journal of Health Services Research Policy* 14: 168–73.

Ho C-J, Lau H-S. 1992. Minimizing total cost in scheduling outpatient appointments. *Management Science* 38: 1750–64.

Lawrentschuk N, Hewitt PM, Pritchard MG. 2003. Elective laparoscopic cholecystectomy: implications of prolonged waiting times for surgery. *Australian and New Zealand Journal of Surgery* 73: 890–3.

Martin S, Smith PC. 1999. Rationing by waiting lists: an empirical investigation. *Journal of Public Economics* 7: 141–64.

Martin RM, Sterne JAC, Gunnell D, Ebrahim S, Smith GD, Frankel S. 2003. NHS waiting lists and evidence of national or local failure: analysis of health service data. *British Medical Journal* 326: 188–98.

Morton A, Cornwell J. 2009. What's the difference between a hospital and a bottling factory? *British Medical Journal* 339: 428–30.

NHS Modernisation Agency. 2002. Step Guide to Improving Operating Theatre Performance. www.modern.nhs.uk/ theatreprogramme.

Pandit JJ. 2008. Gambling with ethics? A statistical note on the Poisson (binomial) distribution. *Anaesthesia* 63: 1163–6.

Pandit JJ, Dexter F. 2009. Lack of sensitivity of staffing for 8 hour sessions to standard deviation in daily actual hours of operating room time used for surgeons with

long queues. *Anesthesia and Analgesia* 108: 1910–5.

Pandit M, Mackenzie IZ. 1999. Patient satisfaction in gynaecological outpatient clinic attendances. *Journal of Obstetrics and Gynaecology* 19: 511–5.

Rabiei R, Bath PA, Hutchinson A, Burke D. 2009. The National Programme for IT in England: clinicians' views on the impact of the Choose and Book service. *Health Informatics Journal* 15: 167–78.

Rogers H, Warner J, Steyn R, Silvester K, Pepperman M, Nash R. 2002. Booked inpatient admissions and hospital capacity: mathematical model misses the point. *British Medical Journal* 324: 1336.

Roland M, Morris R. 1988. Are referrals by general practitioners influenced by the availability of consultants? *British Medical Journal* 297: 599–600.

Schoenmayer T, Dunn PF, Gamarnik D, et al. 2009. A model for understanding the impacts of demand and capacity on waiting time to enter a congested recovery room. *Anesthesiology* 110: 1293–304.

Silvester K, Lendon R, Bevan H, Steyn R, Walley P. 2004. Reducing waiting times in the NHS: is lack of capacity the problem? *Clinicians in Management* 12: 105–11.

Stordhal K. 2007. The history behind the probability theory and the queuing theory. *Telektronikk* 2: 123–40.

Street A, Duckett S. 1996. Are waiting lists inevitable? *Health Policy* 36: 1–5.

Strum DP, Vargas LG, May JH. 1999. Surgical subspecialty block

utilization and capacity planning: a minimal cost analysis model. *Anesthesiology* 90: 1176–85.

Taylor TH, Jennings AMC, Nightingale DA, et al. 1969. A study of anaesthetic emergency work. Paper 1: the method of study and introduction to queuing theory. *British Journal of Anaesthesia* 41: 70–5.

The Joint Commission, USA. 2009. Public Policy: Reducing Waste in Health Care and Improving Efficiency. www.joint commission.org/PublicPolicy/ Efficiency_Waste_Reduction. Htm, accessed 04 / 08 / 2009.

Umeh HN, Reece-Smith H, Faber RG, Galland RB. 1994. Impact of a waiting list initiative on a general surgical waiting list. *Annals of the Royal College of Surgeons of England* 76: 4–7.

Willig A. 1999. *A Short Introduction to Queuing Theory.* Telecommunication Networks Group, Technical University Berlin. www.tkn.tu-berlin.de/curricula/ ws0203/uekn/qt.ps.

Winch S, Henderson AJ. 2009. Making cars and making health care: a critical review. *Medical Journal of Australia* 191: 28–9.

Worthington D. 1991. Hospital waiting list management models. *The Journal of the Operational Research Society* 42: 833–43.

Zhou J, Dexter F, Macario A, Lubarsky DA. 1999. Relying solely on historical surgical times to estimate accurately future surgical times is unlikely to reduce the average length of time cases finish late. *Journal of Clinical Anesthesia* 11: 601–5.

Staffing and Contracts

Jaideep J. Pandit

Introduction

Staffing – and particularly the contracts under which staff are employed – underpins many aspects of performance hitherto discussed. Other than physical constraints such as numbers of theatres, staff are the most important determinants of capacity, and in turn, the capacity they can offer is determined wholly by their contracts of employment. Contracts also influence satisfaction and can create incentives or disincentives that can influence human behaviour; if managed well, contracts can generate goodwill that so often drives healthcare organisations.

It is not the aim of this chapter to create a model contract or discuss ideals of remuneration – this is beyond the scope of any book, and these matters are often settled through politics and individual or trades union negotiation. Theatre managers rarely, if ever, actually hold or create contracts. However, it is important for a theatre manager to understand those elements of a contract that influence the delivery of theatre services.

Contracts and Incentivisation

Substantive Employment

The broad aim of a substantive employment contract is to offer the employee a stable, predictable income (which of course may rise with inflation, pay awards or career progress, etc.). Through the contract and any incentives it contains, a sense of loyalty and goodwill may be engendered (e.g., the thinking that, if the employer does well, that will be translated to improved terms and conditions). The advantage to an employer of a substantive contract is a reliable, stable workforce around which future planning can occur. Incentives can be used to promote certain behaviours or actions over others, so as to attain employer goals within the contract. Other than pay awards, another common incentive is the work-based pension,

wherein a proportion of salary is deducted at source, often enhanced by the employer or even the government, and invested in or set aside for a pension that pays out a regular income and/or lump sum on retirement. Such schemes help retain workers for long periods, or even their lifetimes, and are not available to non-substantive employees.

Substantive employees also need time within the contract to help manage or develop the organisation. Because long-term employees represent the 'memory' of the organisation, they are best placed to see where improvements in practice or process can be made and so often are best placed to hold leadership positions to help implement the necessary policies for advancement. That said, outsiders can also bring fresh perspectives from other organisations, which may be necessary, especially in times of change. However, the time spent in management, committees, audits, research, innovation or professional development means time away from direct patient care. So in keeping substantive staff and making best use of their insights, the employer must accept that these staff need investment in the form of non-clinical time to pursue these other necessary activities.

Implicit in a substantive contract is limitation on hours of work. Contractual relationships are regulated by law, so safe limits of working are imposed (e.g., compulsory break periods). While superficially these rules would seem to limit an employer's flexibility in using the workforce, they also add clarity to help in accurate planning. Rather than guess if staff will stay late, depending on their goodwill, and then trying to plan around this uncertainty, the planner will know for sure that they cannot stay late.

The principle that the employer pays the substantive employee a fixed salary brings other tensions. It is then necessary to define the hours of work associated with that salary. Regardless of professional behaviours, a fixed salary makes it generally in the interest of an employee to do as little work as possible (same pay, less work, thereby enhancing their hourly rate of pay). Equally, it is in theory generally also in the interest of an employer to squeeze as much work as possible out of the employee without additional pay (same pay, more work, thereby increasing hourly productivity). These opposing interests have the potential to create tensions. However, these are short-term views because if taken to their extremes, they will lead to catastrophe for all. If all employees did as little as possible, the organisation might collapse, and the employees themselves would become redundant and lose in the long run. If the employer squeezed too hard, the resulting dissatisfaction would be counterproductive and lead to recruitment difficulties. Hence, fairness is important, and the objective analyses in this book help in making that transparent.

Temporary Staffing

The potential tension created by such opposing interests might theoretically all be avoided by the alternative to a substantive contract on a fixed salary, which is a locum or temporary contract where salary is directly linked to the hours worked. This may be short term or even *ad hoc* (i.e., as and when needed). The advantages to the employee are flexibility; the employee can work whenever they like for as many hours, varied according to their needs, or they can choose the job offer that best matches their needs. Hourly rates of pay may be higher in absolute terms because the employer is not contributing to a pension scheme and also because many such arrangements are finalised at the last minute when the employer urgently really needs staff to cover work. The advantage to an employer is avoiding complex contracts, other staff incentives, and the guarantee that the whole of the temporary employee's work hours will be devoted to clinical care (i.e., temporary employees are rarely if ever paid for non-clinical administrative duties). The employee will not be seeking to do as little work as possible, but instead to impress the employer so that they may be employed again. Unlike substantive contracts, many temporary contracts are not subject to limitations on hours of work (e.g., it might be impossible for one employer to know how many hours an individual has worked that week or month for another employer). This might increase flexibility for the employer, but can also raise concerns about safety. This last may be coupled with uncertainty as to the professional status or career development of the temporary employee, unless there is a robust record kept of appraisals, qualifications, etc. Another problem for the employer in relying wholly on such short-term contracts is that it constrains the ability to plan long-term; there is no guarantee that there will be any workforce to meet the organisation's objectives.

In practice a mix of substantive and temporary staff are invariably needed.

The Role of Contracts in Setting Capacity

We can understand how contracts ultimately determine theatre capacity by considering the UK NHS Consultant Contract, introduced in 2003. In fact, in broad outline this contract merely updated principles that had been in existence since the creation of the NHS in 1948, and it is unlikely that the core principles of this 2003 Contract will change very much in the future.

For surgeons, it is recognised within the Contract that in addition to their theatre lists (which is the main focus of this book), they also need to undertake several other duties: ward rounds, clinics, administration (e.g., dictating letters, reviewing results), multidisciplinary meetings to plan surgeries, on-call activity and professional activity (such as audit, research, innovation, committees, etc.). In our analysis, surgeons can be viewed as the source of the work being generated for theatres, through the bookings for surgery they make in their clinics. Notwithstanding the role of primary care physicians in referring patients to surgeons in the first place, surgeons are the initiators of the operating room (OR) process, not the rate-limiting step.

The elements of an anaesthetist's work, in addition to theatre lists, have similarities to a surgeon's, but also differences: pre- and post-operative ward rounds, pain ward rounds, preoperative clinics, some administration (but perhaps less so than surgeons), possibly multidisciplinary meetings to plan surgeries, on-call activity and professional activity (such as audit, research, innovation, committees, etc.). In contrast to surgeons, anaesthetists can be viewed as one of the potential rate-limiting steps to the OR process. Surgeons may book as many patients for surgery as they can physically operate on for years to come, but the rate at which this work is completed will depend on how much anaesthetic time is available.

The 2003 Contract defines a full-time contract as 40 hours work per week, and Table 6.1 shows how

Table 6.1 Direct clinical care activities. The sum of these should average 30 hours/week. The second column illustrates estimates reasonable estimates applying to most anaesthetists.

Actual work performed on-call	~4–6 hours
Operating sessions	~20 hours
Pre- and post-operative care	~4–6 hours
Other patient treatment*	~30 min
Multidisciplinary meetings about direct patient care	~30 min
Administration related to patient care	~30–45 min
Travel: (a) to and from home for on-call work;	
(b) between sites for elective work	~30–45 min
Professional activity	~10 hours
Total per week	~1,560–2,040 min
	36–44 hours)

this is generally divided for an anaesthetist. These hours can vary because there is scope to work up to 48 hours without breaching national (European Union) limits on working hours.

Thus a full-time anaesthetist will devote ~20 hours per week in theatre, equating to two 10-hour lists spread over 2 days, or perhaps three 8-hour lists spread over 3 days if some additional direct clinical hours are worked.

Leave allocations include the following: (a 'day' is regarded as a weekday; weekends are not regarded as 'normal working days').

1. Annual leave: The basic entitlement is 30 days per year. For consultants with 7 years' or more substantive NHS employment, it is 32 days/year.

2. Study leave: 10 days/year.

3. Professional leave: Over and above annual or study leave, this is best defined as official leave for added responsibilities (e.g., examining, interviewing or representing the hospital or profession).

4. Other leave: This includes sick, maternity and paternity leave. Special leave does not easily fall into any of these categories, and it can be paid or unpaid for any variety of (often discretionary) reasons. Carers' leave is an employee's entitlement to support a relative (usually a child) when care

arrangements (e.g., a nanny) break down. Compassionate leave is granted (normally up to 5 calendar days) where there is a bereavement of a family member.

All this means, when added together, that it is wise for planners to regard that, of 52 weeks of a calendar year, a consultant is likely to be absent from work for up to 10 weeks per year (including public holidays). If working ~20 hours per week in theatre, this means that a full-time consultant anaesthetist has a reliable capacity to deliver ~840 hours of theatre time per year (perhaps up to ~1,008 hours if they take up some additional work within the working hours limits).

These figures can be used to estimate staffing requirements for the theatre suite/department/hospital as a whole (i.e., ten anaesthetists create an annual capacity of ~8,400 hours, 100 anaesthetists ~84,000 hours and so on). However, one additional element to be factored in is the cross-cover of leave. When one anaesthetist is away, unless the hospital wishes to suspend or cancel the associated theatre time, it is important to have a 'spare' anaesthetist who can fill in the vacated slot.

Taking this into account, a simplified formula based on this 2003 national Contract is that for each theatre running 5 days (8 hours per day) per week will require at least ~2.2 full-time anaesthetists to ensure adequate cover. A theatre manager can use this rule of thumb (and the proportionalities that emanate from this) crudely to estimate the staffing requirements. Thus a suite of ten ORs will require at least 22 full-time anaesthetists to be open each day for 8 hours, 5 days a week. The same suite with the OR day extended to 10 hours will need at least 28 anaesthetists, and so on. Of course, these requirements may be met either by employing substantive staff, or by employing short-term temporary staff, or a combination. Appendix 6A outlines a general algorithm to estimate staffing when different contracts are in place.

Like anaesthetists, estimates for other staffing in theatre can also be assessed using the algorithm in Appendix 6A. There is need for one anaesthesia assistant, one theatre scrub nurse, one runner, etc. All these needs can be modelled the same way. Of course, each of these staff groups will have different leave allowances according to their contracts, but the principles of the algorithm remain.

All this seems so simple. All the theatre manager needs to do is know how many ORs there are, and for how long they should be open and for how many days. This will be the prime determinant of anaesthesia and theatre nurse staffing. Yet there is considerable literature from the NHS showing that rarely if ever do NHS hospitals apply such objective analyses to plan staffing. Instead, older methods of needing to 'justify' a consultant-level appointment in a qualitative way are used. When a consultant anaesthetist retires, it would seem a simple matter of advertising the new replacement post, ideally from the time the notice of retirement is given. Instead, for each post a business case for renewal needs to be made, as if somehow the issue was one that the organisation had never encountered before. When an extra consultant surgeon is appointed, it is generally known that they will create demand for additional x hours in theatre per week. This should clearly determine, very simply, how much extra anaesthetic staffing is required (i.e., x hours per week). Rarely, however, are anaesthetic appointments coupled with new surgical appointments in the NHS in a quantitative way. Therefore many if not the majority, of NHS hospitals run with a severe shortage of anaesthetic consultants and theatre nursing staff. This leads to cancellation of theatre sessions, or of last-minute employment of expensive locums to cover the shortfalls.

Staffing in a Typical US List or UK Private List

In the United States, setting the principles for anaesthetists outlined earlier are relevant to a private anaesthetic group, which may be providing a service to one or more hospitals. The group will need to estimate how many anaesthesiologists it needs to cover the work (OR hours) it takes on, whilst allowing each partner some leave. It is also relevant to academic centres where anaesthesiologists are full-time employees along similar lines to the United Kingdom. The private anaesthetic group or university department will need to define its own policies on how many sessions each anaesthesiologist is expected to cover in a week, how much professional time they need, and how much leave they are entitled to. There may be greater flexibility in, say, allowing group members or employees the choice to take less leave for more income or vice versa, but nevertheless the practice manager or department chief will need to know in advance how much absence there is likely to be.

The algorithms described in Appendix 6A apply to US OR staff as much as to the United Kingdom, as

these are generally employed by the respective hospitals, private or academic.

The issues outlined earlier are much less relevant for a UK private hospital setting for anaesthetists, although they are very relevant again for theatre nurse staffing. This is because surgeons will invite their own anaesthetists to staff the list and be wholly responsible for doing so.

Quantity versus Quality

While much of the discussion has been around the quantitative matching of staff numbers, we must emphasise that quality is of paramount importance. Not only do all staff need proper training and to adhere to professional regulatory requirements, but there should also be appropriate attention to skill mix. This means that it may be necessary to apply the algorithms for staffing in Appendix 6A not only to the unit as a whole, but also to each subunit or subspecialty in question.

For example, cardiac, obstetric or neurosurgery may require specific skills of theatre staff (and anaesthetists) and even if hospital-level algorithm application suggests there is 'sufficient staffing' (i.e., 100 anaesthetists), lack of skills may mean that cross-cover is impossible. What should happen then is that the staffing needs of the subunit/subspecialty should be assessed in isolation. So the rule of thumb still applies – for every subspecialist OR working 5 days per week, ~2.2 suitably skilled staff of each group (anaesthetist, assistant, scrub, etc.) are needed to staff it without interruption. If the cardiac unit consists of ten ORs working 5 days a week for 8 hours each, then it needs 'cardiac' ~22 anaesthetists; the fact there are 100 anaesthetists elsewhere is irrelevant.

Timing of Shifts

It is important to ensure that shifts are time-aligned. In the case of theatre nursing staff, a shift refers to the time they need to arrive for work and the time they can depart. Work outside these agreed hours is overtime.

For surgeons and anaesthetists who are on more professional, less time-sensitive contracts (even when employed by the hospital as in the NHS), there is greater flexibility in the collective understanding of a 'shift'. Nevertheless, their contracts are certainly time-aligned or time-limited. For example, the European Working Time Directive limits work to 48 hours per week (although there is an opt-out for consultant staff, it is not clear yet whether working longer than these hours exposes these doctors to medicolegal sanction in the case of an adverse event). In other words, although contracts for surgeons and anaesthetists are not defined by 'shift', the hours they work are recognised and compensated in one way or another. If a surgeon or anaesthetist is contracted, say, for 40 hours per week and finds that one list regularly overruns by, say, 2 hours, then they are entitled to seek recognition within their contract for the extra 2 hours (i.e., they then become remunerated for 42 hours per week).

However, in order to calculate whether they are in fact working those extra 2 hours (or indeed to know what hours they are working) it is necessary to define what the (virtual) 'shift' – or list – length actually is. We have touched upon this already in Chapter 2 in discussion of what is a 'start time'. Let us expand on this examination.

If the start time for a list is defined by the arrival of surgeon for surgery ('knife to skin') then the surgeon's contractual period for reckoning their hours of work starts at that time. However for reasons we have seen in Chapter 2, the anaesthetists' actual start time may then be a full hour earlier. And the theatre nursing and portering staff shift will need to start even before that, to prepare the necessary equipment and perform all the due checks. Similarly, at the end of the list, the surgeon may have opportunity to leave immediately after the WHO 'sign out', but clearly the patient needs to be awoken and transported to recovery/post-anaesthesia care unit (PACU) or intensive care for further management of fluids, pain, etc. Again the anaesthetists' contract needs to recognise this additional time. And theatre nursing and portering staff will need to clean and perform stock checks, etc. Also, the surgeon may need to return perhaps as part of a 'post-operative ward round' hours later to check that all is well with the patients after surgery or to discharge some of them.

In summary, contractual time needs to recognise all relevant work related to the operating list, and not just the list time. While this seems obvious consider this real-life example from the NHS:

Example. A theatre manager decided that a surgical list duration should be increased from 8 hours per week on a given day to 9 hours. The contracts of all staff (surgeons, theatre nursing staff, porters) were duly extended by 1 hour. However, because the hospital had decided that the anaesthetic department had overspent its budget the previous year, and its pay budget was capped to force financial savings, the contracted hours of the anaesthetist were not increased. Although the anaesthetist initially volunteered to extend the working day by an hour, the expected contractual changes never occurred, and he was advised by contract lawyers to cease this practice, otherwise it would constitute formal acceptance of the new arrangements without pay. Consequently, he curtailed the list at 8 hours, as before, cancelling any remaining patients booked. This happened for over a year until proper contracts were implemented. The hospital made no savings and indeed lost income overall as a result: the additional hours of surgeon and nursing staff being paid for were wasted.

Another way that shift timings can be mismanaged is by misaligning the handovers in shifts. Thus, given a single operating list, it is wise to schedule the same team to work the whole duration (notwithstanding rest breaks). The less-effective alternative is to schedule a new team to arrive at some point in the middle of the list. Consider this real-life example from the NHS:

Example. A long surgical list is scheduled from 08.00 to 20.00 (12 hours). The mean duration of each operation is an hour, including anaesthesia and turnover time, so approximately 11–12 cases could reliably be completed. The same anaesthetist and surgeon are assigned to this list. However, theatre nursing staff are scheduled to change shifts at 18.00. What happens at ~17.30 when usually 8–9 cases are complete is that the first shift refuses to start the next case, as they need to perform their final handover checks and paperwork. Similarly, when the new shift arrives, they need 15–20 min to perform their checks, computer logins, etc. So the next patient cannot be sent for until ~18.30 at the earliest. Then, given that the list cannot be allowed to overrun for safety reasons, only one more case can be completed, to finish at ~19.30, making 9–10 cases in total rather than the expected 11–12. Over an hour has been wasted by misaligned handover.

Summary

How an employer handles contracts reflects their fundamental values. The theatre manager should recognise, and advise against, employer attempts to misinterpret contracts to seek inappropriate gains. The theatre manager is in a key position to know when expensive short-term contracts are better replaced by substantive contracts that add value in the long run. Equally, how an employee approaches their contract reflects their professionalism. They should be guided by their advisers and professional societies to work flexibly (e.g., not count every minute of time) and use non-clinical time in ways that add value to the service. The theatre manager is in a key position to suggest areas of focus for audit, research or innovation work in this domain.

Appendix 6A A General Algorithm for Theatre Staffing by Senior Anaesthetists

The following equation estimates anaesthesia staffing capacity with the 2003 NHS Consultant Contract for each consultant:

$$Theatre\ sessions\ per\ year = \left(\frac{[252] - [total\ absence\ in\ days]}{5} \right) \times (direct\ elective\ care\ sessions\ per\ week)$$

Equation 6.1

The equation uses 'session' (a 4-hour block of time or half-day) rather than 'hours'. Whereas 'hours' is useful for overall demand-capacity planning (Chapter 5), it is not useful when assigning days of work across staff. This is in part because leave is awarded in 'days' rather than 'hours' (and the list duration in any given day may consist of 1–3 sessions). The equation also focusses only on the elective surgery sessions and not emergency sessions (or non-clinical professional activitiy sessions) because the remit of the theatre manager is primarily to manage elective theatre sessions.

For most full-time consultants, the total absence in days is ~52 (including all annual, study, professional, estimated sick leave, etc.). For most consultants, the number of direct care sessions is 5–7 per week withint their contract. Equation 6.1 works also for part-time consultants by adjusting these quantities. The constant 252 represents the weekdays, which are the working days. If ever the service moves to 6- or 7-day workweek, then this constant can be suitably adjusted. The constant 5 represents the 5 working days of the week (i.e., if the service moves to 6- or 7-day workweek, then this constant will change to 6 or 7, respectively).

Consider now that a new consultant-led hospital is planned, with four ORs, each running all day (arranged as 2 sessions or 8 hours per day) for 252 working days per year. The demand is 2,016 sessions/year. Our algorithm predicts a need for 8–10 full-time consultants. However, this reflects what is needed at any one time, assuming the hospital does not wish to suspend service during anaesthetists' leave.

Therefore the hospital cannot get away with the lower estimate of eight consultants. The hospital might then consider employing nine anaesthetists and allow no more than one to be absent in any week. But, this leads to another constraint. As we have shown earlier, each anaesthetist is predictably entitled to up to 10 weeks of leave per year (even disregarding other types of unanticipated leave that might be needed). Imagine a leave diary – a calendar in which the anaesthetists write their name against the day to signify they are taking leave for that day. There will be 252 weekdays of leave available (the 'leave slot'). However, nine anaesthetists are collectively entitled to 90 weeks leave (450 days), if taken consecutively, so the proposed solution does not allow all consultants their predictable leave (i.e., it is a potential breach of contract on the part of the employer).

A more workable model is for the hospital to employ ten consultants (which more reliably will cover the expected work) and offer two 'leave slots', which more than encompasses the collective annual/study leave entitlement. Note that at times over the year, there will be more consultants present than are perhaps strictly needed, but this is inevitable and is a flexibility that also helps manage the unforeseen absences.

As a general rule, a department will need one leave slot per five consultants to enable each consultant to take their due leave.

These calculations are replicated in a 'Staffing tool' (an Excel spreadsheet) that is accessible at www.cambridge.org/9781316646830. Readers can adapt the calculations for each cell to their own situation, so the tool provides a template to assess staffing levels.

Appendix 6B Common Problems with Contracts – and How to Avoid Them

Taking of Annual Leave

The contract will stipulate how many 'days' or 'weeks' of leave a consultant is entitled to. However, many contracts (e.g., the UK NHS 2003 Consultant Contract) do not in fact stipulate what a 'day' is. In simplest terms the question is: Does a day in this sense include or exclude weekends? So, if an employee is abroad on vacation from a Monday, and returns to work the following Monday is that 7 days (Monday through to Sunday) or is it 5 (Monday through to Friday)? Generally, if this is unspecified, the contract is assumed, at least in the United Kingdom, to refer to weekdays only. So a leave allowance of 30 days means 6 calendar weeks, if taken in whole weeks. If the employee is on-call for a weekend day, it is customary for them to arrange a swap of duty with a colleague, and formal leave is never taken for this.

However, this interpretation leads to another problem. Because, as explained earlier, UK NHS consultants are in theatre for only 2–3 days of the week (and undertaking other non-clinical duties for the remaining days), some choose to take as leave only their clinical days. This is an artificial (and unsanctioned) means of maximising leave at the expense of colleagues and of the employer. Thus a consultant who is scheduled to be in theatre Mondays and Tuesdays and chooses to take as leave 15 Mondays and 15 Tuesdays, thereby being claiming to be within the contractual entitlement by taking 30 days total, is in fact effectively absent from clinical duties for 15 calendar weeks of the year, rather than the expected 6 weeks. This practice can be restricted by imposing one or a combination of the following rules:

(a) At the end of the leave year, it is expected that an employee will take an approximately equal number of weekdays as leave. If the allowance is 30 days, then the expectation is that 6 of each of the days Monday to Friday should be registered taken as leave. Some tolerance limits should be built in (e.g., ± 2 days, i.e., 4–8 days of each weekday).

(b) The clinical duties are 'annualised' in respect of leave. As explained earlier, ~10 weeks of absence are expected each year, leaving ~42 weeks at work. Therefore, it can be expected that there will be ~42 of each clinical session or clinical day present at work over the year. This way, the actual days' leave are effectively unmonitored – consultants can come and go as they like, with the due notice – but it is the days present that are counted. Again, tolerance limits should be built in (e.g., as few as ~40 allowed, with allowances of course for any sick leave). This can also be applied to non-clinical duties such as committees, etc.

(c) It is stipulated that leave must be taken in whole weeks. However, such a policy must be introduced with great care, as employees often do need the odd day off and are entitled to take it (e.g., leave on a Monday but work on the Tuesday). Such policies are generally unenforceable, but agreement might be reached that a certain proportion of leave (e.g., 2 weeks per year) should be taken as whole weeks.

There is another common problem with leave affecting those clinical days consisting of longer-scheduled lists. Let us consider two colleagues, Drs A and B. Dr A works a 12-hour list on Monday and 12-hour list on Tuesday (24 hours per week). Dr B works 8-hour lists on Monday, Tuesday and Wednesday (also 24 hours per week). On top of this, they are both contracted to cross-cover leave within the department. The hospital adopts an annualised leave policy such that Dr A must deliver 42 Mondays and 42 Tuesdays per year; while Dr B must deliver 42 Mondays, 42 Tuesdays and 42 Wednesdays per year.

So far so good – leave is equitable for both Drs A and B. However, when Dr A goes on leave, Dr B (or another colleague) suddenly finds they have to cover a day on which there is a 12-hour list. In contrast, when Dr B goes on leave, Dr A (or another colleague) finds they have to cover only an 8-hour list. In other words, Dr A's absence on a clinical day imposes more work demands on the department than does Dr B's, even though from each of their perspectives they are correctly taking their apportioned leave. There is no universal solution to this problem. It is something to be recognised and, if possible, factored into the wider contract of employment or through individual negotiation.

Management of Non-theatre List Time within a Contract

Taking the UK NHS 2003 Consultant Contract as an example (see earlier discussion), the recognition of clinical duties for surgeons and anaesthetists is rarely a matter of dispute. List schedules are published, and if a list is x hours long, then x hours must be recognised in the contract. Even when the list schedules are incorrect – i.e., lists always overrun their schedules – it is an easy matter for the real timings to be recognised over the fictional ones. However, disputes can arise over the 'softer' aspects of the contract, namely, the time recognised for clinical administration, ward rounds (for surgeons) or perioperative care (for anaesthetists: the time when they visit the patient pre-and post-operatively). The problem is simple. If x hours are allocated, and in fact the consultant is suspected to undertake in fact $x - y$ hours for any of these, the employer is aggrieved. If, on the other hand, the consultant in fact claims they take $x + y$ for these activities, the employee is aggrieved.

In this situation, a poor management strategy is to impose an arbitrary time. Real examples will help illustrate this.

Example. In one NHS hospital, surgeons were allocated inadequate time for clinical administration. This induced behaviours that led to a massive backlog of certain types of paperwork (i.e., immediate clinical paperwork was prioritised, but coding and billing paperwork was ignored). This led the hospital to employ specialist temporary staff to clear the backlog, with no financial gain overall – they might as well have granted the surgeons the time they felt they originally needed.

Example. At another hospital, anaesthetists were no longer allocated sufficient pre- or post-operative time to assess and review patients. The anaesthesia group responded by (a) disengaging with the preassessment service (because they were not paid for that service), so that they only offered preoperative advice on patients on the very day of surgery, which was sometimes too late and led to last-minute postponement for further tests and (b) curtailing all overrunning lists strictly to time so they could properly and safely assess patients post-operatively. The additional costs as a result of both these reactions more than outweighed any savings to the organisation of reducing their contracted hours. .

To avoid repeating the mistakes in these examples, objective approaches should be sought. Weekly diaries can inform managers as to how long on average these activities take. Evidence from other hospitals can be used to help benchmark the norms. Specialist and professional organisations (e.g., in the United Kingdom, the Royal Colleges) could be asked for national guidance on the expectations for these activities. Any values agreed on should be set by the median or mean times for these activities and not by extreme times (i.e., the fastest or slowest should not set the reference value).

Managing Non-clinical Time and Incentives

Perhaps the most vexed of all discussions is around the management of non-clinical time. This is the paid time within a contract for professional duties, committees, teaching, examining, audit, research and innovation. Some contracts, like the UK NHS 2003 Consultant Contract, will set typical values (10 hours per week stipulated as typical), and national professional societies can set benchmarks (6 hours per week stipulated as the very minimum). However, the disputes are often around whether a particular individual is actually performing or delivering within this time allocation. A question is whether to look at inputs (e.g., simply sitting at a desk reading) or outputs (e.g., publication or presentation of work). Another question is what the benchmarks for either of these should be (if reading, then how much is read and what is the evidence? If publishing, how many papers and where published? etc.).

The non-clinical time allocations are viewed by some as incentives. If the hospital or wider health service needs experienced consultants to sit on a committee or advance the field in other ways, then ring-fencing time away from clinical duties is one way of ensuring this activity gets done. For those who find such non-clinical work as less arduous, stressful or more intellectually fulfilling, then this ring-fencing is an incentive by itself, even if there is no additional monetary gain (it is merely replacing activity, not adding to income). Other employees may not find such non-clinical work an incentive at all, if they find committees dull and uninspiring. All else being equal, this difference of opinion is not a problem – individuals can then freely choose the balance of their own duties. However, any consultant activity that becomes devoted to non-clinical work places a cost on the hospital because the clinical work of that consultant needs to be filled.

An ideal funding system would remunerate hospitals not only for direct clinical work (e.g., number of operations performed) but also by quality markers, which in part would be met by involvement in essential non-clinical committee, audit, innovation and research work.

Financial Incentives – and Data That Could Support Them

Financial incentives for individuals can – and should – also exist and be used to good effect. These will motivate staff to produce the outcomes desired by the organisation. However, the organisation itself needs to be clear on its own goals if such incentives are to be used well, and great care is needed. Consider the consequences of some misapplied incentives:

1. If a 'no overrun' policy is encouraged and teams are rewarded if they finish within time: this will lead to underbooking of lists and underrun, with wasted resources.
2. If a 'full utilisation' policy is introduced, such that teams are rewarded by utilisation of the list alone: this will lead to overbooking of lists, overruns, additional unbudgeted expense, organisational chaos and cancellation (there being no penalty for the last).
3. If a 'no cancellation' policy is adopted, teams will again overrun to avoid cancellation and then claim additional payments for overtime whilst also claiming the reward under the incentive scheme.
4. If a 'no post-operative mortality/morbidity' target is to be rewarded, which seems superficially sensible, then teams will only operate on fit patients, referring all others elsewhere.

The problem with these sorts of incentives is that they are too crude to be effective. An example of misplaced use of the second, utilisation, incentive is from a US hospital, where a surgeon was rewarded for high utilisation under both the incentive scheme and by allocating him additional lists. The problem was that his casemix was already creating a bottleneck in the intensive care unit, so the extra list time simply exacerbated the problems at the hospital. Moreover, the situation further worsened the apparent performance of other surgical teams, impairing their ability to meet their own utilisation incentives.

The first three incentives listed would work better if, instead, the goal was to achieve efficiency, defined by ε (see Chapter 2), as this measure is virtually impossible to 'game'.

The fourth incentive could be improved by using risk-adjusted mortality/morbidity instead of crude data. The principle of this is as follows. First, identify the outcome or event to be measured. The event could be an adverse one (mortality at some time point such as in-hospital, 30-day etc.; or a morbidity or complication); or a positive one (e.g., symptom-free outcome). This data can be presented as unadjusted, or adjusted by any number of factors that represent the risk (e.g., patient age, gender, coexisting disease). Second, calculate the volume of the caseload or activity (e.g., number of patients). This process can be applied at the level of an individual practitioner, team, ward, department, hospital or nation. When plotted, a scatter of data results and from this can be estimated the mean value (a horizontal line) and 95%, 99% (or other percentage) confidence intervals, which are a set of curved lines that asymptote to the mean value, as the volume/caseload increases. These curved lines are mathematically estimated from the binomial expansion (Figure 6.1). What the plot reflects is the reality that as the number of data points for any hospital/unit increases, the precision of its estimate should gravitate to the mean of a 'true representative' value for the population as a whole. If, despite a reasonable caseload, that unit's outcomes are outliers in an adverse direction, then there is a potential problem – either with the data collection or with the practices at that unit.

The basis of any incentive scheme should be 'SMART' (the goal should be 'specific', 'measurable', 'agreed as attainable', 'realistic' and 'time-limited'). The notions of 'agreed-as-attainable' and 'realistic' encapsulate the fact that the targets set for the incentive should be under the control of the individual. There is no point in setting as an individual incentive the goal that 'the organisation must end the year with

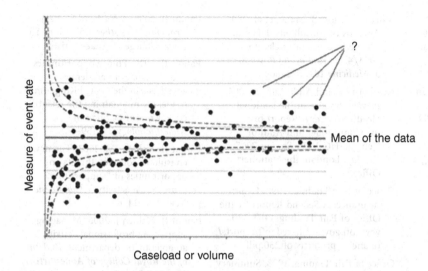

Figure 6.1 An example of a risk-adjusted or standardised event plot. Each point represents the data from a unit. Derivation of lines explained in text. The points marked ? are in the group of potential interest or concern, as their event rate is well outside the confidence intervals.

a financial surplus', as there is no way the individual can influence this outcome, or know if their actions are contributing in a positive way or not. For similar reasons, 'arriving to work on time' may be a SMART target, but 'starting the list on time' is not because so many other factors beyond individual influence are involved.

Different incentives should also not work against each other. If too many things are incentivised, then it means in effect nothing is incentivised. Imagine two separate incentive streams running in parallel, one rewarding full utilisation of the list and a separate one rewarding finishing before time. What might happen is that one person or group, perhaps randomly, chooses one incentive – say the goal of utilisation. Another individual or group, equally randomly, chooses the other – finishing before time. Their subsequent behaviours will then be in opposition. As an example, at one UK NHS hospital, consultant staff were paid extra for weekend waiting list initiatives (see Chapter 5) but in different ways. The surgeons were paid at a fixed hourly rate, per hour of time, so their natural inclination, perhaps subconscious, was to work as slowly as possible to maximise their overall gain from the day. The anaesthetists were paid a fixed amount for the list, regardless of how long or short the day was, so their incentive was to work as quickly as possible. They did not work together, and so the lists were poorly used – they either suffered high cancellation or under- or overran, depending on whether the surgeon's or anaesthetist's tactics prevailed on the day.

Bibliography

Abouleish A. 2008. Productivity-based compensations versus incentive plans. *Anesthesia and Analgesia* 107: 1765–7.

Abouleish AE, Apfelbaum JL, Prough DS, et al. 2005. The prevalence and characteristics of incentive plans for clinical productivity among academic anesthesiology programs. *Anesthesia and Analgesia* 100: 493–501.

Abouleish AE, Prough DS, Whitten CW, et al. 2002. Comparing clinical productivity of anaesthesiology groups. *Anesthesiology* 97: 608–15.

Abouleish AE, Prough DS, Zornow MH. 2001. Is average base units per surgical specialty indicative of billing productivity? *Anesthesiology* 95: A1107.

Abouleish AE, Prough DS, Zornow MH, et al. 2001. The impact of longer-than-average anesthesia times on the billing of academic anaesthesiology departments. *Anesthesia and Analgesia* 93: 1537–43.

Barker SJ. 2001. Lord or vassal? *Academic anaesthesiology finances* in 2000 *Anesthesia and Analgesia* 93: 294–300.

Becker KR, Cohen NH. 2007. Update on alternate payment methodologies workgroup. *American Society of Anesthesiologists' Newsletter* 11: 8–12.

Bowie R. 2005. Private surgical fees in New Zealand. *The New Zealand Medical Journal* 118: 1–3.

British Medical Association. 2003. *The New NHS Consultant Contract (England)*. London: British Medical Association.

Brown P, Windsor J, Law M. 2005. Dollars and sense: is there a better way to determine private surgical fees in New Zealand? *The New Zealand Medical Journal* 118: 1–3.

Chapman B. 2004. Private practice in the United Kingdom. *British Medical Journal Careers Focus* 328: 15.

Datamonitor. 2007. UK Private Medical Insurance 2006 – An In-Depth Analysis of the Private Medical Insurance Market in the UK. DMFS 1990, Datamonitor March 2007. www.datamonitor.com.

Harrop-Griffiths W. 2008. AAGBI private practice fee survey. *Anaesthesia News* 257: 31–3.

Lubarsky DA. 2005. Incentivize everything, incentivize nothing. *Anesthesia and Analgesia* 100: 490–2.

Monopolies and Mergers Commission. 1994. Private Medical Services: A Report on Agreements and Practices Relating to Charges for the Supply of Private Medical Services by NHS Consultants. February. London: the Stationery Office.

Morris S, Elliott B, Ma A, et al. 2008. Analysis of consultants' NHS and private incomes in England in 2003/4. *Journal of the Royal Society of Medicine* 101: 372–80.

Northern Ireland Audit Office. 2006. Private Practice in the National Health Service: A Report by the Comptroller and Auditor General. *HC 1008, Session 2005–6, 18 May*. London: the Stationery Office.

Office of Fair Trading. 1998. Health Insurance: A Second Report by the Office of Fair Trading. OFT 230. www.oft.gov.uk/shared_oft/reports/financial_products/oft230.pdf.

Office of Fair Trading. 1998. Summary of non-infringement decisions made under the Competition Act 1998 in respect of complaints concerning the activities of various groups of anaesthetists. www.oft.gov.uk/advice_and_resources/resource_base/ca98/decisions/anaesthetists-groups.

Pandit JJ. 2003. The new consultant contract and anaesthesia: practical implications of the new terminology. A personal view. *Anaesthesia News* 195: 16–7.

Pandit JJ. 2005. *A National Strategy for Academic Anaesthesia*. London: The Royal College of Anaesthetists.

Pandit JJ. 2010. Future opportunities and challenges in academic anaesthesia in the United Kingdom: a model for maintaining the scientific edge. *Current Opinion in Anaesthesiology* 23: 159–66.

Pandit JJ, Fielden JM. 2003. The new consultant contract: threats and opportunities of "supporting professional activity." *Anaesthesia News* 197: 24–6.

Pandit JJ, Fielden J. 2006. Managing supporting professional activity in an anaesthetic department. *Bulletin of the Royal College of Anaesthetists* 35: 1754–7.

Pandit JJ, Tavare A, Millard P. 2010. Why are there local shortfalls in anaesthesia consultant staffing? A case study of operational workforce planning. *Journal of Healthcare Organisation and Management* 24: 4–21.

Toledo P. 2007. Residency and economics: why you need to pay attention. *American Society of Anesthesiologists' Newsletter* 12: 42–3.

Theatre Finances

Jaideep J. Pandit

Introduction

Cost pressures across health services worldwide are well known. The true cost of healthcare is inexorably rising due to rise in absolute demand as more people rightly seek care, and also due to factors like earlier diagnosis, screening, an ageing and more obese population with expensive-to-treat comorbidities, and ever complex technology. Yet at the same time, governments and insurers who collectively fund healthcare costs constantly seek to drive down payments for care interventions, creating significant cost pressures for hospitals. In other industries whose products' demand is rising, the result is enormous profits for workers, managers and especially executives. Even in banking, massive dividends can be made by supporting and sustaining large deficits. Yet somehow in healthcare these rules do not seem to apply, and neither rising demand nor deficit budgets are seen as desirable or even tolerable.

In a manufacturing industry, introduction of a new product is predicated on the product being profitable. That is, the roughly the same level of utility is offered by the product (regardless of whether it is a car or a phone or a fizzy drink) for a higher price – and everyone is happy, including the consumer, with this deal. Even in other service industries the best lawyers, accountants, even artists are those who charge and profit the most. Not so in healthcare, where the onus is on cost savings to the consumer – the same or even higher-quality care for less and less cost. The aim of all is that, unlike the best law firms, the best hospitals should also be the cheapest.

The economics of healthcare – at least in many countries – is therefore topsy-turvy. There are several fundamental reasons for this. First and foremost – and the clue is in the name – is that healthcare is not about the profit motive. It is about 'care'. Historically it is based upon acts of altruism – one person (or teams) caring for another driven by motivations to heal and relieve pain, regardless of the cost or effort. Second, and perhaps to a large extent connected with the first, the greatest burden of ill health falls upon the poor and elderly; i.e., those not necessarily regarded as part of conventional economic markets. Healthcare has to be 'cheap' in that restricted sense, if those who most need it are to afford it. Hospitals originated from the Middle Ages as charities, often religious foundations, and therefore the profit motive is historically a low priority, with care being first.

Outline of Revenues and Expenditure

The theatre manager does not need to manage the finances of the whole organisation, or the nation's health service, but does need to be aware of how the system is funded.

Theatre Revenue

As outlined earlier, many hospitals in fact run at an operating loss. In the United States, hospital profit margins were estimated to be just 2–4% between 2004 and 2010, with about 40% of hospitals reporting negative margins. In the United Kingdom (UK), the majority of National Health Service (NHS) hospitals have been in deficit for many years, such that the total deficit at 2017 stands at ~£2.5 billion.

Revenue accrues to the hospital as a whole from a range of outpatient and inpatient activities. In the context of theatres, what is generally important is the payer and the type of contract under which services are provided by them. Generally, government tariffs for procedures are very low and often lower than any true cost of providing the service (this is explored later in the chapter). This is as true for the US Medicaid system as it is for the system of UK NHS tariffs. Medical insurers, however, pay at a more reasonable market rate: in the United States the most profitable organisations have a high proportion of commercial income. In the United Kingdom there are set limits as to how much an NHS hospital can earn from private, insurer or fee-paying work. Generally, therefore, contracts are of several types:

1. Service level agreements (SLA). In this arrangement, the provider (hospital) simply agrees to provide a service (surgery) of whatever volume is agreed or necessary, at a fixed cost. In this arrangement, any increase in demand means less per-case revenue for the hospital. This was generally the arrangement across the NHS for most of its existence; hospitals were responsible for simply doing the work that was necessary for the public.

2. Block contract. This arrangement has greater specificity than the SLA: it is agreed that the provider will undertake a certain number of cases for a fixed, agreed total price. While there is certainty of income, there is a pressure on the provider to reduce its costs so that the revenue generates profit (or at least breaks even). There is a risk when real demands exceed the volume of work agreed: the hospital may not be in a position to turn patients away, and so these cases are done 'for free'. In the NHS this is sometimes referred to as 'overperformance against budget'.

3. Fee-for-case. This is simplest to understand: each case carries with it a set or agreed fee. The issue is then what that fee is and how it is set, as this will be a crucial factor in determining whether the arrangement results in profit-per-case. Under such a system there may be competition between hospitals, perhaps based on quality of care. The patient, or the person or body responsible for their healthcare, or their insurer can use the fee as a driver to direct the case to one provider or other. If individual negotiations are possible, price for a given case might be adjusted.

All three types of methods can coexist in any system, in different proportions. Often it is claimed that the key determinant of operating profitability is the number of cases completed per list, but this is not strictly true. If, as shown in the earlier section on revenue, each case is priced differently, then the per-minute income of the case might differ, but the per-minute cost of theatres will be constant. It might therefore matter more which type of case is undertaken than how many cases are done: it is the per-minute profit that matters. This is explored in greater detail later in the chapter.

Theatre Expenses

Labour Costs. Labour costs are by far the biggest proportion of expense, making up >60% of total costs (see also Chapter 6, 'Staffing and Contracts'). When viewed as per-patient costs, theatre costs can be very high because so many staff are involved in each case (at a minimum: surgeon, anaesthetist, anaesthesia assistant, scrub nurse, runner, porter; but often many more).

Training Costs. Added to this should be the added costs of training, especially medical training. Trainees do offer some element of service, but regulations generally dictate that they need constant supervision. They also need added time for teaching (which is non-productive to the service). The productivity of the consultant is therefore in a sense reduced, not enhanced, by having a trainee present. Yet, trainees bring income into the hospital by virtue of the organisation and funding of training programs. In the United Kingdom, the body is known as Higher Education England (HEE), and the hospital will receive ~ £40,000 per year per trainee in income (2017 figures). This in part underwrites the added costs of training, but in turn must be managed carefully.

Consumables. Supplies can make up ~20% of theatre expenses, with costs enhanced by new technologies and equipment. The need for these is especially high in innovative, academic or teaching centres.

Capital Costs. This represents the cost of building and maintaining the physical space, and some of these costs might overlap with consumables and supplies. For example, replacing a gas cylinder on an anaesthesia machine is a consumable cost; replacing all the anaesthesia machines in the operating room (OR) suite is a capital cost. Replacing a light bulb is a supply cost, but renewing all the theatre lighting system is a capital cost.

Depreciation Costs; Interests on Loans. In accounting, depreciation is the yearly reduction in value of a tangible asset such as equipment. It has the effect of reducing net profit as recorded in the accounts. Loans that a company takes will have to be repaid with interest; this interest also affects net profits. In the NHS one of the largest loans taken collectively by hospitals is the Private Finance Initiative (PFI) scheme, used to modernise and build new hospitals. However, the interest payments create a debt burden. These factors place hospitals in an accounting deficit, with pressure to save money elsewhere, such as in the provision of clinical services to service the debt.

Where the Theatre Manager Fits; Management Accounting

Finance accounting is the presentation of an entity's finances for external review or consumption (such as shareholders, auditors, etc.). A theatre manager is unlikely to be involved at all in that. Management accounting is the way accounts are held or created for internal consumption to help run or develop the organisation. To some extent a theatre manager may be involved in this, but in different ways in different organisations.

Key will be the extent to which the theatre manager (or close colleague) actually holds or manages an identified theatre budget (e.g., £X per year). Second will be the question of how that theatre budget is actually set, and third what activities it encompasses. The answers to these questions are not straightforward.

At one extreme, a hospital might organise each of its departments as quasi-independent units, each raising its own income and managing its own expenditure. Only *post hoc*, at a higher level of accounting or at the end of a financial year, will the budgets (profits and losses) be merged across departments to create a broader picture and set of financial accounts for the organisation as a whole. In this scheme, the units' budgets are in real-time, but units do not know where the organisation as a whole stands until and unless they are told.

At another extreme, the single budget is held centrally, all income is received centrally and each department or unit simply makes a regular declaration of its costs and expenses. The balances are calculated and apportioned centrally with information returned to each department, say, at the end of the year. In this scheme, the organisation only views the units' costs, and there are no budgets assigned to those units; the units do not know where they stand until and unless they are told.

In between these two extremes, theatres may be assigned a virtual annual budget, with responsibility to work within it for the year. It should be made clear what expenses that nominal budget is for and ideally, how that budget was calculated in the first place. Generally, budgets are set historically with at most, annual adjustments for inflation. Otherwise, budget setting is used by the organisation to try to influence managerial behaviour. For example, if the hospital decides to make

a 10% saving overall, this might lead to each department's budget for that year being reduced by 10%. The expectation is that each department will reduce its expenses (or increase its income) in its own way, by this amount to meet the expectation.

Assigning costs to theatres is not a simple matter. First, the bulk of actual costs are staffing, yet 'theatres' may not hold the contracts of any of the staff who work there. Surgeons' and anaesthetists' contracts are most likely held by their respective departments. Those departments (of Surgery and Anaesthesia, respectively) and those individuals may have other contractual responsibilities and commitments for their staff unrelated to theatres. Nursing staff contracts may be held by the nursing department, and even porters may be contracted centrally. Costs of locum or temporary staff may be assigned to the respective departments, rather than to theatres. Even where some staff costs are assigned to theatres (e.g., porters), their activities might be shared with other departments – porters might be used flexibly to transport patients or equipment in radiology, pathology, etc. An example of how this matters is if, say, a surgeon is tasked to sit on a hospital committee and reduce their commitment to operating theatre lists by 4 hours per week. This has a potential impact on apparent theatre income (less surgery, fewer operations, less income) and also possibly on apparent theatre costs (finding and paying someone else to cover the hours vacated by the surgeon).

Even if it is possible to account for a portion of each staff member's costs within a real or virtual theatre budget, theatres rarely have control over salaries (e.g., in the United Kingdom these are set according to national scales). So a 5% increase in national salaries will instantly translate into a 5% increase in theatre costs. Factoring in the costs of pensions, superannuation etc., makes such calculations extremely complex.

Second, the status of off-site work may be unclear. Many radiology or cardiology interventional procedures need to be performed within specialist suites in those departments. Should this be a 'theatre cost' or a 'department of radiology cost'? Similarly, equipment is also often shared with other departments within the hospital, so again it can be arbitrary or unclear as to whose budget this should fall under.

Third, in defraying costs against income, it is rare for theatres as a unit itself actually to receive the income from surgical operations. Generally these are assigned as income either to the surgical department or to the hospital as a whole. If so, then theatres can be regarded purely as a loss-making or service department (i.e., one with no income at all). Anaesthetics, pathology and radiology departments can also fall into a similar category. The danger of being assigned in this way is that, there being no perceived income, the expectation is that the sole available strategy is cost-cutting (e.g., through employing lesser-trained, cheaper staff or using less-expensive or outdated equipment). In fact, these departments and theatres can successfully argue that any increase in surgical income is correctly assigned at least in part against their running costs such that if there is a net gain, it is because of (and not despite) the expenditure made within theatres, anaesthetics, etc.

In summary, management accounting is extremely complex and often arbitrary. There is no 'correct' way of creating internal budgets or managing them within an organisation. While some theatre managers may be very adept at completing financial spreadsheets, this should not detract from the main principles governing financial interrelationships within an organisation. Theatre managers should use their financial and accounting knowledge to maximise the position of theatres within the politics of the wider organisation. Finally, we should not forget the savings that can be made through safety and avoidance of litigation, or income via education, innovation and research.

Some examples are given following:

1. Surgeons wish to start a new procedure which is estimated to bring in income £10,000 (to the surgical department). The theatre manager is able to schedule an additional theatre, fully staffed list at cost £5,000. It is alleged that theatres have overspent their budget by £5,000, but the manager shows that because £10,000 is greater than £5,000 this is an example of good theatre management.

2. The anaesthetic department appoints three new consultants, able to cover a total of nine lists per week (at cost £300,000 to the anaesthetic budget). Previously those lists were covered by temporary locum staff at cost £600,000. Being locum staff, these costs were assigned to a different, central budget. It is now suggested that the anaesthetics department has overspent its budget by £300,000, but the theatre manager can argue that there is in fact a saving here of £300,000 overall, i.e., the difference between locum and substantive salaries.

3. A theatre manager identifies that within theatres are hosted a total of 100 medical students and estimates that, given the portion of the time they spend there, this is equivalent to £100,000 of the training tariff. The manager argues that this should be used in managerial accounts as income assigned to theatres.

4. Theatre loans a machine (capital cost £100,000) to radiology for several weeks each year. The theatre manager argues that the proportion of capital cost is defrayed against theatre costs as a 'sale' or 'loan' to radiology.

5. The theatre manager identifies that there have been 10% fewer adverse incidents within theatres and, from the previous year's cost of litigation related to such incidents, estimates a cost saving of £100,000.

In these ways, the manager is maximising the perceived gain from theatres and acting as its champion. Also in each of these examples, the detailed accounting is left to more senior accountants, and it is the principles of income and expenditure that are handled by the theatre manager.

Balancing Theatre Costs and Income

One area where the theatre manager can make a contribution is providing information on detailed costs. Such 'service line reporting' seeks to make improvements through better information available to financial and performance managers. It assessed the income generated and the costs associated with providing a service to patients, for each department or operational unit. This section provides an overview of how those detailed results can be analysed.

The Link between Efficiency ε and Cost

In Chapter 2 we stressed the need to achieve efficiency ε as defined by Equation 2.2, reproduced here:

$$\text{Efficiency}, \varepsilon = \left[\begin{pmatrix} \text{fraction of} \\ \text{scheduled time} \\ \text{utilised} \end{pmatrix} - \begin{pmatrix} \text{fraction of} \\ \text{scheduled time} \\ \text{overrunning} \end{pmatrix} \right] \times \begin{pmatrix} \text{fraction of} \\ \text{scheduled cases} \\ \text{completed} \end{pmatrix} \qquad \text{Equation 2.2}$$

We explained why this was important, amongst other things, because a fixed amount of theatre time is budgeted in advance, so the optimum point is to utilise this budgeted time. Underrunning carries extra cost in the investment that is wasted; overrunning carried extra cost in unbudgeted expenditure, and cancellation clearly carries the cost of no income from the case (plus any fines imposed by the funder). Because each minute of underutilised time costs money, each minute of overrunning costs money, and cancelling cases costs money, the notion can be expressed by an equation very similar to Equation 2.2:

$$Extra\ cost = £(mins\ of\ underutilized\ time) + K£(mins\ of\ overrunning) + £(cost\ of\ cancellation)$$

Equation 7.1

The factor K incorporated the idea that overrunning likely costs more than underrunning.

Balancing the Costs

For theatres, income derives from performing operations. To break even financially for any single operation, income must equal expenses. If income from an operation is £X, the operation lasts Y minutes and an operating theatre costs Z £/min, potential profits are only possible if $X / Y > Z$. However, this potential profit from theatre activity will only translate to actual profit for the hospital if this difference between X / Y and Z is larger than other hospital costs, W.

We now develop a more formal model demonstrating the relationships between these different costs. Income is derived from a tariff (in £), which is fixed and specific to the procedure (Equation 7.2). Expenses can be regarded as consisting of

(a) 'Theatre' costs ($Costs_{theatre}$, e.g., equipment, consumables, personnel)
(b) Hospital or 'ward' costs ($Costs_{ward}$, e.g., administration, nursing care, food, etc., which can all be bundled into a single value; Equation 7.2)

The theatre costs are time dependent. The longer a single case takes (including the time wasted in unproductive gaps before or after the case), the greater the costs; Equation 7.4). Ward costs are also time dependent, usually over days (i.e., the longer a patient stays in hospital the more it costs that

hospital). However, for a day case (i.e., a patient who is discharged any time before the ward closes for the day), the ward costs are fixed. The relevant equations for a single case are

$$Profit = Tariff - Expenses \qquad \text{Equation 7.2}$$

$$Expenses = Costs_{ward} + Costs_{theatre} \qquad \text{Equation 7.3}$$

$$Costs_{theatre} = (Theatre\ cost/\min) \times (procedure\ time) \qquad \text{Equation 7.4}$$

$$Profit = (Tariff) - [(Costs_{ward}) + ((Theatre\ cost/\min) \times (procedure\ time))]$$

Equation 7.5 (combining Equations 7.2–7.4)

These relationships can be plotted on a universal set of graphs (Figure 7.1). These are universal because the shapes apply in any system, anywhere in the world regardless of actual prices or currency (i.e., the £ sign can be replaced by $ or Euros with the same result).

These equations, and the graphs they create, lead to an interesting result. Every minute by which procedure time is reduced (e.g., by faster anaesthetic induction, more rapid turnover, prompt surgery) yields the same increment of profit, regardless of prevailing ward costs (Figure 7.1A) or of prevailing tariff (Figure 7.1B). By contrast, reducing a minute of procedure time gains more if prevailing theatre costs are high, as compared with when they are low (Figure 7.1C). We can conclude that altering ward costs or tariff do not influence the potential to increase profits by reducing procedure time; these measures simply help attain more absolute profit. By contrast, reducing theatre costs magnifies the potential profitability of reducing procedure time. In mathematical modelling terms, reducing ward costs or increasing tariff is *additive* to increasing efficiencies in operative time to the overall profit. Reducing theatre costs, on the other hand, is *synergistic* to increasing efficiencies; it increases the overall 'gain' of the system.

Creating Strategies for Profit in Theatres

It is not at all helpful to state that 'operating more quickly' (including eliminating non-productive gaps on the list) or 'reducing ward costs' or 'increasing tariffs' can all help. Obviously they will. However, we need to go beyond such platitudes and show precisely how these measures can influence profit.

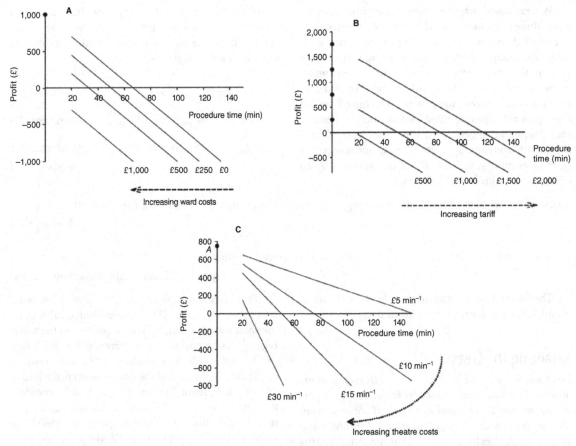

Figure 7.1 Panel A: Effect of ward costs on profit for any single case. Profit declines linearly as procedure time increases (e.g., slow anaesthetic induction, slow surgery or gaps before or after the case). Changing ward costs shifts this linear relationship in a parallel manner (i.e., it affects the intersection on the y-axis, but not the slope). The maximum possible profit that can be made is shown at the point on the y-axis when ward costs are eliminated is always simply the value of the tariff. To plot the panel, the assumptions for these examples were tariff = £1,000, theatre costs = £15/min and ward costs of range £0–1,000 as shown; but the same relationships hold regardless of the values used – all that changes is the actual absolute profit. Panel B: Effect of tariff on profit for any single case. Profit declines linearly as procedure time increases. Changing the tariff shifts this linear relationship in a parallel manner (i.e., affects the intersect on the y-axis, but not the slope). The maximum possible profit that can be made are shown as points on the y-axis, for each of the tariffs shown. The assumptions for these examples were ward costs = £250, theatre costs = £15/min and tariff range between £500 and 2,000; but the same relationships hold regardless of the values used (all that changes is the actual absolute profit). Panel C: Effect of theatre costs (£/min) on profit for any single case. Profit declines linearly as the procedure time increases. Changing theatre costs changes the slope of this relationship (but not the intersect on the y-axis). The maximum possible profit (point A) is always the same (i.e., the difference between tariff and ward costs). The assumptions for these examples were ward costs = £250, tariff = £1000; but the same relationships hold regardless of the values used (all that changes is the actual absolute profit).

The graphs show that setting the tariff sets the overall 'envelope' under which profits can be made. The higher the tariff, the higher will be the likely profit, regardless of prevailing efficiency. (The truth of this is readily seen by considering an infinitely high tariff; it would not matter how inefficiently one worked). Reducing ward costs is akin to increasing tariffs because the difference between the two determines the 'envelope' (i.e., reducing expenses is the same as increasing income in its overall effect). We regard this as an envelope because the tariff (or expenses) set the maximum that can be achieved (i.e., we cannot possibly gain more income than is being paid for the operation). Raising tariffs or reducing ward costs is analogous to giving a runner a 100-m advantage in a 200-m race. (The race is always going to be 200 m, and not any other distance).

By contrast, reducing theatre costs changes the 'conditions' (rather than envelope) by which work can be translated to profit. Lowering theatre costs makes each minute of work more profitable (e.g., than if conducted under high theatre costs). It is like making the machine more efficient – or akin to a 100-m runner racing downhill against a 100-m runner running uphill; the distance or envelope is the same but the conditions are different.

In these analogies, both things are advantageous – changing the running distance and increasing the slope – they both influence the finish time, but in specifically different ways.

This more precise knowledge enables the theatre manager to focus efforts on where it is needed. If surgery and anaesthesia are inefficient (see Chapter 2 for efficiency), increasing tariff or reducing ward or theatre costs only resolves a financial issue, but the fundamental problem (of inefficiency) will always remain. Indeed, it can be argued that increasing tariff in this scenario is throwing good money after bad – like keeping an old, inefficient car going at great expense. Thus if a theatre manager has inefficient ORs and argues for cuts in ward or other hospital costs, they find themselves unpopular if little or nothing changes after those other departments have gone through cutbacks and pain. If the manager argues for an increase in tariffs, there may be criticism if theatres remain inefficient despite the increased funding.

If, on the other hand, surgery and anaesthesia practices are already efficient, increasing tariff or reducing theatre costs (e.g., by reducing equipment costs, running costs or staffing levels where possible) is key to translating good practice into profit. In this last case, increasing tariffs may be essential and proper if hospitals are to break even. In other words, attaining efficiency (as described in Chapter 2) is key to further development of theatres and of the organisation.

Advising on 'Profitable' Operations

One of the most unfortunate aspects of hospital remuneration worldwide is that tariff levels are not related to the actual time it takes to perform the surgery. Table 7.1 shows some common operations, the UK NHS tariff (which changes every year, marginally) and the income per minute. There is no reason why the rates of income per minute should differ so markedly for these cases.

In contrast, UK insurers do seem to recognise that procedure time is a factor (Figure 7.2). Although

Table 7.1 Some UK NHS tariffs for certain common operations along with published times to complete the operations (2011 data).

Operation	Tariff (£)	Mean time (SD)	Income (£/min)
Inguinal hernia	1015	63 (11)	16
Unilateral cataract	750	32 (6)	23
Unilateral varicose veins	953	86 (19)	11
Circumcision	633	46 (11)	14
Cystoscopy	444	33 (6)	13
Breast biopsy	791	54 (10)	15
Hydrocoele	703	52 (7)	14

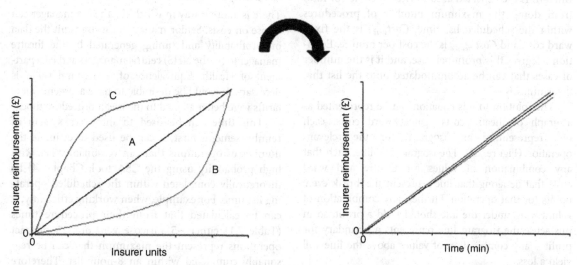

Figure 7.2 How UK insurers reimburse hospitals and consultants. First (left panel), different insurers A, B, C 'unitise' each operation where each unit carries a fixed reimbursement price. The relationship of absolute price to the units varies by insurer, with some exhibiting a linear price-unit relationship (A), and others curvilinear (either exponential or asymptotic; B and C). Second (right panel), if these prices paid are plotted against procedure time, there is in fact a linear and equivalent relationship for all insurers.

absolute rates of reimbursement differ across insurers, there is a clear relationship to time.

What this means is that, illogically, some operations by government tariff are inherently profitable and others loss making, but not on average, for those private operations funded by insurers. The theatre manager is in a key position to identify which these are. This does not mean that hospitals must cherry-pick only the profitable procedures, or only undertake private insurer–funded cases. If all did so, clearly profits would rise, but nobody would ever do the unprofitable surgeries, and hospitals would not be doing what they were supposed to. However, senior managers will be better informed as to the balance of procedures to undertake overall, so that they can match their duty to provide financial stability whilst also meeting their social responsibilities.

Equally, for those operations in which the tariff is low, particular attention might then be devoted to assessing if or how hospital costs could be further reduced. For example, by reducing the cost of equipment, or where possible performing as day cases (if not already) or assigning more junior staff (if safe).

Specifically, the data can be used to calculate target values required to break even. From Equation 7.5, for any single type of operation this is derived as:

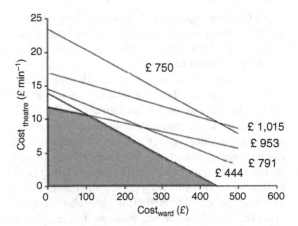

Figure 7.3 Calculating the maximum ward and theatre costs for a hospital or theatre suite. For each procedure, the line represents the combination of points where the costs will break even financially, given the tariff for the procedure (which is shown), for a hypothetical, maximally efficient operating list consisting solely of the procedures shown (calculated from Equation 7.6). Combinations of costs lying anywhere within the shaded sector will yield a profit for all operations in this cohort.

be drawn for all the operations. The boundary of the lowest lying lines then represents the upper boundary for costs.

$$Target\ value\ 0 = (Tariff \times B) - (Cost_{ward} \times B) - (scheduled\ list\ time \times Cost_{theatre})$$

Equation 7.6

where B is the expected accumulated income (or loss) from doing the maximum number of procedures within the scheduled list time, $Cost_{ward}$ is the fixed ward cost, and $Cost_{theatre}$ is the cost per minute. Equation 7.5 gives this profit per case, and it is the number of cases that can be accommodated onto the list that determines B.

The solution to this equation can be represented as a graph of theatre costs against ward costs, each line representing an 'isogram' for the relevant operation (Figure 7.3). The isogram is a line, such that any combination of values for theatre and ward costs that lie along that line represent the 'break even' points for that operation. Further, any combination of values lying under the line should yield a profit, so in this sense the isogram line represents a boundary for profit – any combination of values above the line will yield a loss.

If a hospital wishes to make a profit on all the types of surgery it performs, then isograms need to

Creating New Funding Systems

There is another way in which the theatre manager can advise on costs. Senior managers can transmit the data on profitability and timing generated by the theatre manager to (in the NHS) central managers at the Department of Health. Equivalence of 'procedural value' is necessary. It would be desirable to have a system where tariffs were better aligned to the mean procedure time.

This time can be used to inform a system of reimbursement, First, it can be used to estimate the number of operations that can reasonably (i.e., with high probability using the CSA tool; Chapter 4) be theoretically completed within the scheduled operating list time. For example, when working efficiently, it can be calculated that from their procedure times (Table 7.1) either ~5 varicose vein or ~15 cataract operations represent the maximum that can be reasonably completed within an 8-hour list. Therefore the income from completing these 5 and 15 operations, respectively, should be equal. This could form the fundamental basis for calculating reimbursement. Cancellations and overruns could be penalised to discourage deliberate overbooking of lists.

A second method would be to reimburse only for the period of time that anaesthesia or surgery occurred (and for agreed ward costs) but not for any wasted or unutilised time in theatre, up to a predetermined maximum of, say, 8 h (to discourage overruns). This tariff would be the same for all types of surgery, with enhancements for costs of any unusually expensive, but necessary, equipment or consumables. In other words, this would be a system that rewarded productive operating time (see Chapter 3. 'Defining Productivity') and paid per minute, but disregarded payment for non-productive time in theatre.

Bibliography

Abbott T, White SM, Pandit JJ. 2011. Factors affecting the profitability of surgical procedures under 'Payment by Results'. *Anaesthesia* 66: 283–92.

Audit Commission. 2008. *The Right Result? Payment by Results 2003–07.* London: Audit Commission, Health Summary.

Basso O. 2009. Cost analysis of a system of ad hoc theatre sessions for the management of delayed trauma cases. *Journal of Orthopaedics and Traumatology* 10: 91–6.

Chakladar A, White SM. 2010. Cost estimates of spinal versus general anaesthesia for fractured neck of femur surgery. *Anaesthesia* 65: 810–4.

Department of Health. n.d. NHS reference costs 2008–2009. www.dh.gov.uk/en/ Publicationsandstatistics/ Publications/ PublicationsPolicyAndGuidance/ DH_111591.

Department of Health. n.d. Tariff information: confirmation of Payment by Results (PbR) arrangements for 2009–10. www.dh.gov.uk/en/ Publicationsandstatistics/ Publications/PublicationsPolicyAnd Guidance/DH_094091.

Department of Health. n.d. Tariff information: confirmation of Payment by Results (PbR) Arrangements for 2009–10. http:// webarchive.nationalarchives.gov.uk/ +/www.dh.gov.uk/en/ Publicationsandstatistics/ Publications/ PublicationsPolicyAndGuidance/ DH_094091.

Dixon J. 2004. Payment by results – new financial flows in the NHS. *British Medical Journal* 328: 969–70.

Epstein D, Mason A. 2006. Costs and prices for inpatient care in England: mirror twins or distant cousins? *Health Care Management Science* 9: 233–42.

Finkler SA, Ward DM. 1999. *Cost Accounting for Healthcare Organisations: Concepts and Applications*, 2nd edn. Gaithersburg, MD: Aspen.

Garattini L, Giuliani G, Pagan E. 1999. A model for calculating costs of hospital wards: an Italian experience. *Journal of Management in Medicine* 13: 71–82.

Hearnden A, Tennent D. 2008. The cost of shoulder arthroscopy: a comparison with national tariff. *Annals of the Royal College of Surgeons of England* 90: 587–91.

Lewellyn S, Northcott D. 2005. The average hospital. *Accounting, Organisation and Society* 30: 555–83.

Malcomson JM. 2007. Hospital cost differences and payment by results. *Health Economics, Policy and Law* 2: 429–33.

Mangan JL, Walsh C, Kernohan WG, et al. 1992. Total joint replacement: implication of cancelled operations for hospital costs and waiting list management. *Quality and Safety in Health Care* 1: 34–7.

Mannion R, Marini G, Street A. 2008. Implementing payment by results in the English NHS: changing incentives and the role of information. *Journal of Health Organisation and Management* 22: 79–88.

Needham PJ, Laughlan KA, Botterill ID, Ambrose NS. 2009. Laparoscopic appendicectomy: counting the cost. *Annals of the Royal College of Surgeons of England* 91: 606–8.

O'Connor RJ, Neumann VC. 2006. Payment by results or payment by outcome? The history of measuring medicine. *Journal of the Royal Society of Medicine* 99: 226–31.

Pollock A, Shaoul J, Vickers N. 2002. Private finance and 'value for money' in NHS hospitals: a policy in search of a rationale? *British Medical Journal* 342: 1205–9

Street A, Maynard A. 2007. Activity based financing in England: the need for continual refinement of payment by results. *Health Economics, Policy and Law* 2: 419–27.

Stubbs D, Ward ME, Pandit JJ. 2010. Estimating hourly anaesthetic and surgical reimbursement from private medical insurers' benefit maxima: implications for pricing services and for incentives. *Anaesthesia* 65: 396–408.

Chapter 8

Preoperative Patient Preparation

Jaideep J. Pandit

Scope and Limits of 'Preassessment'

Preassessment encompasses the optimisation of patients for elective surgery, so that when they arrive on the day of surgery there are no medical conditions that have not been addressed or for which treatment has not begun. Preassessment is large part of what is also referred to as 'perioperative medicine' (United Kingdom) or 'surgical home' (United States). It is not our purpose to detail exactly what the preoperative clinic does in terms of tests and the evidence for them. This is a book on practical operating theatre management, not a detailed clinical text on how to run a preoperative clinic. It is, however, important for the theatre manager to know in principle what a good preassessment clinic is about in terms of its philosophy.

It is important to distinguish preassessment from the anaesthetist's preoperative visit on the day of surgery. Preassessment is the opportunity for anaesthetists, physicians or nurses to review the patient, ideally as soon as possible after surgery is booked, and ensure that any ongoing medical problems are optimised. It is also an opportunity to provide – in broad outline – the anaesthetic (or surgical) plan. Preassessment is most decidedly **not**:

1. The specification of the anaesthetic plan (this is for the anaesthetist on the day of surgery to decide)
2. The occasion for anaesthetic or surgical consent (this is for the primary anaesthetist or surgeon to finalise)
3. The place where it is decided that proceeding with surgery is appropriate or not (this is for the primary anaesthetist, surgeon and patient to decide, after any test results arising out of preassessment are known)

Preassessment **is** instead:

1. The opportunity to ensure that all test results will be in place for the team to review on or ideally before the day of surgery

2. The time to start booking intensive care or other specialist perioperative care interventions (cell salvage, haemofiltration, high-dependency care bed, etc.) as are judged likely (these can always be cancelled later, but before day of surgery, if not needed)
3. The opportunity to risk-assess patients by quantitative scoring systems based on their functional capacity (this may inform the primary team to make a decision as to the wisdom of surgery and be important in audit)
4. The place to conduct some specialised tests, notably exercise testing or echocardiography (again, the results may inform the primary team to make a decision as to the wisdom of surgery)
5. The point from which to refer to other specialist services to diagnose identified symptoms or signs, or to optimise preexisting conditions (e.g., cardiology, respiratory, haematology)
6. The occasion to introduce preoperative optimisation therapies such as exercise training, cessation of smoking, oral or intravenous iron therapy, antibiotics, etc.

Philosophy of Risk Reduction and Risk-Benefit Analysis – The Fallacy of 'Fit for Surgery'

Elective surgery concerns a surgical intervention planned to improve the patient's condition or quality of life but that is not of itself immediately lifesaving (in contrast to emergency surgery). Elective surgery can therefore always be planned for a time which suits the patient (or the patient's medical condition), the surgeon, the anaesthetist, and the healthcare organisation in which the surgical intervention takes place. Therefore, a fundamental tenet is that optimal treatment of all coexisting medical problems should minimise perioperative risk. If the patient can wait, then they should wait until health matters are optimised or resolved because that would reduce their risk.

An example of an elective operation is an inguinal hernia repair. The operative risks for this operation will be higher in an untreated hypertensive patient, as compared with the risks for a treated patient (we make no comment on the degree of hypertension or the threshold for treatment). Because the hernia operation itself does not in any sense contribute to increased survival, a superficial risk-benefit analysis clearly favours prior treatment of the hypertension, rather than urgently proceeding with surgery without any treatment. In contrast, an example of a corresponding emergency operation is a strangulated, obstructed hernia. Again, the risks of surgery will still be greater in an untreated hypertensive patient than in an appropriately treated patient. However, here the risks of delaying surgery for antihypertensive therapy will far exceed any additional risks of proceeding with surgery.

These simple examples demonstrate that the goal – or sometimes clinical dilemma – is a risk-benefit balance. The choice is between whether or not delaying surgery outweighs the benefits of delay for medical optimisation.

The terms 'fit for anaesthesia' or 'fit for surgery' must be abandoned as being both uninformative and misleading. A further illustration reinforces this point. Let us imagine a young professional athlete scheduled for elective varicose vein surgery. She is found, surprisingly, to have left bundle branch block and a diastolic murmur, all uninvestigated. Let us now imagine a patient scheduled for the same varicose vein surgery, but one who is very elderly and in severe heart failure on maximal treatment. If we ask: 'Who is the 'fitter'? it is obviously in one sense the athlete, who only yesterday ran a near record-breaking race. But let us pose a different question: 'Who is not optimised?' It is obviously also the athlete because all these cardiac findings are new, and we do not know what degree of risk these initial findings might pose. The elderly patient, on the other hand, is fully optimised. Yes, in a bad shape, but as well as he can possibly be. If we now ask, 'Whose surgery should be postponed?' then the answer is, of course, the underoptimised athlete.

This example highlights the problem with the term *fitness*, as it strongly implies that there is some threshold, absolute value of physical fitness, above which anaesthesia or surgery is safe and below which it is unsafe. The reality is that 'fitness' is a continuum,

and the challenge is to know at any given moment in time, when a decision needs to be made, whether the risk-benefit balance supports proceeding with surgery on the day or postponing pending further investigations or treatment.

Unfortunately, objective, high-quality evidence in support of this philosophy of risk reduction is sparse for each and every medical condition. Large, controlled trials for all possible coexistent diseases do not always exist to guide us. So for any given medical condition, we cannot quote a precise numerical value indicating perioperative risk. Scoring systems have been used by clinicians for some diseases (most notably cardiac), and also exercise testing can provide a global assessment of function, but all these approaches can be misleading. Amongst the reasons for these limitations include ethical issues in conducting some trials; the heterogeneity of the patient population; the variability in surgical methods; and the variability in anaesthetic management. Therefore it also impossible to plan risk reduction in a meaningful way for every medical condition. However, that is the long-term goal of research.

Communication in Preassessment

From the preceding considerations we can define the following aims of the preoperative evaluation (in no particular order of importance).

First, that a possibly inadequately treated condition (e.g., angina or heart failure) is suitably optimised. The relevant specialists are best placed to comment on this, and they might conclude that the condition is already optimally treated, and no further intervention is warranted. Even if this is the case, this is valuable input or reassurance to the anaesthetic/surgical plan.

Second, that an undiagnosed condition (e.g., new-onset atrial fibrillation or a heart murmur) should be investigated. Again, it is possible that once diagnosed, this condition may not need any treatment. Alternatively (though perhaps less commonly), medical investigation reveals an abnormality that not only needs attention but also is judged to need attention before the surgery that resulted in the referral.

Third, that objective data should be provided to help guide anaesthetic management or provide an index of risk. One increasingly common such index is the preoperative exercise test (e.g., assessing anaerobic threshold), or a specific request for left ventricular ejection fraction or ischaemic threshold of tachycardia on exercise test. In this context, if some tests are referred to physicians, then the physician to whom the patient is referred is (to some extent) simply providing only a support service to the anaesthetic/surgical team. The final decision as to whether to proceed with surgery and, if so, in what manner (e.g., extent of invasive monitoring to be used, or the need for elective post-operative intensive care admission) must rest with the anaesthetic/surgical team, based upon data provided by the physician. In other words, the physician is **not** providing an opinion on 'fitness for surgery' but data to their colleagues to help inform their decisions.

This last point brings with it the importance of communication from the preoperative team to the physicians or others to whom it is referring the patient. If the referral request states simply, 'Please assess fitness for surgery,' there will be a completely different answer than if instead the question was: 'This patient has severe heart failure: can it be improved or not before surgery so that we can make a decision on whether or when to proceed?'

If a patient attends medical clinic with only the vague request that they be assessed for 'fitness', the physician may not know the precise nature or implications of the planned surgery. For example: what does a transvaginal tension-free tape operation actually involve? What are the physiological implications of a bimaxillary osteotomy as opposed to a repair of zygomatic fracture? Second, the physician may not be familiar with the details of all anaesthetic techniques: How should the blood pressure best be managed during laparoscopic adrenalectomy? What are the indications or contraindications for a combined spinal-epidural technique? Thus, apart from some exceptional circumstances, it is truly impossible for a cardiologist to make any useful comment on the practical conduct of surgery or anaesthesia. Advice such as 'the heart rate should be monitored during surgery', or 'low blood pressure should be avoided during surgery', are clearly useless. Equally, from a cardiologist's perspective, the patient may be 'fit' in the sense that they are maximally treated: this different perspective can be a cause of misunderstanding if the term 'fitness' is used. The outcome of the medical referral can only be as useful as what is asked of it; hence the importance of the preassessment clinic to ask precise questions in its referral to other services.

Structure: Types of Preassessment, Patient Selection and Staffing

These three things are interrelated. Preassessment models exist as various types, crudely from superficial assessment to intensive examinations; some patients need more preassessing than others, and these requirements in turn determine the staffing composition.

Types of Preassessment: Staffing

Questionnaire. Perhaps the simplest form of preassessment is a questionnaire. This might be a core set of questions completed at the first surgical clinic booking, or soon after; or it may be posted to the patient. It might be coupled with a nurse-led telephone questionnaire, or even be internet- or website-based. Appendix 8A indicates some core questions. The questionnaire can then be used to direct further investigations, if they are not already present in the patient's case notes. For example, cardiac or blood pressure history might dictate an ECG, echocardiogram, or exercise test. Respiratory disease would require lung function tests. Thus a team, which could be nurse led, is required to assess the results of this screening questionnaire information and collate any additional results from it. Those patients who have few or no positive answers to the questionnaire may not need any further preassessment, so in this way the tool acts as a filter or triage. Nurse-led teams may also benefit from the responses to each question being scored to assess disease severity.

Nurse-Led Preassessment Clinic. This is a clinic to which the patients selected for further preassessment (perhaps after a screening questionnaire) attend. Over and above the questionnaire, the clinic might offer an opportunity to see the patient face-to-face and identify additional issues or requirements. Amongst these are specific patient needs related to mobility, additional nursing care (e.g., learning difficulties, manual handling), the opportunity to measure height, weight and blood pressure, and actually to take the blood tests dictated by the screening questionnaire.

One purpose of the nurse-led clinic is then to identify the cohort of patients who needs more intensive investigation in a doctor-led clinic, notably the need for exercise testing. Another purpose (with physician oversight) is to confirm that the place and timing of surgery is suitable and that additional arrangements are made. For example, it may be unwise to schedule a high-risk patient to have surgery at an isolated or satellite site, where there are limited resources, or to an extra waiting list initiative on a weekend (when there are fewer staff and backup available). Or, to ensure that a high-dependency or critical care bed has been booked. Or that cross-matched blood will be available on the day.

The question is whether this clinic should be combined with (e.g., run in parallel with) the next type of preassessment clinic (doctor-led) or be a separate stage on the pathway.

Doctor-Staffed Clinic. Physicians (usually anaesthetists) require some oversight of the preassessment process, and ideally an anaesthetist lead or faculty should be identified. The advantage of the nurse-led clinic is reduced cost – e.g., several nurses reporting to one anaesthetist lead. However, a potential disadvantage is that it if the two clinics are separate, then it adds yet another barrier or bottleneck in the patient pathway (see following). One solution is to run a doctor-staffed clinic in parallel with the nurse-staffed clinic, so that (a) medical advice is on hand immediately and (b) more sophisticated tests can be performed immediately if needed. The latter might include preoperative exercise testing (and the prescription of any exercise training programs).

Patient Selection: Demand-Capacity Balance

It is clear from the preceding that unless there is some sort of patient selection for being seen in the clinic, there could be huge demands on the preassessment service. The different types of preassessment listed earlier will take different times to complete and assess, and it is important that locally time estimates are made in order to plan the services. There is little or no published literature about demand-capacity analysis of preoperative clinics, but we might speculate that a questionnaire-based assessment takes (per patient) on average 15–30 min of service time; a nurse-led clinic possibly 30–45 min, and a doctor-led episode 45–60 min. Therefore, a 4-hour clinic staffed by one doctor and two nurses has a capacity for a maximum of twenty patients (just four of whom receive the more sophisticated interventions).

Therefore, the demand profile created by surgical clinics will determine the required capacity of the clinics. A surgical team specialising in oesophagectomies will create more demands for high-level preassessment than, say, an ophthalmic team specialising in cataract surgery.

Nevertheless, investment in preassessment is designed to reduce the risk of expensive cancellation for medical reasons on the day of surgery. The philosophy is that if all medical conditions are identified and optimised, and the risk profile has put in place bookings to intensive care unit, etc., the anaesthetist has all the information on the day of surgery to proceed. There is no stone left unturned, no questions remaining unanswered. The anaesthetist can then focus on discussing the anaesthetic plan and taking consent for this.

Therefore just as the theatre manager needs to assess the demand-capacity balance for operating theatres (see Chapter 5), the preassessment lead (or theatre manager if it falls within their responsibility too) needs continually to assess the demands imposed on the preassessment service. Again, *time* (not number of patients) should be crucial unit of currency for any calculations. Key questions will be: What is the mean (SD) time to see a patient in clinic (this statistic may vary by staff type in clinic)? How many patients are referred? How many patients who were administered a screening questionnaire need additional investigations? What proportion of patients seen in a nurse-led clinic need physician review? What proportion of patients seen in a doctor-led clinic need referral to other specialties?

Audit and Research

The preassessment clinic is an important focus for audit (of its own performance) and also innovation and research (to improve services).

One question is whether the capacity of the service is meeting demands (see earlier section). Clearly a rise in the waiting list for the clinic will require a review of (a) the filters being applied to patient selection, including the questions being asked at screening or the protocols followed by nurses or doctors to refer onwards and (b) the capacity of the clinic.

Another question is whether the decisions of the clinic are 'correct'. 'Failure' of preassessment can be measured in several ways, depending on the scenario, and can include the following:

1. Unplanned admission of a patient to intensive or high dependency care, when preassessment did not identify this need.

2. Unplanned transfer of a patient from an isolated site to a major centre, when preassessment judged that surgery at that remote site was suitable.

3. Discovery of preexisting medical conditions by team on the day of surgery, overlooked at preassessment.

4. Failure of test results to materialise on day of surgery, although requested from clinic.

5. Patient cancellation on day of surgery despite preassessment. The point of interest is not cancellation due to lack of beds or overrunning, but due to difference of opinion about suitability for surgery between the anaesthetist on the day of surgery versus judgement made at clinic. There is no 'right answer' here; it is the fact there is a difference of opinion that is of interest for further exploration.

Continuously measuring these outcomes helps assess, and so improve, the performance of the clinic.

Research is also important because for many additional tests and interventions being requested there is still no hard evidence that they are strictly necessary (or how they should best be interpreted). For example, what are the exact indications for echocardiography in non-cardiac surgery? Is the anaerobic threshold the best endpoint for an exercise test, or are other parameters more useful? What is the most suitable threshold for preoperative haemoglobin before iron therapy? Should iron therapy best be delivered pre- or post-operatively? There are often national guidelines for each of these, but there is always the need for their refinement. It is even more important to use these guidelines (if they exist) as a baseline and then develop local adaptations based on known outcomes. The philosophy is that, where sophisticated tests can be rationalised or targeted to only those patients who need them, the demands on the preassessment service can be reduced.

Summary

Managing the preassessment service is rarely if ever the sole remit of the theatre manager. However, the theatre manager should know the principles by which this service works. The concern for theatres is if there are last-minute cancellations due to failure of preoperative assessment. Hence, the philosophy of optimisation, the tests undertaken, as well as the demand–capacity balance of the preassessment service are important to appreciate. Indeed, the theatre manager is in a key position to feed back relevant information that might help the preassessment clinic improve and develop in a way that better matches the needs of the operating theatres.

Appendix 8A Some Core Questions in a Preassessment Questionnaire

1. Do you have any of the following conditions?

   a. Cardiac problems
   b. Respiratory problems
   c. High blood pressure
   d. Diabetes
   e. Blood disorders
   f. Renal or kidney problems
   g. Problems with the liver
   h. Epilepsy, or other problems related to the brain

2. List any other medical conditions.
3. List your medications.
4. List your allergies.
5. If you were walking briskly on the flat, roughly how far would you get before you had to stop?

   a. A few hundred yards or less
   b. A quarter mile
   c. A half mile
   d. A mile
   e. A mile or more

6. What would stop you if you had to stop at the end of the walk (tick as many as relevant)?

   a. Nothing stops you
   b. Breathlessness
   c. Tiredness
   d. Chest pain
   e. Leg pain or weakness
   f. Other

7. Do you have any allergies to medicines?

The STOP-BANG questionnaire is also useful:

1. Snoring: Do you snore loudly (louder than talking or loud enough to be heard through closed doors)?
2. Tired: Do you often feel tired, fatigued, or sleepy during the daytime?
3. Observed: Has anyone observed you stop breathing during your sleep?
4. Blood Pressure: Do you have or are you being treated for high blood pressure?
4. BMI: Is BMI > 35 kg/m2?
5. Age: >50 years old?
6. Neck Circumference: >40 cm?
7. Gender: male?

   If three or more 'Yes' responses, there is high risk of obstructive sleep apnoea.

Appendix 8B Investigations Available to or Instigated by a Preassessment Clinic

The following should be regarded as essential, within or accessible to a clinic (FEV1/FVC are forced expiratory volume in 1 second/forced vital capacity, respectively):

1. Height, weight measurements
2. ECG
3. Spirometry (FEV1, FVC, peak flow at a minimum)
4. Blood gas machine (for both arterial bloods if necessary and immediate electrolytes on site)
5. Blood glucose measurement

The following are ideal:

6. Exercise testing for anaerobic threshold and other parameters

7. Transthoracic echocardiography
8. Facilities for iron infusion, if indicated according to local protocols

The following may need to be requested (if not already available):

9. Chest X-ray or other imaging
10. Full blood complement of tests and cross matching
11. Sleep studies (for sleep apnoea)

Appendix 8C Example of Guidelines to Perform Additional Tests at Preassessment

The following is adapted from the UK National Institute of Health and Care Excellence (NICE). Tests are performed on basis of a combination of ASA grade and severity of surgery. The latter is broadly graded as:

Minor: excising skin lesion, draining breast abscess

Intermediate: primary repair of inguinal hernia, excising varicose veins in the leg, tonsillectomy, knee arthroscopy

Major/complex: total abdominal hysterectomy, endoscopic resection of prostate, lumbar discectomy, thyroidectomy, total joint replacement, lung operations, colonic resection, radical neck dissection

Table 8.1 shows the NICE advice for routine testing. While evidence based there are some areas for debate. For example, an ECG is such a simple test that it could/should be performed more widely. Both lung function (spirometry) and blood gases are grouped as if they are one and the same, yet spirometry is a simple test that can be done easily, whereas blood gases are invasive specialist investigations. Kidney investigations really ought to include the glomerular filtration rate, which is also a specialist test, whereas electrolytes are very easy to do. Note, however, that these are guidelines only for routine investigations, and very often the patient with the condition warrants a test dictated by that, and not just by their ASA (American Society of Anesthesiologists') score.

Table 8.1 Routine testing advice (adapted from NICE). FBC = full blood count; INR = international normalised ratio, signifying all haemostasis tests; C+E = creatinine and electrolytes, including kidney function tests; ECG = electrocardiogram; lung/ABG = lung function test and arterial blood gas. ASA = American Society of Anesthesiologists' classification. The shading code is: black = routine test not necessary; white = routine testing can be considered' grey = routine testing should be performed. Note that the table only applies to 'routine' testing, which may not apply to any given patient, and that there is debate as summarised in text.

Test	Minor			Intermediate			Major		
ASA	1	2	3/4	1	2	3/4	1	2	3/4
FBC									
INR									
C+E									
ECG									
Lung/ABG									

Bibliography

Asimakopoulos G, Harrison R, Magnussen PA. 1998. Preadmission clinic in an orthopaedic department: evaluation over a 6-month period. *Journal of the Royal College of Surgeons of Edinburgh* 43: 178–81.

Association of Anaesthetists of Great Britain and Ireland. 1998. *Risk Management*. London: The Association of Anaesthetists of Great Britain and Ireland.

Association of Anaesthetists. 2010. *Preoperative Assessment and Patient Preparation: The Role of the Anaesthetist*. London: The Association of Anaesthetists of Great Britain and Ireland.

Association of Anaesthetists. 2010. *The Anaesthesia Team*. London: The Association of Anaesthetists of Great Britain and Ireland.

Association of Anaesthetists. 2017. *Consent for Anaesthesia*. London: The Association of Anaesthetists of Great Britain and Ireland.

Audit Commission. 1997. *Anaesthesia under Examination*. Abingdon, UK: Audit Commission Publications.

Audit Commission. 2003. *Waiting for Elective Admission: Review of*

National Findings. London: CW Print Group.

Barnes PK, Emerson PA, Hajnal S, Radford WJP, Congleton J. 2000. Influence of an anaesthetist on nurse led, computer-based, preoperative assessment. *Anaesthesia* 55: 576–80.

Basu S, Babajee P, Selvachandran SN, Cade D. 2001. Impact of questionnaires and telephone screening on attendance for ambulatory surgery. *Annals of the Royal College of Surgeons of England* 83: 329–31.

Dix P, Howell S. 2001. Survey of cancellation rate of hypertensive patients undergoing anaesthesia and elective surgery. *British Journal of Anaesthesia* 86: 789–93.

Down MP, Wong DT, McGuire GP. 1998. The anaesthesia consult clinic: does it matter which anaesthetist sees the patient? *Canadian Journal of Anaesthesia* 45: 802–8.

Eagle KA, Berger PB, Calkins H, et al. 2002. ACC/AHA Guideline Update for Perioperative Cardiovascular Evaluation for Noncardiac Surgery – Executive Summary: A report of the ACC/AHA task force on practice guidelines (Committee to Update the 1996 Guidelines on Perioperative Cardiovascular Evaluation for Noncardiac Surgery). *Journal of the American College of Cardiology* 39: 542–53.

Fischer SP. 1996. Development and effectiveness of an anesthesia preoperative evaluation clinic in a teaching hospital. *Anesthesiology* 85: 196–206.

Hardy JJ, O'Brien SV, Furlong NJ. 2001. Information given to patients before appointments and its effect on nonattendance rate. *British Medical Journal* 323: 1298–300.

Katz RI, Barnhart JM, Ho G, Hersch D, Dayan SS, Keehn L. 1998. A survey on the intended purposes and perceived utility of preoperative cardiology consultations. *Anesthesia and Analgesia* 87: 830–6.

Kelion AD, Banning AP. 1999. Is simple clinical assessment adequate for cardiac risk stratification before elective non-cardiac surgery? *Lancet* 354: 1837–8.

Kleinman B, Czinn E, Shah K, Sobotka PA, Rao TK. 1989. The value to the anesthesia – surgical care team of the preoperative cardiac consultation. *Journal of Cardiothoracic Anesthesia* 3: 682–7.

Koay CB, Marks NJ. 1996. A nurse-led preadmission clinic for elective ENT surgery: the first 8 months. *Annals of the Royal College of Surgeons of England* 78: 15–19.

Lee TH, Marcantonio ER, Mangione CM, et al. 1999. Derivation and prospective validation of a simple index for prediction of cardiac risk of major noncardiac surgery. *Circulation* 100: 1043–9.

Mangano DT, Browner WS, Hollenberg M, et al. 1990. Association of perioperative myocardial ischemia with cardiac morbidity and mortality in men undergoing noncardiac surgery. *New England Journal of Medicine* 323: 1781–8.

Mangano DT, Wong MG, London MJ, Tubau JF, Rapp JA. 1991. Perioperative myocardial ischemia in patients undergoing noncardiac surgery – II: incidence and severity during the 1st week after surgery. *Journal of the American College of Cardiology* 17: 851–7.

National Confidential Enquiry into Perioperative Deaths. 2002. *Functioning as a Team? The 2002 Report of the National Confidential Enquiry into Perioperative Deaths*. London: The Association of Anaesthetists of Great Britain and Ireland.

Pandit, JJ. 2004. Maximising the benefit from pre-operative cardiac evaluation for elective, non-cardiac surgery. *British Journal of Cardiology* 11: 468–473.

Pandit MJ, MacKenzie IZ. 1999. Patient satisfaction in gynaecological outpatient attendances. *Journal of Obstetrics and Gynaecology* 19: 511–5.

Park KW. 2003. Preoperative cardiology consultation. *Anesthesiology* 98: 754–62.

Poldermans D, Boersma E, Bax JJ, et al. 2001. Dutch Echocardiographic Cardiac Risk Evaluation Applying Stress Echocardiography Study Group. Bisoprolol reduces cardiac death and myocardial infarction in high-risk patients as long as 2 years after successful major vascular surgery. *European Heart Journal* 22: 1353–825.

Rai M, Pandit JJ. 2003. Day of surgery cancellations after nurse-led preassessment in an elective surgical centre: the first 2 years. *Anaesthesia* 58: 684–711.

Reed M, Wright S, Armitage F. 1997. Nurse led general surgical preoperative assessment clinic. *Journal of the Royal College of Surgeons of Edinburgh* 42: 310–3.

Royal College of Surgeons of England. 1992. *Guidelines for Day Case Surgery* (Revised Edition). London: The Royal College of Surgeons of England.

Stinson DK. 2003. An abbreviation of the ACC/AHA algorithm for perioperative cardiovascular evaluation for noncardiac surgery. *Anesthesia and Analgesia* 97: 295–6.

Vaghadia H, Fowler C. 1999. Can nurses screen all outpatients? Performance of a nurse-based model. *Canadian Journal of Anaesthesia* 46: 1117–21.

van Klei WA, Moons KGM, Rutten CLG, et al. 2002. The effect of outpatient preoperative evaluation of hospital inpatients on cancellation of surgery and length of hospital stay. *Anesthesia and Analgesia* 94: 644–9.

Vicenzi MN, Ribitsch D, Luha O, Klein W, Metzler H. 2001. Coronary artery stenting before noncardiac surgery: more threat than safety? *Anesthesiology* 94: 367–8.

Wallace A, Layug EI, Tateo I, et al. 1998. Prophylactic atenolol reduces postoperative myocardial ischemia. *Anesthesiology* 88: 7–17.

West R, Galasko CSB. 1995. Medical audit. The role of an orthopaedic

preoperative clinic. *Annals of the Royal College of Surgeons of England* 77(Suppl): 134–5.

Wijeysundera DN, Duncan D, Nkonde-Price C, Virani SS, Washam JB, Fleischmann KE, Fleisher LA. 2014. Perioperative beta blockade in noncardiac surgery: a systematic review for the 2014 ACC/AHA

guideline on perioperative cardiovascular evaluation and management of patients undergoing noncardiac surgery: a report of the American College of Cardiology/ American Heart Association Task Force on practice guidelines. *Journal of the American College of Cardiology* 64: 2406–25.

Chapter

9

Operating Theatre Management in New Zealand
A Case Study of Applying Efficiency Principles at Waikato Public Hospital

Cameron C. R. Buchanan

Introduction

New Zealand is predominately a state-funded health-care service that is funded by taxation and levies. The Accident Compensation Corporation (ACC) is a separate state entity responsible for provision of payments to support people who are injured as a result of an accident. Medications and medical devices are procured through a centralised state-operated purchasing agency called Pharmac.

Primary care is predominately provided by private medical practitioners and is funded by the user and state. There is also a substantial private healthcare service. The public (state) hospitals provide emergency, acute and elective surgical care, whereas the private hospital focus is elective surgical care.

There are twenty District Health Boards (DHBs), whose responsibility includes public hospital care and primary care. These DHBs are state-owned enterprises with governance boards that report to the Minister of Health.

The private hospitals are funded by private health cover insurance, out-of-pocket payments, the ACC and third parties such as DHB contracts with the private hospital. Payments to the hospital are per day and per item. The private hospitals are owned by charities, companies, insurers, community trusts or publicly listed entities. Private hospitals contribute substantially to national elective surgical productivity. Medical practitioners that work in these facilities require visiting rights that are conferred by the organisations credentialing committees, and these practitioners can also have a substantive appointment at a public hospital (as with private practice in the United Kingdom).

Medical practitioners in public hospitals receive a salary, whereas those in private hospital care or consultation receive a fee for service. Primary care practitioners

are paid a fee for service with capitation. There are no performance incentive systems for public hospital employees. Base employment contracts for doctors are usually determined by two national unions representing senior and resident doctors. The DHBs have a position description for every job that lists expectations.

The revenue stream to the DHBs includes government funding from taxation (known as Vote Health), ACC, overseas paying patients, sidearm Ministry of Health (MoH) contracts, invoices to other DHBs and sundries. The MoH amount of funding is determined by population indices such as age, ethnicity and socio-economic indicators. This revenue is received by the DHBs' funding arm and is divided between the internal providers (hospitals, mental health, older persons, rehabilitation services, laboratory and radiology) and the external providers (primary care, non-government organisations, pharmacy and community laboratory).

The funder arm allocates funding to the internal provider based on a price volume schedule, which is a contract of volumes of care and services that will be delivered. These volumes are principally based on historic levels but also any known treatment or capacity changes and standardised intervention rates. The DHB should have alignment between the cost budget and the production plan (e.g., the price volume schedule includes all hospital services for which the greater proportion is for emergency care (80%) and the minority for elective care (20%). The DHB's surgical service gets its split of price volume schedule, which details cases and case weights but has a greater proportion for elective care (45%). However, the surgical focus is on the elective deliveries due to financial incentives of the elective service patient flow indicators (ESPIs). Failure to meet compliance, results in non-payment of revenue that has been included in the DHBs budget. The most important ESPI for a theatre service is ESPI 5, which requires elective patients to have surgery within 4 months of acceptance for surgery. Non-delivery of the agreed volume targets by the DHB provider arm means that potential income is not earned from the DHB funder.

Theatres are part of a DHBs surgical service and have a budget primarily based on staffing and consumable costs. The amount that is available to spend on replacement capital items is the value of the depreciation expense in a financial year. All replacement and new items require a capital request and for items over $50,000 a business case.

Waikato DHBs' share of Vote Health is $NZ 1.1 billion (~£550 million) of which NZ$ 650 million (~£325 million) of funding goes to the internal provider arm (e.g., Waikato Hospital). Waikato Hospital Surgical Services have a budget of NZ$ 240 million (~£120 million), of which NZ$ 90 million (~£45 million) is allocated to the hospital theatres' budget. In this chapter, we will describe the key elements of Waikato hospital in relation to operating theatre management and show how it is already adopting to good effect many of the principles described in earlier chapters of this book.

Waikato Hospital Organization

Waikato Hospital is the largest hospital within the Waikato DHB. It provides acute and elective care to surgical and medical patients, including paediatrics and obstetrics. It is both a regional hospital and a tertiary referral hospital for some services with referral population of up to 900,000.

All surgical specialities are present except transplant and paediatric cardiac surgery, and all reside on a single campus. The surgical services perform approximately 25,000 operations per annum, of which half are acute (unplanned). There are twenty-three operating theatres, and general anaesthesia is provided for interventional radiology, endoscopy, oncology, MRI, CT, ECT and cardiac catheter suites. Waikato Hospital is the base for the regional level-one trauma service and receives about 240 major trauma cases per annum.

The theatre suite is arranged as a hub of acute theatres next to specialist theatres of services that also have an acute demand. All services have dedicated 'home' theatres, and where there is more than one elective theatre, they are generally colocated. There is no separate day case facility, and day case surgical patients are mixed with surgical inpatients. Day case patients are discharged home from a second-stage

post-anaesthesia care unit (PACU). The same day of surgery admission unit is within the theatre suite. High-dependency care, cardiac catheterisation suites, invasive radiology, endoscopy and the emergency department are all closely located.

Waikato Hospital Surgical Services Cluster has three business units, one being theatre that includes the Department of Anaesthesia and Pain Medicine.

Departments are a mixture of full- and part-time senior medical officers (SMOs, otherwise known as consultants or specialists), some of whom may work in private practice. Departments have resident medical officers (RMOs), which include house officers and registrars. The RMO workforce is resident outside routine working hours and provides first response to emergency work. The SMO workforce is predominately scheduled to routine hours with on-call duties. However, SMOs have a greater out-of-hours on-the-floor presence, both in supervision and service delivery, than before.

The office hours operational management of the clinical theatre service is the joint responsibility of the duty anaesthetist, an SMO and a nursing coordinator. The duty anaesthetists have regular days and are expected to have, or develop, operational expertise. All medical requests for service are made via the duty anaesthetist. Out of hours the operational roles are undertaken by the on-call staff.

The administration of the theatre service is through a service and business manager with a small resource of administrative staff.

A theatre and interventional governance group, with representation from surgery, anaesthesia, operational management and senior management is responsible for the quality, safety, performance and strategy of the theatre service. This group maintains the master surgical schedule and writes theatre policies and procedures. A separate theatre operational group meets weekly and is responsible for staffing to the master theatre schedule.

Training and Research

Training of future health professionals by the public hospitals is a core activity and function. Health Workforce New Zealand, a division of the MoH, is responsible for some of the workforce production pipeline. It is also funded by Vote Health but only partially funds training, which reduces as training advances for medical specialists. The funding goes to the DHBs units' operating budget and is allocated on the basis of full-time equivalents (FTEs) in training programmes. The funding shortfall is made up by the DHBs with a premise that there will be a greater contribution to service with experience.

Trainees are desirable by the DHB because they are a source of future specialists, attract a workforce that wants to be associated with training and are relatively inexpensive. The national specialty colleges (equivalent to Royal Colleges in the United Kingdom) accredit departments within hospitals as suitable for training. Cyclical review of the departments by the colleges ensures that they remain fit for purpose.

Universities that have medical schools pay DHBs that have clinical schools a student access fee that again goes into the operating budget. This fee ostensibly covers the use of the facility and teaching from non-university employed staff. DHB SMOs often have contractual non-clinical time, where teaching would count as part of that time. The DHB must provide an appropriate clinical teaching environment with exposure to teaching and learning situations. The university also employs some clinical staff part-time and offers honorary positions to others. With this comes teaching and research expectations by the university.

Research has not been traditionally funded by the DHBs, but this is changing with the emerging recognition of improved patient outcomes, long-term financial returns and use as a recruitment incentive. Research at Waikato DHB has been included as a recent key strategic imperative. The Maori phrase 'Pae taumata' reflects the objective of being a centre of excellence in learning, training, research and innovation. The DHBs have contributed in various ways to research, such as provision of office space, administrative support, funding of individual projects and part funded academic salaries.

Research organisation and activity is *ad hoc* across the DHBs with no blueprint or national strategy. Research within departments is by individuals, or occasionally a research team may exist. Funding is usually met by grants from various organisations, or revenue generated from device or pharmaceutical trials. Clinical trial networks that acquire funding from national funding bodies exist and organise multicentre trials within the DHBs. All research activities within DHBs require ethical and DHB approval. This approval is to mitigate patient risk, organisational reputation and unknown financial impact.

Patient Pathways

Public hospitals have two patient streams, acute (unplanned) and elective (planned). Elective patients are divided into those that require hospitalisation following surgery and those that can be discharged the same day as surgery (day case).

Acute surgical patients are mainly referred to hospitals from primary care or present via the emergency department. Some may be referred from private surgical rooms, clinics or another DHB. The acute demand (both volume and procedures) has been found to be reasonably predictable. Figure 9.1A and B show the data used to help assess the required operating theatre capacity (notwithstanding this data is expressed as number of patients rather than in hours of surgery needed, as is the main principle of this book). Most acute presentations to hospital occur between, 12.00 and 20.00 hours.

Elective surgical patients are mainly referred from primary care to the surgical service within the DHB. Other referral ports include surgeons' private rooms, from within the hospital service or other DHBs. Elective demand (complexity and numbers) has been found to be much more variable. This variance appears secondary to predictable leave for school holidays and conferences.

ESPIs are used to monitor and report to the MoH the performance of the DHB in delivery of elective surgical services required by the state. Standard intervention rates allow benchmarking of one DHB against another. ESPI 1 requires an acknowledgement of whether the referral for specialist opinion within 15 days of receipt is required. ESPI 2 requires all patients that are accepted for first specialist assessment be assessed within 4 months. What determines a first specialist assessment acceptance varies between DHBs, but all require attendance and oversight of an SMO.

Patients that require a specialist assessment are seen in the DHB clinics by the appropriate service and or specialist. Access to surgery varies between DHBs and services within a DHB. Patients in whom surgery is indicated join the waiting list with an expectation of surgery within four months. For other services that have a wait list pressure, a prioritisation tool is used. Triaging or rationing patients for treatment is achieved with a clinical prioritisation assessment criteria score, indicating a severity score for underlying surgical condition. If this score

A

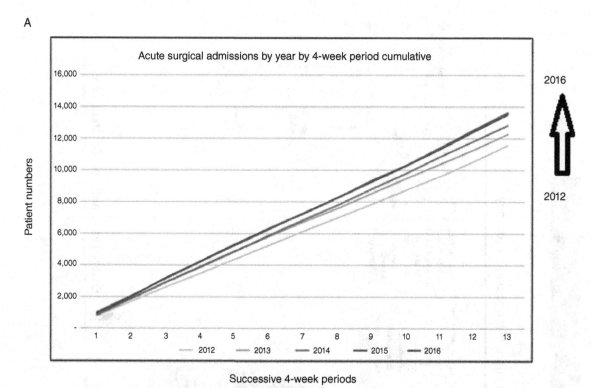

B

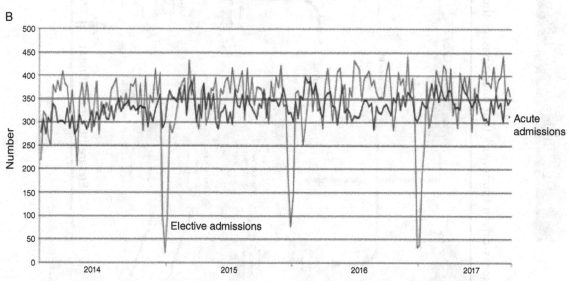

Figure 9.1 (A). Acute case presentations by successive 4-week periods over the year, for successive years (cumulative; shown by arrow for years in question). (B) Weekly surgical admissions over successive years by elective (paler line with sharp drops) and acute (darker line with less variation).

meets the DHBs' threshold they join the waiting list. This severity scoring tool is generic, without validity and subject to scoring variance, Thus access to surgery varies across the DHBs, leading to inequities and unmet needs. Those patients that do not meet the threshold score are returned to primary care. There is no active review for patients that are near threshold.

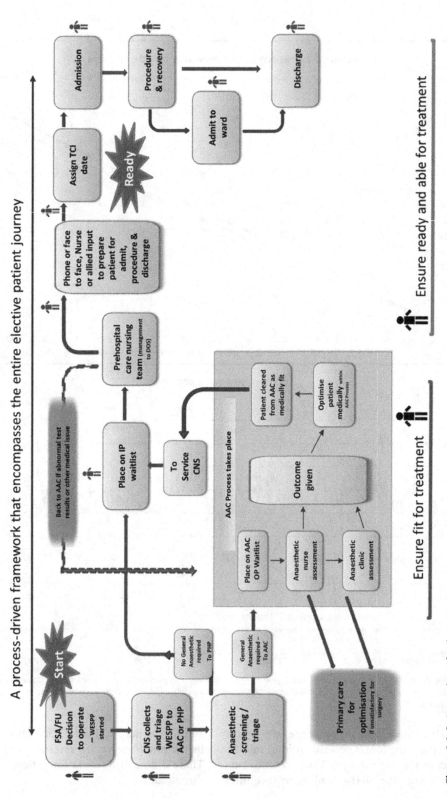

Figure 9.2 Patient pathway for elective surgery.

New Zealand also has MoH health targets of which access to elective surgery and faster cancer access (treatment to diagnosis within 62 days) are included. Both impact on theatre service, but do not currently have a financial penalty.

Once the decision to operate is made, the Waikato elective surgical and procedure pathway document is generated, and the Waikato elective surgical pathway commences (Figure 9.2). The pathway captures surgical booking details, a health questionnaire and social details. An electronic version would offer greater utility than the current paper version. All patients that require Anaesthesia must be processed by the anaesthesia assessment clinic. Some require no anaesthesia assessment (20%) until the day of surgery, while most require either a nurse or doctor assessment.

Most patients (>80%) are admitted on the day of surgery via the day of surgery admission unit. A relatively low same day of surgery admission rate is partially explained by the geographical size of the DHB and the socioeconomic status of its population. It represents a trade-off between minimising unnecessary bed occupancy and ensuring surgery takes place the following day.

The hospital's aim is to see patients for non-urgent surgery within 1 month, for urgent surgery within 1–2 weeks and those on faster treatment cancer pathways, within a week of booking. Preoperative routine laboratory testing guidelines specify required investigations and are performed before arrival at the clinic. Any specialised tests are requested as a result of the anaesthesia assessment and also reviewed by the anaesthesia assessment clinic. Although not seen by scheduled list anaesthetist, anaesthesia consent is taken at the AAC when seen by a medical practitioner (although the clinic anaesthetist may not actually anaesthetise the patient for surgery, they will usually take consent for anaesthesia in the clinic).

Patients are not allocated to the surgical waiting list until they are optimised or properly prepared for surgery. Those on 'hold' pending investigations or workup represent a trade-off between the risk of surgical delay and the risk of being poorly prepared. The patients on hold are reviewed on a weekly basis by the anaesthetic assessment clinic in conjunction with the surgical nurse coordinator. The MoH ESPI 5 target only commences when the patient has been cleared as suitably optimised for surgery. This front-end assessment takes place often 3–4 months in advance of surgery, which means that a patient's status may change. This risk is mitigated with a preoperative structured phone review just prior to the admission date.

It is arguably the case that the efficiency of a hospital is best assessed by the way it manages its elective cases. In fact, Waikato's experience is that a hospital that manages its acute demand effectively and efficiently will deliver on its elective delivery plan more predictably.

Theatre Efficiency: Implementing ε

Theatre Utilisation

The dilemma of balancing the often-conflicting demands of the different operating theatres' metrics are now well understood at Waikato. Common metrics used to reflect theatre efficiency include start times, theatre utilization (or gap time), patient cancellations and finish times. These metrics are monitored using run charts, and Figure 9.3 shows how this can be used to show real improvements over time.

Cancellations on or Near to Day of Surgery

It is one of the priorities at Waikato to avoid elective patient cancellations, as these do not reflect a patient-centric service. The intention is therefore to ensure the capacity plan matches the delivery plan and has some built-in redundancy to manage any demand variance. Yet patient cancellation is still unacceptably high ranging from 6 to 11% (Figure 9.4): indeed, the corresponding trend does not match the improving trend in utilisation shown in Figure 9.3. The consistently top reasons for elective patient cancellation are list overrun, patient unwell, substituted for an emergency case, patient did not arrive and no staff available.

Start Times and Gap Times

As outlined in Chapter 3, Waikato start times have not correlated with finish times; the impression is that start times are a symptom not a cause of inefficiency. The hospital finds that gap times are more useful when used to compare the same teams doing the same work, but less useful for comparisons across teams: a high turnover children's ENT list and an elective cardiac surgical list gap times will predictably differ.

Efficiency ε Plots

Waikato has adopted the measure of efficiency ε (see Chapter 2) for elective services and generated for each service and its surgical-anaesthesia teams

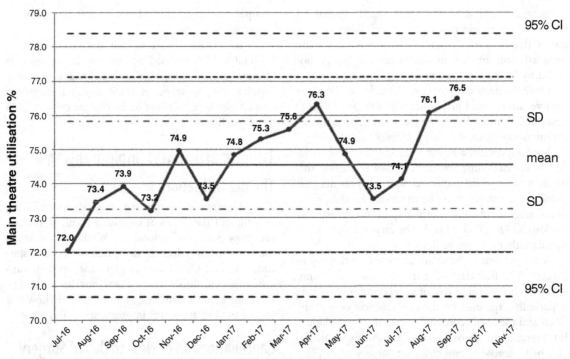

Figure 9.3 Plot of utilisation (%) of all main operating theatres over time. The numbers show the actual values for the month; the mean and ± SD lines and the ± confidence limit (95% CI) lines are also shown.

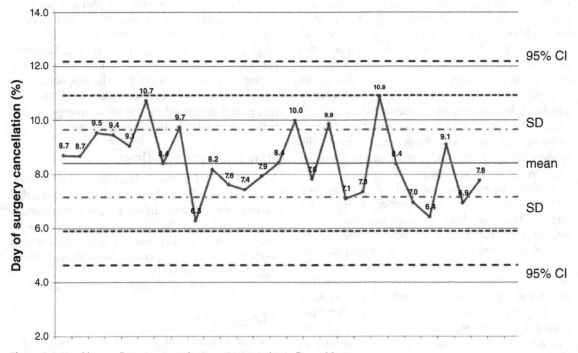

Figure 9.4 Monthly cancellation rate over the same time period as in Figure 9.3.

retrospective efficiency plots. The efficiency of a theatre is regarded as that of a team as a whole and not reflective of surgeons alone. Underruns or over-runs are defined as being plus or minus 30 minutes from the scheduled finish time.

The plastic surgical theatre at Waikato represents a good microcosm of the adoption of efficiency ε as a guide to improvement. Details of these plots and how to interpret them have been explained in Chapter 2. The cases are almost exclusively elective and must also accommodate some planned overruns for certain operations. However, the efficiency plots show (a) too many overruns and (b) too many cancellations (Figure 9.5).

The distinction between efficiency and productivity is also well understood at Waikato. A list that finishes on time with no cancellations but that has low prod-uctivity will have a better efficiency ε measure than one that finishes late, cancels a patient, but has a higher productivity. The efficiency formula ε does not account for productivity or quality, which has different indica-tors. At Waikato productivity is estimated predomin-antly using case numbers completed, where similar operation types are performed, but there is less need to compare productivity across dissimilar teams using the Φ metric discussed in Chapter 3.

Demand-Capacity Matching and Challenges

For Waikato, monitoring the clearance of emergency cases (acute bookings) is an important performance indicator. As a rule of thumb, the hospital tries to clear 80% of acute surgical bookings in 24 hours and 100% within 48 hours. Ideally all acute surgical book-ings would be treated within 24 hours. Timely access to theatre for emergencies improves patient outcomes and releases bed days. This goal is monitored through use of run charts for the 24- and 48-hour clearances, the numbers of patients booked per speciality and treated within 24- and 48-hour targets (Figure 9.6). However, this data illustrates the hospital still has some way to go properly to set its acute capacity to meet emergency demand. Moreover, surges in demand (for example, due to multiple trauma cases) disrupt this performance and usually take 2–3 days to correct. Knock-on effects include delays in expected acute delivery for those patients already in the queue, disrup-tion of the elective service and bed block.

So there is need to map capacity in the manner described in Chapter 5. To implement this fully the

data will need to be represented as demand in terms of hours of surgery rather than patient numbers, and Waikato has yet to implement that change in data collection. Nevertheless Figure 9.6B does help indicate the capacity required. This shows that, given the fluc-tuations in admissions, the lowest performance attained was ~85% when 100% was desired. Because demand–capacity matching is a question of probabil-ity, this indicates a capacity gap of ~15% for acute/emergency surgery. The organisational challenge is, of course, to create this increased capacity through investment, but at least the analysis helps show the degree of additional capacity that is necessary to achieve 100% compliance. Of course, such an increase in capacity will result in greater waste of unused capacity but that is a balance discussed in detail in Chapter 5.

Scheduling

The master surgical schedule is the basis for organ-ising all surgical procedures and (Blake & Carter, 1997) is a repeating timetable (Waikato's is four weekly) that allocates time in the available operating rooms to surgical specialities and defines their hours of operation. It is based on forecasts of acute and elective surgery demand and consists of blocks of time to which surgeons, anaesthetists, nursing tech-nical and other staff are ultimately added. Once staffing is in place, it constitutes capacity for patient treatment.

Capacity in the master surgical schedule must be maintained by making sure it is used. That means ensuring surgeons on leave are replaced by others - perhaps not necessarily from the same specialty, i.e., the operating room time is offered up to other speci-alities. This means that leave requests must be sub-mitted well in advance (e.g., 6 weeks). A weekly theatre operations group scheduling meeting is held to confirm surgical, anaesthesia and nursing staff are allocated to sessions in 4 weeks' time. Anaesthesia, anaesthesia technicians (also known as operating department assistants, ODAs) and nursing staff need to be managed appropriately to allow each employee leave such that leave plans do not disrupt the smooth running of theatre sessions (see chapter on staffing and contracts, Chapter 6).

Waikato uses an enterprise-wide SMO scheduling tool AMION (www.amion.com/; Figure 9.7). Who works, where and when can be easily identified in real

A

All plastic surgery

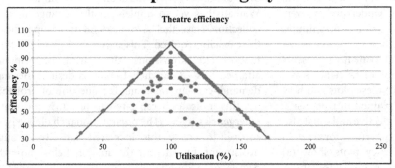

Total sessions	353
Cancelled cases	79 (6%)
Acute cases	52 (4%)
Sessions with 100% efficiency	106 (30%)
Sessions with >85% efficiency	179 (51%)
Overrunning sessions (>17.30 finish)	64 (18%)

B

'A surgeon's team'

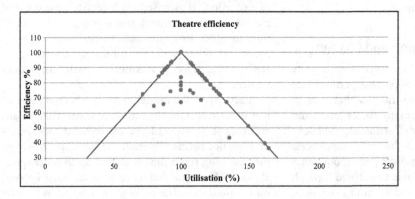

Total sessions	64
Cancelled cases	16 (7%)
Acute cases	11 (5%)
Sessions with 100% efficiency	16 (25%)
Sessions with >85% efficiency	31 (48%)
Overrunning sessions (>17.30 finish)	9 (14%)

Figure 9.5 (A): Efficiency plots for the plastic surgery unit as a whole, with the numerical data below. (B): A single representative surgeon's efficiency data within the team, with numerical data below. Despite overlap of data points the density of data on the downslope (overruns) and within the triangle (cancellations) is evident.

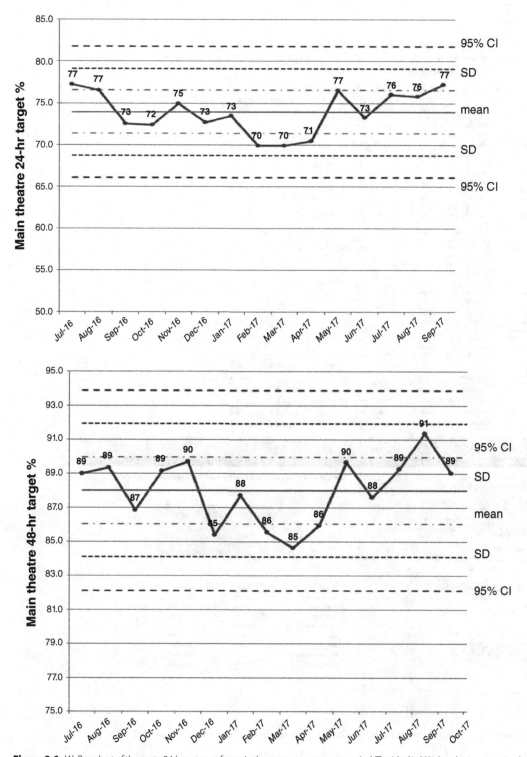

Figure 9.6 (A): Run chart of the acute 24-hour target for main theatres over a one-year period. The ideal is 80%, but this is not attained in any month. (B): Run chart of the acute 48-hour target for main theatres over a 1-year period. The ideal is 100%, but this is not attained in any month

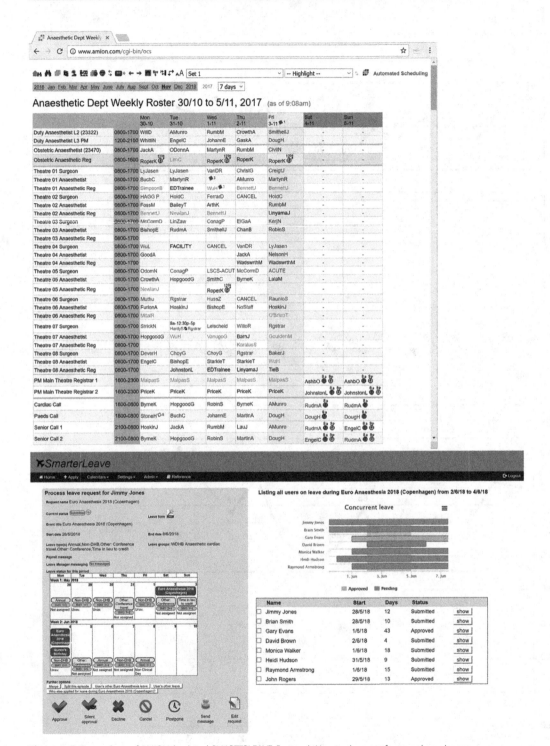

Figure 9.7 Screenshots of AMION (top) and SMARTERLEAVE (bottom). Names do not refer to real employees.

time including an individual's leave status. Leave modules that allow leave booking online and give real-time leave availability status and leave approval likelihood are in use (www.smarterleave.com/).

All day, 8-hour lists are the routine in Waikato and on average represent about 6 hours of actual surgical 'cutting' time (taking into account anaesthesia induction and gap times). Procedures that will exceed 6 hours require notification, 4 weeks in advance, at the weekly scheduling meeting. These bookings are made in context with other demands across the service and hospital to avoid overloads any one aspect of service (e.g., high-dependency beds).

Patients are allocated to lists usually based on patient need (highest score prioritised) and the longest waiting, as assessed by the surgical services booking clerks. However, the engagement of surgeons in the planning process appears variable, from no input at all, to being actively engaged in all aspects of the list construction. Although the system uses the surgeon-estimated operation duration, there is scope to challenge this if it is unrealistic, using the objective data from previous theatre records.

Most lists are finalised in the preceding week, with some services achieving this up to 3 weeks in advance. Lists changes thereafter occur due to a variety of circumstances and remain a source of ongoing frustration. The operating theatre lists are finalised at midday on the day before scheduled surgery. Any later changes, of which there are too many, are made by using the acute surgical booking process. At this point the nursing staff prepares the bill of materials (e.g., consumables) for the list and pick up potential problems. A 1-month horizon of list seems pragmatic.

One challenge in a multiroom operating suite is the competition for the availability of frequently shared resources (e.g., image intensifiers). Waikato has advocated a 'list building' environment whereby theatre stakeholders can anticipate the future demand for shared resources so that clashes can be resolved ahead of time. This would mandate the use of standardised unique identifiers for all surgical procedures instead of the free text statements currently used. This would allow the requirements of the procedure to identify the consumables, equipment (routine and non-routine) required and to estimate the likely procedure duration.

An electronic list building tool could identify a list that is likely to overrun, have resource clashes or have other logistical challenges that need to be identified and remedied before the day prior to surgery. This opportunity is lost when list contents are only confirmed the day before.

An important aspect of the master surgical schedule is the allocation of time for emergency surgical procedures. Orthopaedics, general surgery and plastic surgery generate most acute surgical demand, so they are allocated dedicated daily capacity for the expected workload. It is important (and not that easy) to get this acute/elective split correct and regularly review it. The ability to clear or deal with acute surgical patients quickly prevents them from waiting their turn in ward beds, where they can affect the ability to admit elective surgical patients.

Acute orthopaedics, general surgery and plastics are allocated named theatres every day of the week: their scheduling thus resembles the 'typical NHS UK list' described in earlier chapters. All other elective services are assigned different named theatres on specific days, and they also have access to book to free slots within elective theatre time that prioritises cases on urgency, waiting times, staff and equipment availability. These therefore resemble the 'typical US list' model described in earlier chapters. Batching of cases is favourable as it avoids constant staff changes. Some specialties like neurosurgery and vascular, may require specific theatres because of limited access to specialist staff or equipment.

The first scheduled case for each acute theatre is identified on the preceding day. This is the 'pole' patient and is selected by the surgical team and is ideally a straightforward case. This facilitates a prompt start whilst it also gives the surgical team on the wards to order the subsequent patients, with most urgent and longest waiting being prioritised. The acute theatres are assigned specialist anaesthetists paired with a named consultant surgeon.

Acute cases are prioritised within the theatre schedules with regard to allocation of resources and elective cases planned accordingly around the spare capacity remaining. This is certainly a clinically effective policy but creates its own operational problems in meeting elective contractual obligations if the required elective capacity is unavailable.

There is recognition that variance should be managed. Variance for the elective service comes in the form of seasonal (e.g., winter illness) and annual events (school holidays). The acute service must accommodate emergency cases (multitrauma) and surges in demand. Unfortunately, the policy to prioritise the acute cases inevitably means that the elective surgical schedule acts as a buffer or 'shock absorber' for surges in acute demand (i.e., acute cases displace the elective). This in large part explains both the theatre overruns and the high cancellation rates where they occur (Figures 9.4 and 9.5). These issues may be compounded by capacity reductions such as short notice leave (e.g., sick on the day). Ideally this requires the schedule to have some built-in redundancy to avoid cancellations. The team brief before the day's work is another opportunity to check that the required consumables and equipment are available.

Scheduling and the Challenge of Overruns

List overruns are a longstanding operational issue for Waikato Hospital with 50% exceeding the designated finish time (Figure 9.8A) and 20% exceeding the finish time by 75 minutes (Figure 9.8B). Lists are 8 hours duration with a scheduled finish time of 4.15 pm (standard start time 8.15 am). There is a grace interval of ±30 minutes that defines an overrun or underrun. List overruns are either 'planned' (i.e., a scheduled extended list time) or, more commonly, unplanned.

Planned overruns are almost exclusively single-case lists that are identified 4 weeks in advance and resourced independently; i.e., the duration of the list is officially increased for the case. These lists are spread across the week to even out the resource requirements. Split shifts for nurses and anaesthesia technicians are required if there are not volunteers for overtime or the list duration is excessive. The surgical demand for these lists has steadily increased as more complex surgery is offered.

List overruns that are unplanned and not resourced result in one or more of: patient cancellations, staff dissatisfaction, overtime payments and the interruption of the evening's planned acute service. Whether to cancel or overrun is made on a case-by-case basis, day-by-day, with the operational decision made by the clinical operational staff. The listed finish time is 'wheels out of theatre' and does not include a lot of staff activity that continues after this time (e.g., in PACU).

Unplanned overruns come in two categories, unexpected and expected. Expected overruns means that the published list is likely to overrun its allotted time (see Chapter 4 for probabilistic case scheduling). Unexpected overruns occur when the published list appears reasonable but some other unpredictable factors conspire to cause overrun. The duration distribution of a procedure is often skewed to the right and often bimodal. Despite similar mean and median times, there is a considerable range in the time taken to complete elective cholecystectomies for all surgeons, so some operations are just harder and take far longer to do than expected. Figure 9.9 shows the distributions for what should be a reasonably predictable operation, laparoscopic cholecystectomy, by several surgical teams (although this is ascribed by 'surgeon', the timings are total theatre times and represent team performance).

There are some particularly challenging lists to manage. One is that of an expected or predicted overrun on a list with just two cases. The only alternatives are (a) either scheduling just one case and underrunning the list or (b) scheduling two cases and overrunning the list. The latter requires resources to meet demand and be staffed accordingly; the former requires that the team decides on an early finish, with appropriate adjustment in compensation.

Multiple case lists that repeatedly overrun reflect poor list construction and a failure to identify that risk and act before the day of surgery. A review of median, mean and finish time range for service and individual teams is helpful. When the efficiency graph and session duration bar graph are plotted together the issues emerge (see Appendix 9A).

Determining Session Length

The norm at Waikato is 8-hour lists. However, some routinely exceed this scheduled duration (e.g., by more than 9 hours). Waikato has adopted the method of Pandit and Dexter (2009) to help determine when a list needs additional time (see Chapter 5). Thus, although general surgery might occasionally overrun 9 hours, these lists are left unchanged. On the other hand, the actual list duration for cardiac surgery requires a scheduled and resourced longer day (Figure 9.10).

Lists that are routinely overbooked require better booking methodology and using the known median procedure times and standard deviation. A review of the list's contents in advance is required to avoid cancellation on the day of surgery.

A

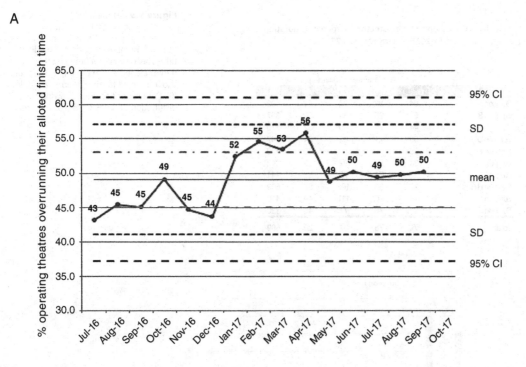

B

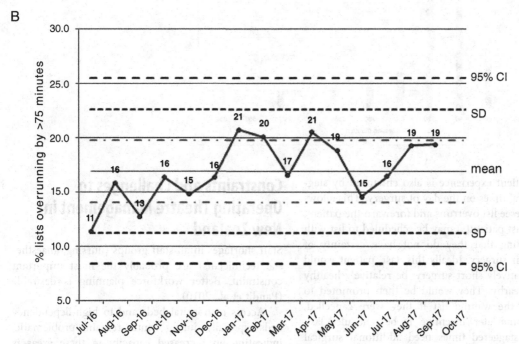

Figure 9.8 (A): Proportion of all lists overrunning by 30 minutes their allotted finish times. (B): Proportion of all lists overrunning by >75 minutes.

A

Elective laparoscopic cholecystectomy procedure duration
FY 2015 – 2018 YTD Sep 27

Surgeon - Top 10	Procedure duration (Minutes)				
	Cases	Median	Average	Min	Max
Surgeon A	64	82	89	41	192
Surgeon B	51	78	89	36	337
Surgeon C	44	76	80	32	170
Surgeon D	39	71	82	24	247
Surgeon E	35	77	80	46	129
Surgeon F	34	81	92	26	212
Surgeon G	33	71	75	28	141
Surgeon H	29	85	106	57	609
Surgeon I	27	96	112	49	410
Surgeon J	26	76	77	46	120
Total	562	78	87	20	609

Figure 9.9 (A): Table of numerical data for a single operative procedure by 10 different teams. The columns show, in turn, the number of cases, the median time, mean (average) time and the minimum and maximum times. The totals show the data for the group as a whole. (B): Data for one team (I) showing the distribution of times for the procedure.

B

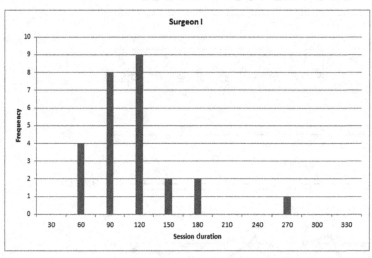

The patient experience is also enhanced by staggered arrival times on the day of surgery. This allows staff to foresee list overruns and forewarn the patient. Thus the last patient(s) may be scheduled to list with understanding that they do not have certainty of having their surgery. Ideally this 'last' patient would require relatively short surgery, be relatively healthy and live nearby. They would be then promoted to higher up the waiting list if they were cancelled, creating some later 'incentive' to be scheduled last. However, staggered times need additional surgical and anaesthesia staff to review and consent the later-arriving patients (i.e., the staggered arrival times do not work well with single-handed anaesthetists and/or surgeons).

Constraints and Challenges to Operating Theatre Management in New Zealand

Staff shortages in all staff groups (nursing, anaesthesia, technicians) are probably the most important constraint. Better workforce planning is desirable (Pandit et al., 2010).

Access to hospital beds and to high-dependency beds especially during winter remains problematic, indicating an increased capacity in these areas is necessary. Any delay in access to post-operative inpatient beds increases the length of PACU stay, ultimately causing a bed gridlock and cancellations in operating theatres. Any increase in capacity should

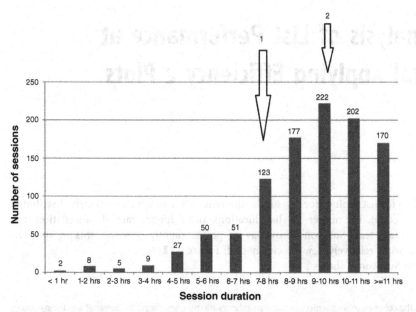

Figure 9.10 Histogram of actual list duration for cardiac surgery. If scheduled duration was held at 8 hours, the majority of lists would overrun (arrow 1). However, extending the scheduled list duration to, say, 10 hours captures the majority of lists (arrow 2).

also take into account the need to absorb unexpected demands due to urgent complex surgery such as multiple trauma cases.

Even in hospital there can be frustrating waits for patients before arrival in theatre due to shortages of porters/orderlies or poor execution of processes (e.g., failing to send for the patient appropriately early). To mitigate this, it is common to transfer the first listed patient of the day for each list to PACU at 07.30 am for an 08.15 am prompt start. Subsequent patients are called for 'early' and held in a theatre transfer area before surgery, where the required checks can be undertaken.

Delays in surgery can afflict even acute/emergency patients, and as they occupy hospital beds waiting for surgery, this can interrupt the elective surgical activity, so that the acute backlog can be cleared. Patients may also be occupying hospital beds waiting for investigations, discharge or other services. The most concerning aspect of this is patient deterioration as a result of excessive delay, especially for emergency patients.

Beds are only one limiting factor. Shared resources such as access to image intensifiers and a radiographer are a constraint. Elective lists need to be planned and scheduled in advance to manage this shared resource, especially at weekends.

Appendix 9A Analysis of List Performance at Waikato Hospital Applying Efficiency ε Plots

Table 9.1 shows the numerical data for list timings for fourteen teams (listed by 'surgeon' code). The numerical data do not make clear that in fact, team Surgeon A has a tendency to overrun, with relatively few cancellations (Figure 9.11). Team Surgeon F shows a subtle difference with much more widely distributed list durations and a higher rate of cancellation (the overlay of points slightly obscures this in the efficiency plot; Figure 9.12).

Table 9.1 List timings for 14 teams. The columns show the median duration in hours and minutes, the mean (average) and the minimum and maximum duration over 50–70 lists.

Session owner	Session duration (hours)			
	Median	Average	Min	Max
Surgeon A	8:35	8:33	5:33	11:17
Surgeon B	8:28	8:24	6:49	10:36
Surgeon C	8:23	8:26	6:14	11:45
Surgeon D	8:09	8:12	6:19	10:08
Surgeon E	8:02	8:00	6:22	10:00
Surgeon F	8:01	8:23	5:35	13:30
Surgeon G	7:50	7:59	6:20	10:53
Surgeon H	7:45	7:45	5:25	12:17
Surgeon I	7:35	7:21	2:27	10:33
Surgeon J	7:36	7:56	6:00	11:31
Surgeon K	7:27	7:41	6:24	9:36
Surgeon L	7:14	7:22	5:05	11:25
Surgeon M	7:46	7:42	5:45	12:24
Surgeon N	7:06	7:15	1:22	10:16

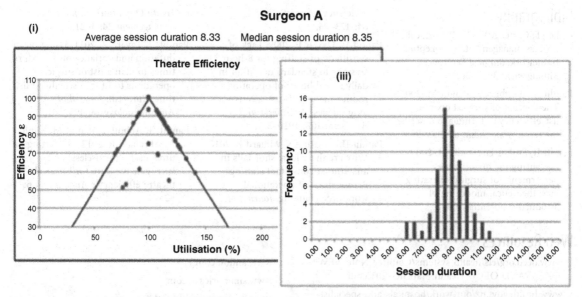

Figure 9.11 Efficiency ε plot for team Surgeon A (i) showing that many lists lie on the descending limb of the triangle, and relatively few lists lie in the middle, indicating a tendency to overrun but cancel little. This is borne out by the team's numerical analysis, with 26% of lists overrunning but only 3% cancellations for electives and just 1% for acute cases (Table 9.1). Overall efficiency is not too bad (63% of lists have efficiency > 85%) but could be improved through better scheduling. Plot (iii) is a histogram of the duration of lists: these should be clustered close to 8 hours, but are clearly skewed to >8 hours.

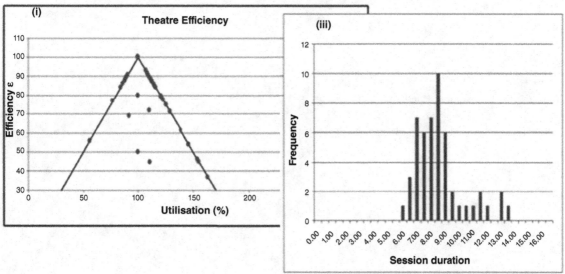

Figure 9.12 Efficiency ε plot for team Surgeon F (i) showing that many lists lie on both the ascending and descending limbs of the triangle. Although relatively few lists lie in the middle, there is some overlay of points, and some lie much lower in the triangle than in Figure 9.11, indicating a higher rate of cancellation. This is borne out by the team's numerical analysis (Table 9.1), with 7% and 11% cancellation rate for electives and acutes, respectively. There is a wider splay of both underruns and overruns (iii) such that overall efficiency is poorer than team Surgeon A, with just 52% of lists with efficiency >85%.

Bibliography

Blake JT, Carter MW. 1997. Surgical process management: a conceptual framework. *Surgical Services Management* 3: 31–36.

Pandit JJ, Westbury S, Pandit M. 2007. The concept of surgical operating list 'efficiency': a formula to describe the term. *Anaesthesia* 62: 895–903.

Pandit JJ, Stubbs D, Pandit M. 2009. Measuring the quantitative performance of surgical operating lists: theoretical modelling of 'productive potential' and 'efficiency'. *Anaesthesia* 64: 473–86.

Pandit JJ, Dexter F. 2009. Lack of sensitivity of staffing for 8-hour sessions to standard deviation in daily actual hours of operating room time used for surgeons with long queues. *Anesthesia and Analgesia* 108: 1910–5.

Pandit JJ, Tavare AN, Millard P. 2010. Why are there local shortfalls in anaesthesia consultant staffing? A case study of operational workforce planning. *Journal of Heath Organisation and Management* 24: 4–21.

Pandit JJ, Tavare A. 2011. Using mean duration and variance of procedure times to plan a list of surgical operations to fit into scheduled list time. *European Journal of Anaesthesiology* 28: 493–501.

Pandit JJ, Abbott T, Pandit M, Kapila A, Abraham R. 2012. Is 'starting on time' useful (or useless) as a surrogate measure for 'surgical theatre efficiency'? *Anaesthesia* 6: 823–32.

Web Resources

www.oecd.org/els/health-systems/Country-Note-NEW%20ZEALAND-OECD-Health-Statistics-2015.pdf

www.health.govt.nz/our-work/hospitals-and-specialist-care/elective-services/elective-services-and-how-dhbs-are-performing/about-elective-services-patient-flow-indicators

www.amion.com

www.smarterleave.com

www.commonwealthfund.org

Chapter 10

Operating Theatre Management in Japan

Yoshinori Nakata

Introduction

Teikyo University Hospital offers an example or microcosm for the Japanese healthcare system. Teikyo University Hospital is located in metropolitan Tokyo, Japan, serving a population of ~1,000,000. It has 1,152 beds and has a surgical volume of ~9,000 cases annually. It has thirteen surgical specialty departments (thoracic surgery, cardiovascular surgery, neurosurgery, obstetrics & gynaecology, plastic surgery, orthopaedics, general surgery, urology, emergency surgery, oral surgery, ophthalmology, dermatology and otolaryngology).

Japan has maintained a universal health insurance system for more than half a century. The services covered and the fees set for physicians and hospitals have been uniform across the nation since 1959; i.e., the same operation is reimbursed equivalently regardless of where in the country it is undertaken. Most healthcare providers are reimbursed on a fee-for-service basis according to the fee schedule that sets prices uniformly at the national level. Although patients might select different insurers, depending on their jobs or places of residence, the same fee schedule is enforced for all plans and healthcare providers.

The surgical fee for each surgical procedure is classified by a 'K code (K000–K915) in the Japanese surgical fee schedule. The fee is identical regardless of who performs surgery (e.g., a senior surgeon or a surgical trainee as long as they have medical licensure), how many assistants they use, or how long it takes to complete surgery. This all means there is some theoretical incentive to use a lower grade of surgeon (by rank or training), use fewer staff, and encourage quicker operating, but as we shall see later, this theory is rarely translated into practice.

Hospitals are owned by 'management bodies', which function like independent companies. National and municipal governments or universities also directly own some hospitals. Private companies and private universities also own hospitals. Some of them form a hospital network owned or sponsored by the same management body. They are not linked to medical insurers and they compete for patients with each other in the healthcare market.

All Japanese patients are covered by the universal health insurance system. Typically, the insurance covers 70% of medical expenditure, but the out-of-pocket cost above a certain limit is covered by the subsidies from the government. Thus patients usually pay US$ 500–1,000 a month depending on their incomes.

Hospital Budgeting

The budget for the operating theatre suite is not easily defined within the larger budget of the hospital; the two are generally merged and inseparable. The current fee-for-service reimbursement system does not formally define which cost components are covered by the surgical or anaesthetic fee – rather, it is simply regarded as an overall fee to the hospital (Ishi, 2012). This lack of detail or impenetrability gives surgeons and physicians the impression that the reimbursement system is unfair. In fact, it is uncertain whether the prices are appropriate or not. In some ways, therefore the reimbursement system is similar to the Payment-by-Results described for the United Kingdom in Chapter 7. It can be supposed that those principles might apply equally to Japanese hospitals. However, what is different from the United Kingdom is that in Japan *all* insurers also use the same fee schedule. As we saw in Chapter 7, in the United Kingdom different insurers reimburse different rates (i.e., they are in competition with each other), and also all insurers pay a different rate from the NHS tariff.

All the surgeons and anaesthetists are employees of the management body of the hospital and are paid salaries (e.g., they are paid by the university if the hospital is owned by the university). Typically, doctors have one free day a week, and they can choose to work in other hospitals for extra income or to do some research (or choose to have free time). Salaries, of course, differ across hospitals, so there is competition for recruitment of staff in this way.

There are few if any salary incentive schemes in hospitals. Because both surgeons and anaesthetists are employees of the hospital, paid at equal rates, they have an equal relationship. The relationship between surgeon/anaesthetist and the hospital is that of employee–employer.

Hospital Departmental Structure

Teaching is a part of the mission of a hospital if the hospital is designated as a clinical training hospital by the government. Academic activity is a part of the mission of a hospital if it is a university hospital. Generally speaking, monetary incentives for these activities are very small, and they do not cover any part of the reimbursement for their clinical activities of the hospital. Promotion to higher academic ranks is virtually the only incentive for these activities, but with promotion comes increased salary, which is itself an incentive.

The Patient Pathway

All patients in Japan have absolutely free access to any doctors at any healthcare facilities of their choice, including direct access to a specialist without recourse first to a general practitioner. Some patients will see family doctors in the clinics near their homes, and others will directly see specialists at the outpatient services in the large-scale university hospitals. Which of these they choose is entirely the patients' preference. If the doctors in these clinics feel their patients need advanced care, they refer them to the appropriate hospitals.

Not all patients have an anaesthetic preassessment before surgery. If they need further preoperative tests, anaesthetists refer them back to the surgeons, and surgeons arrange tests by other (medical) specialists. This happens quite frequently because the more preoperative tests that are done, the larger is the revenue to the hospital. Therefore there is a tendency to conduct more than fewer tests.

The average length of time from referral to surgery varies widely depending on the demand for surgeons and their specialties. Some established orthopaedic surgeons may have waiting lists of several months. However, long waiting lists have never been a major

social problem in Japan because all the patients in Japan have absolute freedom of choice and access and they can easily switch to less-congested hospitals or doctors. Although there is no publicly accessible information to guide this choice, if patients feel the initial waiting time they were given was too long, they can by trial and error consult other specialists to obtain shorter wait times.

Operating Theatre Activity

The struggle for efficiency has never been much of an issue in the operating theatre in Japan because almost all surgical patients are inpatients; there is very little day surgery. There is a much greater emphasis on safety rather than volume or throughput of surgery. Therefore, the concept of efficiency is only qualitatively and subjectively measured in Japan. Perhaps the author's own research using data envelopment analysis is virtually the only one that has quantitatively measured the efficiency of surgery in Japan.

There are 'surgical slots' designated for each surgical department. For example, only general surgeons, neurosurgeons, orthopaedic surgeons and dermatologists might operate on elective cases that require anaesthetists' care on Monday (Table 10.1). On a Tuesday it might be a different combination of specialties, and so on.

To this extent, the arrangement seems similar to a 'typical UK NHS list', discussed elsewhere in this book. But within each slot, the allocation of operating time by surgeon is decided solely by that department. Thus, for the neurosurgery slot on a certain day the slot may be allocated to Surgeon A, then B, then C, etc. Surgeons D, E and F may be granted time the following week. So this aspect in fact resembles more a 'typical US list'. The scheduling within this scheme is *ad hoc*, and there is little or no use of time information in the manner described in Chapter 4 ('Case Scheduling'). Notably, independent operating theatre managers are not involved in the decision making. However, the head nurse in the operating theatre finally approves the schedule 3 to 5 days before surgery, although it is rare for any schedule not to be approved.

The operating theatre management committee of the hospital monitors in advance the utilisation of each of the surgical slots on a biannual basis (as a snapshot). The utilisation is calculated by the ratio of time when patients actually occupy the slots

Table 10.1 Example arrangement of surgical slots with anaesthetists' involvement in the main operating theatre in a typical Japanese hospital. The columns can be regarded as a single operating room (OR), wherein the listed specialties are allocated their slots.

Day	Surgical specialty		
Monday	General surgery General surgery Orthopaedic surgery Neurosurgery	General surgery General surgery Orthopaedic surgery	General surgery Dermatology Orthopaedic surgery
Tuesday	General surgery Obstetrics & Gynaecology Cardiovascular surgery	General surgery Urology Cardiovascular surgery	Orthopaedic surgery Urology Plastic surgery
Wednesday	General surgery General surgery Otolaryngology Trauma surgery	General surgery Orthopaedic surgery Otolaryngology	General surgery Orthopaedic surgery Plastic surgery
Thursday	General surgery Orthopaedic surgery Ophthalmology	Neurosurgery Obstetrics & Gynaecology Cardiovascular surgery	Orthopaedic surgery Urology Plastic surgery
Friday	General surgery Obstetrics & Gynaecology Cardiovascular surgery Ophthalmology	General surgery Obstetrics & Gynaecology Orthopaedic surgery	Orthopaedic surgery Otolaryngology Oral surgery
Saturday	General surgery	Orthopaedic surgery	Urology

divided by the total time of the slots given. If a specialty has underbooked its time slots, then the underused time is given to overbooking specialties. For example, if after 6 months general surgery has used only 80% of its allocated time, while neurosurgery has used 20% more than allocated, neurosurgery is allocated 20% more time, and general surgery allocations are cut. This creates a potentially perverse incentive to overbook and overrun lists so that specialties do not lose their allocated time. Thus teams generally work until all work is completed, regardless of the time it takes. The last patients are almost never cancelled because most of them are inpatients anyway, so there is no drive for a reasonable finish time to discharge patients in a timely manner. All this is counterbalanced only by the fact that surgeons do not want to work for too long, as there is little incentive to do so (other than the drive to keep their slots).

This system understandably creates pressures for the anaesthetic department, which is serving all the specialties. In this way, a bottleneck to service delivery is probably the number of anaesthetists and operating theatre nurses, although this problem is resolving gradually through training and recruitment and expansion of these specialties. If this is overcome, then the physical number of operating theatres may next become the bottleneck.

Future Pressures and Developments

As in all other countries the demand for surgery is increasing with an aging population with increasingly complex requirements. Japan faces the most rapidly aging society in the world, and the demand for surgery will dramatically increase at least until 2040. In the face of this increasing demand, Japan has to think seriously about the efficiency of its healthcare system as well as the financial viability of universal health coverage (this last being a problem perhaps in common with the UK NHS). Operating theatres are one of the most expensive parts of the system, so their efficiency is key to any future healthcare strategy.

Currently, however, a lack of data is inhibiting progress in this field in Japan. It is one of the paradoxes that one of the most technologically advanced societies is also the one that lacks the data that that technology could so easily handle, in respect of operating theatre services. As a circular explanation, one of the reasons why operating theatre efficiency has not attracted attention as a focus for academic enquiry in Japan is that there is not sufficient data available to analyse.

From a different perspective, because almost all patients stay in the hospital at least one night, there is little focus on making operating theatres more efficient: any small gains in efficiency will be limited or negated by the fact that the patient is utilizing an expensive overnight stay anyway. A shift towards day case surgery would then properly increase the focus on operating theatre performance.

Clinical Training: Workforce Implications

The Japanese Medical Specialty Board (JMSB) aims to start a new board certification process for all medical specialties in April 2018. Each medical specialty board that is affiliated with its medical specialty society has hitherto been allocated its certified trainees, but from April 2018 JMSB will take over the certification processes from medical specialty boards. However, JMSB does not have any expertise in each medical specialty, and it only provides education on general medical safety and ethics. Moreover, at time of writing (2017–18), not much has been finalised, and the current trainees are left with many uncertainties, which threatens workforce planning. Hence, Chapter 6 in this book embedding the principles of staffing and contracts will become very relevant.

Key Areas of Concern and Need for Development

Because finance drives development, there are some essential anaesthetic practices that are not reimbursed by the fee schedule in Japan.

Postanesthetic Care Units and Holding Areas

Few hospitals in Japan have post-anaesthesia care units (PACUs) and holding areas (i.e., areas where patients come to, just before surgery, for insertion of regional blocks or invasive lines before induction of anaesthesia). PACUs are normal in the United Kingdom, but holding areas are rare; both are common in

the United States. This is because Japanese fee schedules do not directly reimburse their costs. Therefore, patients come directly from their inpatient hospital rooms to the operating theatres, undergo anaesthesia and surgery, and go directly back to their rooms.

This current practice has several cost consequences. First, there is the cost of the (potentially unnecessary) prior admission to an inpatient bed. Then, there is the time delay (adding to cost) of starting intravenous lines, regional blocks and other invasive lines in the anaesthetic room/OR just prior to surgery, which adds to anaesthetic time. Then, all patients must be fully recovered from anaesthesia in the operating theatre so that they are ready for the care at the hospital wards. In other words, what in many other countries would be 'PACU time' is transferred to 'total operation time'. In the scenarios described for efficiency and total operative times in Chapters 2 and 3, Japanese data would be very long indeed for all operations.

There is clearly potential to transfer costs of inpatient admission to PACU and/or holding area investment and thus increase the productivity of ORs in Japan.

Day Case Surgery

Day case surgery in Japan is uncommon. The rate of outpatient surgery in Teiko University Hospital is <10% of all surgeries. The unique funding system means that hospitals in Japan can make more revenue by keeping patients in the hospital before and after surgery than by offering outpatient surgery programs. This is even the case with patients for minor ophthalmic surgery and simple orthopaedic surgery (Ichimura et al., 2003). Anecdotally, some patients become so bored of this regimen in the ward that they sneak out of the hospital to smoke or drink beer in nearby parks, at times leading to their cancellation for non-fasting. All this is a waste of medical resources, but requires extensive culture change across the whole system.

Emergency Cases and Late-Running Cases

There is a significant conflict of schedule between emergency cases and late-running cases, so the principles of Chapters 2–4 are important to reduce late-running cases whilst managing emergencies.

Restricted Use of Medications

There is an unusual aspect of the Japanese fee schedule that only reimburses post-operative pain management with continuous epidural analgesia, and not for intravenous patient-controlled analgesia or continuous peripheral nerve blocks (see: http://japanhpn.org/en/finan2/). This policy significantly limits options for post-operative pain management and creates perverse incentives. For example, coupled with extra revenues for inpatient admission it means there is arguably excessive use of neuraxial blockade that requires longer inpatient stays, when in fact this could all be avoided by early mobilization.

Second, although dexamethasone and ondansetron have long been proven to be effective antiemetic medications for post-operative nausea and vomiting, the fee schedule only allows these drugs for nausea and vomiting after chemotherapy for malignant tumors. If these drugs are administered perioperatively in absence of chemotherapy, there is no reimbursement. The approach to antiemetic drugs in Japan may have been influenced or skewed by one of the largest sets of scientific journal retractions in biomedical history, concerning a Japanese anaesthesiologist who particularly investigated antiemetic medications as part of his now-retracted research (Carlisle, 2012; Pandit, 2012; Carlisle et al., 2015).

Along similar lines, intravenous nonsteroidal anti-inflammatory drugs (IV NSAIDs) are known to be effective for post-operative pain when administered intraoperatively. However, IV NSAIDs are not reimbursed for costs if administered intraoperatively in Japan, leading to suboptimal pain management.

Even labour analgesia, including epidural analgesia, is rarely provided as part of a formalized protocol or program in Japan because the universal insurance system does not cover its cost. Teikyo University Hospital does not have a labor analgesia program with the result that < 5% of pregnant women receive epidurals, usually obtained through personal approaches to or requests to physicians involved in their care. The only obstetric anaesthesia reimbursed is anaesthesia for caesarean sections. This funding policy not only reduces patient satisfaction and suffering but also increases the rate of operative intervention overall. The rate of cae-

sarean sections has been increasing since 1987 and reached ~25% in 2014 in hospitals according to the data of Ministry of Health, Labour and Welfare (www.mhlw.go.jp/toukei/saikin/hw/iryosd/14/dl/gaikyo.pdf).

Summary

Few healthcare economists in Japan are familiar with the work involving operating theatres. Although the Japanese literature on operating theatre management is sparse, it is clear that operating theatre efficiency is something that should concern planners and hospitals in Japan. The Japanese healthcare system has had universal health insurance for more than a half century but the sustainability of this healthcare system is in question because of the Japanese government fiscal debt. It is inevitable that there will be a focus on making efficiencies across the public and insured sector system, with further impetus provided by the demands of the aging population.

The reference list shows some outputs and conclusions from data in Japan that verify many of the conclusions of chapters in this book, including the following:

1. Efficiency of operating theatres is distinct from productivity.
2. Efficiency is a prerequisite of productivity.
3. Tariffs (the funding for) surgical operations are independent of efficiency but dependent upon surgery type, such that certain subspecialties are inherently profitable, regardless of the efficiency of their ORs.
4. Arbitrarily changing the tariff structure will alter the perception of what are the profitable subspecialties.
5. Data envelopment analysis is a useful means, especially within the Japanese model, to assess operating theatre performance and development.

Although data in Japan cannot yet directly influence the shaping of tactical operating theatre management overall, it is clear that many if not all of the principles in the chapters of this book are directly applicable and could be introduced in Japan.

Appendix 10A Analysis Framework in Our Research

Microeconomic Model of Surgery

Research based on Japanese data has used the following microeconomic model to calculate efficiency and productivity for operating rooms (Figure 10.1), which exploits data envelopment analysis (DEA; see Chapter 3).

In this model, the operating room efficiency and productivity are considered to depend on surgeons' (as opposed to anaesthetists') efficiency and productivity because they usually utilize the longest time portion of the operating room time. A decision-making unit (DMU) is defined as the entity that is regarded as responsible for converting inputs into outputs in DEA. The DMU is defined as the surgeon with the highest academic rank involved in an operation; all the inputs and outputs are under the control of a DMU. 'Inputs' are defined as (a) the number of medical doctors who assist in surgery (assistants) and (b) the time the surgical operation takes from skin incision to skin closure (surgical time). The 'output' is defined as the surgical fee for the operation.

Data Envelopment Analysis (DEA)

As described in Chapter 3, DEA is a non-parametric technique for efficiency measurement that applies linear programing and has been widely used to measure efficiency of various entities, such as national defense, education and healthcare. DEA is particularly relevant because of its ability to manage multiple inputs and outputs and does not require an a priori specification of a function. The efficiency scores are calculated from an 'isogram' curve or 'production possibility frontier', as has been earlier explained.

For example, in a two-input, one-output model we can draw an isogram curve as shown in Figure 10.2. Just as defined in Chapter 3, the efficiency score of point B is defined as:

$$\text{Efficiency} = {OB'}/{OB} \qquad \text{Equation 10.1}$$

The efficiency scores all lie between 0 and 1, and the most efficient DMUs are given the score of 1.

Malmquist Index (MI)

The Malmquist productivity index (MI) represents total factor productivity change of a DMU between two time periods under dynamic observation. It

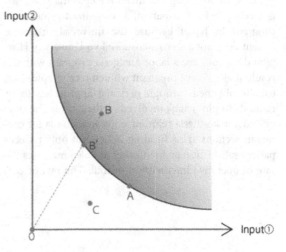

Input②

Input①

Figure 10.2. Isogram curve in a two-input, one-output model. A is an efficient DMU. B is an inefficient DMU because it lies further from the origin. Point C is unattainable because it does not lie on any frontier.

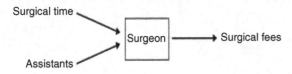

Surgical time

Surgeon → Surgical fees

Assistants

Figure 10.1. For purposes of analysis, the chief surgeon (central box) during an operation is classed as the DMU. The two inputs into the surgeon's functioning are the surgical time and the assistants; the output is the fee generated as revenue.

extends the notion of DEA, which evaluates relative efficiency of DMUs (εDMU) against the efficient frontier under static conditions. By comparing DEA results between two time periods, MI can apportion productivity change into two components, one measuring efficiency change (EC) and the other measuring technical change (TC). MI is defined as the product of the EC and TC terms. The EC term relates to the degree to which a DMU improves or decline in efficiency, while the TC term reflects the change in the efficient frontiers between the two time periods. If productivity change of a DMU is compared between Period 1 frontier (P1F) and Period 2 frontier (P2F), they are mathematically defined as follows:

$$\text{Efficiency change} = EC = \frac{\varepsilon DMU_{P2} \cap P2F}{\varepsilon DMU_{P1} \cap P1F}$$

Equation 10.2

Where ∩ indicates 'with respect to'.

$$\left(\text{Technical change TC} = \sqrt{\left(\left(\frac{\varepsilon DMU_{P1} \cap P1F}{\varepsilon DMU_{P1} \cap P2F}\right) \times \left(\frac{\varepsilon DMU_{P2} \cap P1F}{\varepsilon DMU_{P2} \cap P2F}\right)\right)}\right)$$

Equation 10.3

Then, MI = EC × TC. If instead we choose a different two-input, one-output model (Figure 10.3). EC is defined as:

$$EC = \frac{OA/OB}{OE/OG}$$

Equation 10.4

TC is defined as:

$$TC = \sqrt{\left[\left(\frac{OE}{OG}\right)/\left(\frac{OF}{OG}\right) \times \left(\frac{OC}{OB}\right)/\left(\frac{OA}{OB}\right)\right]}$$

$$= \sqrt{\left(\frac{OE}{OF}\right) \times \left(\frac{OC}{OA}\right)}$$

Equation 10.5

Thus, combining EC with TC, we get

$$MI = EC \times TC$$

$$= \sqrt{\left(\left[\left(\frac{OC}{OB}\right)/\left(\frac{OE}{OG}\right)\right] \times \left[\left(\frac{OA}{OB}\right)/\left(\frac{OF}{OG}\right)\right]\right)}$$

Equation 10.6

where OA, OB, OC, OE, OF and OG are defined as the linear distances from the origin to the respective points.

The actual calculation of efficiency and productivity is performed by a software, 'DEA-Solver'. These tools are freely available from the web (see: Web Resources in bibliography). All the researchers have to do is to define DMU, inputs, outputs and time periods for observation. It is possible to choose any number of inputs and outputs and to choose more than two time periods. It is useful to evaluate time changes of productivity in the operating theatres. The researchers can also identify the causes of change in productivity by dividing it into efficiency change and technical change.

Solving a Practical Problem Using the MI

The MI can be used to track changes in productivity. If a theatre manager finds the productivity of a surgeon has declined using the Malmquist index, they can analyze this further by dividing MI between 'efficiency change' and 'technical change'. As mentioned earlier,

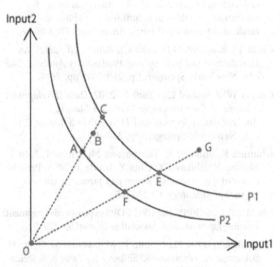

Figure 10.3. The Malmquist index in a two-input, one-output model. A DMU is in G in Period 1, and moves to B in Period 2. P1 indicates the efficient frontier in Period 1. P2 indicates the efficient frontier in Period 2. OA, OB, OC, OE, OF and OG in the text are defined as the linear distances from the origin to the respective points.

Table 10.2 Solutions for reduced productivity

Cause	Interpretation	Examples of solutions
Technique	Frontier regressed	Repair/upgrade obsolete equipment Improve nursing practices
Efficiency	Surgeons regressed from frontier	Change/increase staffing by quality/quantity Change working practices

the efficiency change relates to the degree to which a surgeon improves or worsens their efficiency relative to the respective efficient frontier, while the technical change term reflects the change in the efficient frontiers between the two time periods. The technical change affects all surgeons simultaneously, and even the best surgeons might do worse in this period than in the previous period. The efficiency change depends on individual surgeons. The following is an example of simple solutions for reduced productivity (Table 10.2).

Where finances are modeled using MI, increasing surgical fees will also positively shift the efficient frontier, but this may be outside a theatre manager's control. Although a theatre manager has limited measures to improve individual surgeons' efficiency, they certainly have influence in improving technical regress.

Bibliography

Carlisle JB. 2012. The analysis of 168 randomised controlled trials to test data integrity. *Anaesthesia* 67: 521–37.

Carlisle JB, Dexter F, Pandit JJ, Shafer SL, Yentis SM. 2015. Calculating the probability of random sampling for continuous variables in submitted or published randomised controlled trials. *Anaesthesia* 70: 848–58.

Coelli TJ, Rao DSP, O'Donnell CJ, Battese GE. 2005. *An Introduction to Efficiency and Productivity Analysis*, 2nd edn. New York: Springer. Pp. 289–310, pp. 76–7.

Cooper WW, Seiford LM, Tone K. 2007. *Data Envelopment Analysis: A Comprehensive Text with Models, Applications, References and DEA-Solver Software*, 2nd edn. New York: Springer. Pp. 328–47.

Ichimura K, Ishikawa K, Takanosawa M, Sejima T, Sato T, Makino N, Ishikawa T, Ohta Y, Ishida T. 2003. Present status of day-case nasal surgery in Japan. *Japanese Journal of Rhinology* 42: 138–45.

Ishi M. 2012. DRG/PPS and DPC/PDPS as prospective payment systems. *Japan Medical Association Journal* 55: 279–91.

Ikegami N, Yoo BK, Hashimoto H, Matsumoto M, Ogata H, Babazono A, Watanabe R, Shibuya K, Yang BM, Reich MR, Kobayashi Y. 2011. Japanese universal health coverage: evolution, achievements, and challenges. *Lancet* 378: 1106–14.

Nakata Y, Watanabe Y, Otake H, Nakamura T, Oiso G, Sawa T. 2015. Productivity change of surgeons in an academic year. *Journal of Surgical Education* 72: 128–34.

Nakata Y, Watanabe Y, Otake H, Nakamura T, Oiso G, Sawa T. 2015. The Japanese surgical reimbursement system fails to reflect resource utilization. *International Journal of Health Services* 45: 801–9.

Nakata Y, Yoshimura T, Watanabe Y, Otake H, Oiso G, Sawa T. 2015. Resource utilization in surgery after the revision of surgical fee schedule in Japan. *International Journal of Health Care Quality Assurance* 28: 635–43.

Nakata Y, Yoshimura T, Watanabe Y, Otake H, Oiso G, Sawa T. 2016. Japanese surgeons' productivity change after the revision of surgical fee schedule. *Operations Research for Health Care* 9: 1–6.

Nakata Y, Watanabe Y, Narimatsu H, Yoshimura T, Otake H, Sawa T. 2016. Surgeons' efficiency change is a major determinant of their productivity change. *International Journal of Health Care Quality Assurance* 29: 417–24.

Nakata Y, Watanabe Y, Narimatsu H, Yoshimura T, Otake H, Sawa T. 2017. Predictors of surgeons' efficiency in the operating rooms. *Health Services Management Research* 30: 16–21.

Nakata Y, Yoshimura T, Watanabe Y, Otake H, Oiso G, Sawa T. 2017. Efficiency of inpatient orthopedic surgery in Japan: a medical claims database analysis. *International Journal of Health Care Quality Assurance* 30: 506–15.

Pandit JJ. 2012. On statistical methods to test if sampling in trials is genuinely random. *Anaesthesia* 67: 456–62.

Watanabe Y, Nakata Y. 2018. Association between costs for outpatient orthopedic surgery and scale of healthcare facilities in Japan. *International Journal of Health Care Quality Assurance* 31: 265–72.

Web Resources

Healthcare finance in Japan: http://japanhpn.org/en/finan2/

DEA Solver tools: http://extras.springer.com/2007/978-0-387-45281-4/DEA-SOLVER-LV8(2014-12-05).xlsm (this is an Excel file that goes with the next resource)

http://extras.springer.com/2000/978-1-4757-8313-1/DEA-Solver-LV(V8)/SpringerLV8/User's_Guide_LV(V8).pdf

http://opensourcedea.org/

https://opensolver.org/dea-frontier-for-opensolver/

Operating Theatre Management in Two European Nations
The Netherlands and Switzerland

André van Zundert and Thomas Sieber

Overview

There is no common health service across Europe with many independent nations. This chapter introduces the state of theatre management in two countries. Similarities and differences can be seen with descriptions of operating room (OR) management in other chapters. However, the text underlines the fact that the principles presented in earlier chapters on assessing efficiency, productivity and scheduling are potentially very applicable.

The Netherlands

Introduction

The Netherlands has a population of ~17 million with just three cities of populations >500,000 (Rotterdam, Amsterdam and The Hague). All citizens are covered by a basic, compulsory health insurance scheme, currently with a fixed premium of €108/month per person (children are free of charge). On top of this basic premium there is a salary-dependent premium, deducted direct from income as tax. Those with a very limited income need only pay a very small contribution (e.g., €26/month). In essence this scheme means few people have to pay additional fees for most types of hospitalisation or surgery.

The healthcare insurer produces a list of procedures that are covered by the insurance. This list is available to patients. If covered, the insurer pays; if not, the patient pays (depending on the package that covers the insurance). Almost all care is covered except for contraceptive care, homeopathic care, dentistry and cosmetic/plastic surgery. There is optional private health coverage available on top of the mandatory level of insurance.

National statistics indicate ~1.5 million inpatient operations per year plus ~500,000 day case procedures. There are 82 'institutional' hospitals (i.e., owned by

not-for-profit companies), 8 academic centres and ~270 privately owned hospitals/day care centres, some of whom are listed on the stock market as business concerns (these range in size and by the specialties they manage). There are four large healthcare non-profit insurance companies who negotiate with individual hospitals for the type, quality and volume of surgical interventions, in the manner of a 'block contract'. Even smaller insurers are in a position to negotiate, as they may have clientele concentrated in a particular locality. One of the risks of such contracts is that of 'overperformance', where the hospital undertakes more procedures than contracted for; these extra procedures are not reimbursed. The contracts also provide reimbursement for achieving standards for proportions for inpatient surgery, unplanned admissions, length of stay, postoperative infections, death rate, re-admissions, etc. These standards are set by the government working in close cooperation with the medical specialist societies. There are additional standards for such quality measures set by the government via its regulators. The insurance companies also negotiate the price per intervention. Under the agreements there are clear incentives to achieve the quality goals, but also penalties for failing to do so. The total cost of all negotiated care may not increase more than the allowed budget increase.

The government, which is ultimately paying for healthcare via the mandatory insurance schemes, is able to set managed growth targets for the overall budget. For 2017, for example, the fiscal growth rate was set at 1%. Insurance companies can then apportion this rise (in spending or investment through the negotiated contracts) equally across all hospitals, or invest more in some hospitals or services than others. Companies are also at liberty to invest more in services than the 1% limit, but this will be at the expense of their own profits.

In addition to income from healthcare insurers like all other hospitals, academic hospitals also receive a budget from the ministries of education and health, and also any directly charged services for teaching or research (e.g., fee-paying students or research grants).

Hospitals allocate budgets to different departments, based on activity-based costing. This is the prerogative of the hospital executive director. Budgets for operating theatre are generally determined by hospitals on historic grounds, depending on volume of interventions and type (range) of surgical interventions.

Individual practitioners (surgeons or anaesthetists) work under contract to one hospital with broad parity across the specialties, with enhancements for on-call duties, administration or teaching. There are no enhancements for seniority per se. In the private sector, many physicians 'buy in' to their contract (termed a 'goodwill' payment), which is then returned on retirement or departure from the hospital. Each department works under a service level agreement (i.e., to deliver an agreed number of operations/procedures in a particular year). Private hospitals can be part-owned by doctors (up to 5% of the total share of hospital turnover in the Netherlands), so the budgetary negotiations in turn can determine their income. Academic contracts are somewhat different, being more dependent upon seniority and academic progression. Academic contracts will have time set aside for research and teaching, although the proportion depends both on the specialty and negotiations with the head of the department (who has to balance academic with service commitments). Because the only direct income for academic activity is via research grants (which are very limited by budgetary constraints), in essence academic work has to be undertaken as an investment by a department and as goodwill (i.e., for free) by the individuals undertaking it.

The Patient Pathway

Patients are referred to a hospital by their general practitioner (GP), except emergency cases that may enter a hospital directly via the emergency department. However, due to the overwhelming number of patients that attend the emergency departments in a hospital, a triage system has been set up, whereby both the GP and the hospital checks before a patient can be seen in the emergency department and/or needs to be admitted to the hospital. In fact, GPs are now sited within the hospital (emergency department) and are often the first 'check' for the patient.

There is a quality metric that waiting time to be seen by a specialist for elective surgery should be <3 weeks after referral by the GP, but wait times can be longer for some specialists due to demand. If the patient needs surgery, there is a second quality goal set at 7 weeks after booking for surgery. These wait times are publicly available, to help patients choose their specialist or hospital. Rarely, insurance companies can also use hospitals in neighbouring countries, if a waiting list is deemed too long.

The use of a preassessment anaesthesia clinic is universal, although the basic questionnaire can be completed online, sometimes with the help of the GP, or in the hospital the same day as the specialist consultation. Based on the questionnaire, the need for further assessment is filtered to either a nurse or an anaesthetist. Many hospitals use an electronic registration system that integrates the preassessment, the intraoperative and post-operative anaesthesia records. In such a system, the patient can submit a 'preadmission record', which includes, e.g., medical, surgical and family history, use of drugs and known allergies.

Operating Theatre Efficiency

Surgeons are allocated their fixed block times and try to fill out the list times with as many cases as possible, providing theatres with a list of patients that need surgery (akin to the 'typical UK NHS list' model discussed in earlier chapters). This list has to comply with certain guidelines and agreements regarding type and volume of surgery, and sufficient notice needs to be given for the operation to be performed. In turn, anaesthetists also enter details of their plans, which might assist scheduling (e.g., need for invasive monitoring, regional blocks), and any specialised equipment is also identified. In the Netherlands, all data about surgical interventions, e.g., arrival in holding, arrival in theatre, time-out, start of anaesthesia, start of surgery, end of surgery, end of anaesthesia, is registered in a central hospital system. Each week or month a summary is made with the mean operating times for each individual surgeon. The system can provide information about the mean operating time for a specific procedure by each individual surgeon. These mean times help inform the coordinators in their planning of the list (see following). However, two factors remain that limiting how effective this is in practice, both of which are addressed in Chapter 4 ('Case Scheduling'). One is that hitherto, the mean times have not been used along with standard deviations in a probabilistic manner to assist scheduling.

Second, no account has hitherto been made for non-Gaussian distributions or very uncommon procedures that make the mean alone a poor reflection of reality, as has been earlier discussed.

A floor coordinator theatre manager manages a team of several theatre head nurses (e.g., one nurse unit manager for surgery and one for anaesthesia). The coordinator makes up the operating theatre lists a week in advance, based on the known bookings and also manages any emergency cases. On the day of surgery this coordinator also troubleshoots by moving patients between theatres to maximise utilisation and prevents overruns or cancellations.

As in the United States, but in contrast to the United Kingdom, a single physician anaesthetist can supervise multiple (usually maximum two theatres, which are staffed by nurse anaesthetists, for suitable cases; otherwise a single physician anaesthetist will supervise only one theatre for a major case such as cardiac).

In principle, surgery has a dual management system: (a) 'medical', where a surgeon determines the resources needed to staff emergencies and ICU capacity, and (b) 'business', where a floor coordinator organises the day-to-day running of the resources. The floor coordinator has a good overview. They can shift patients to other theatres provided a surgical team is available to try to manage potential overruns. If that is not possible, patients may have to be cancelled (and scheduled by priority to the next available session – often the next day if the surgeon is available). Cancellation rates are generally 5–10%. Overall there is a pressure not to overrun theatres. Staff are entitled to both enhanced rates of overtime pay and time off in lieu to ensure they rest, and in any case cannot be compelled to stay late (notwithstanding the fact that staying to complete a case is sometimes unavoidable). Only limited use can be made of on-call staff to manage elective overruns, especially if the emergency commitment is large, as it can be in tertiary referral or trauma centres.

Operating teams are generally scheduled between 8 am and 5.30 pm. After 5.30 pm only very few operating theatres still carry on. The night shift team can take over both overrunning elective theatres and emergency cases. After 10 pm the number of active theatres is further reduced so that only one or possibly two teams are still working; after midnight there is generally only one team working. On average, out-of-hours teams probably spend ~70% of the time working between 5.30 pm and midnight, and much less thereafter. The floor coordinator will try to utilise any free space in elective lists with appropriate emergency cases to minimise the workload out of hours. Supporting nursing staff can either be in the hospital or be on-call from outside the hospital (provided they live within a reasonable distance to the hospital).

Bottlenecks and Pressures within the System

Perhaps the main pressure on operating theatres is lack of staff, especially nursing staff, which is itself due to a mix of factors such as constraints on training numbers and attempts by hospitals to save money by employing fewer staff. In part because of this, both post-anaesthesia care unit (PACU) and intensive care unit (ICU) capacity can be a rate-limiting step to smooth patient flow. In turn, these pressures have had increased waiting times for surgery over the years.

The future impetus is likely to be on increased day case surgery, a dedicated increase in ICU bed capacity and better triage by introducing a system of better categorisation, and hence prioritisation of emergency cases.

Switzerland

Introduction

As in the Netherlands, health insurance is compulsory for all Swiss residents (coverage is ~99.5%). Only international civil servants, members of permanent diplomatic missions and their family members are exempted from compulsory health insurance. However, they too can apply to join the Swiss health insurance system within 6 months of taking up residence in the country. Health insurance covers the costs of medical treatment and hospitalization of the insured; however only up to certain limits, and the insured person pays a part of the cost of treatment themselves. The insurance scheme is regarded as a vehicle for avoiding differential standards in healthcare, as the rules are the same throughout the country. Insurers are required to offer this basic insurance to everyone, regardless of age or medical condition. They are not allowed to make a profit from this basic insurance. They can, however, have varying prices on supplemental plans. Approximately 60 private insurance companies are competing to offer these services. Attempts to replace the private insurance system with a single federal insurer have been rejected several times by the Swiss public.

Overall, the Swiss health system is a variant of the highly government-regulated social insurance systems of Europe: private hospitals as well as non-profit health insurers are subject to uniform fee schedules and myriad government regulations for the basic services.

In summary, the insured person pays the insurance premium for the basic plan up to 8% of their personal income. If a premium is higher than this, the government gives the insured person a cash subsidy to pay for any additional premium. In contrast to the United States, where 90% of people get their insurance through their employers or government, in Switzerland everyone buys insurance for themselves. The universal compulsory coverage provides for treatment in case of illness or accident (unless another accident insurance provides the coverage) and pregnancy. The compulsory insurance can be supplemented by private 'complementary' insurance policies that allow for coverage of some of the treatment categories not covered by the basic insurance or to improve the standard of room and service in case of hospitalization. This can include dental treatment and private ward hospitalization, which are not covered by the compulsory insurance.

As far as the compulsory health insurance is concerned, the insurance companies cannot set any conditions relating to age, sex or state of health for coverage. Although the level of premium can vary from one company to another, they must be identical for all insured persons of the same age group and region, regardless of sex or state of health. This does not apply to complementary insurance, where premiums are risk-based. The insured person has full freedom of choice among the recognized healthcare providers competent to treat their condition on the understanding that the costs are covered by the insurance up to the level of the official tariff. There is freedom of choice when selecting an insurance company to which one pays a premium, usually on a monthly basis.

The Swiss healthcare system is, according to WHO, one of the most advanced healthcare systems worldwide, guarantees outstanding medical outcomes to a set standard across the entire country and therefore is often taken as a role model by other countries.

Hospitals are corporations overseen by boards of directors. Non-profit hospitals have boards that often consist of influential members of healthcare and local communities. Educationally affiliated hospitals are often overseen by universities. Therefore, university boards of trustees may double as the board of directors for a hospital. Multihospital systems, particularly for-profit ones, usually have one board of directors overseeing numerous facilities. Traditionally hospitals were organized according to three pillars: administration, nursing facilities and doctor services. Today, hospitals are mostly organised in a departmental structure corresponding to medical specialities. Operating theatres are rarely managed as a single entity, but instead split between different departments, usually surgery and anaesthesia. Therefore, the budget of the operating theatre is usually not managed separately but embedded in the larger budget of the hospital or the affiliated departments of surgery and anaesthesia. This makes it difficult or impossible to assess the operating theatre budget as an independent entity.

In the majority of Swiss hospitals, doctors are employed directly by the hospital. Only a minority of private hospitals have contracts with groups of doctors, e.g., anaesthesiologists or cardiac surgeons. The doctors employed by hospitals receive a basic salary, but most get additional variable reimbursements for treatment of patients for ambulatory care and for patients with additional private insurance plans. This variable part can often be much higher than the basic salary.

For outpatient services, there is a fee-for-service system in Switzerland that comprises dedicated amounts covering the infrastructure and doctor's fees. According to this reimbursement system there is an incentive for doctors to increase their service to patients, especially in the outpatient setting and with patients under private insurance plans.

A teaching hospital is a hospital or medical center that provides medical education and training to future and current health professionals. Teaching hospitals are affiliated with medical schools and work closely with medical students in many cases. Teaching hospitals also offer graduate medical education (GME)/physician residency programs, where medical school graduates train under a supervising physician to assist with the coordination of care. In addition to offering medical education to medical students and physician residents, many teaching hospitals also serve as research institutes.

Most university-affiliated hospitals offer some incentives for staff members involved in academic and teaching activities. These incentives are mostly nonfinancial and include educational opportunities, allotted teaching time, academic appointments and special recognition events. However, as in many other countries, university attending doctors are commonly later recruited by private hospitals due to more attractive financial compensation packages.

The Patient Pathway

The patient pathway from referral to surgery begins with the first contact with their primary care provider. This provider makes an assessment and discusses the best options with the patient, including whether to refer to a surgeon or interventionalist. Patients in Switzerland also have the option to directly contact a specialist such as a surgeon unless they are part of a restrictive healthcare plan that requires the gateway of a primary care physician before a referral to a specialist.

In contrast to the United States and the United Kingdom, where patients often just need a consent for the surgical procedure, a separate written consent for anaesthesia is needed in Switzerland. This consent used to be obtained the evening before surgery in inpatient services, but now there is a shift to preoperative screening clinics where patients get their consent for anaesthesia and/or surgery in an ambulatory setting days to weeks before the planned procedure. For minor surgery, especially in the outpatient setting, a consent for anaesthesia and/or surgery obtained just before the procedure is also acceptable.

Preoperative tests can be done by the primary care physicians, but more often this is done in the hospital according to guidelines issued by the anaesthesia department.

There are no published data on the average length of interval between referral and surgical procedure in Switzerland, but it is well known that this is usually no more than a few weeks for most procedures. For patients with additional private insurance coverage, this period can even be shorter, as they have more choice in selecting centres with even shorter waiting times. This is in stark contrast to countries with highly government-regulated healthcare systems, as Canada and the United Kingdom, where the wait for surgery can last months to even years depending on the procedure.

Managing Theatre Efficiency

It is generally recognised in Switzerland that the broad order of priority governing principles of OR managers should be:

1. Ensure patient safety and the highest quality of care.

2. Provide surgeons with appropriate access to the OR.
3. Maximize operating room utilization.
4. Manage staff and materials to reduce costs.
5. Decrease patient delays.
6. Enhance satisfaction among patients, staff and physicians.

It is notable that while maximizing efficiency (generally understood to relate to utilisation) is very important, this should not compromise patient safety and quality of care; therefore it shows up on the third position in the preceding list of priorities.

The concept of maximizing efficiency is understood to mean maximising the number of surgical cases that can be done on a given day while minimizing the required resources (personnel, materials). Therefore, the most commonly used parameters of efficiency include the following:

1. OR utilization. This is measured in two ways, A or B, that follow. First (A) is the proportion of time in total that the cases sum to (i.e., from time of arrival of the patient for start of anaesthesia, whether this is in OR or in an induction room):

   A: total hours of cases performed ÷ total hours of OR time allocated

   Or, B, the total time that the surgery occupies in the OR (i.e., in essence a statistic restricted to surgical 'cutting' time:

   B: total hours of 'patient in OR' ÷ total hours of OR time allocated

2. Block Utilization. This is a measure of the use of operating room time by a surgeon or group of surgeons to whom given blocks of time have been allocated.

3. Turnover Time. Different definitions exist. Measuring the gap between the time from the previous patient leaving the OR to when the next patient arrives in the OR recognises the time needed to anaesthetise the patient, and any delays are due to factors like portering or transfer from the ward. Measuring the time from end of the previous surgical procedure to the start of next surgical procedure regards anaesthesia as part of the 'gap'.

4. Start times. The proportion of the first cases in each OR that start on time is measured (but not always the extent of delay, and also no account is taken of the possibility that some cases start early).

5. Cancellation Rate: Cancellation on the day of surgery.

The Swiss definitions may differ from those used in other countries, therefore direct comparisons may not be possible.

Theatre Scheduling

In a hospital with an established form of OR management, scheduling is in accordance with a set of local rules agreed upon by all the stakeholders in the OR, i.e., surgery, anaesthesia and nursing. These rules will be centre-specific and cover issues pertaining to short, mid-term and long-term OR planning (e.g., which specialty should take priority in access to certain theatres), or planning on the day of surgery (e.g., which cases should take priority or in which order on any given day; whether inclusion of emergency cases should occur or if cases should be added onto which OR); or OR processes (such as rules governing the transport of patients to and from theatres, timing and type of premedication, positioning of patients. These local rules will also determine the definition of process time stamps for audit and data collection (see 'Managing Theatre Efficiency' section, earlier).

It is common practice to allocate operating room time slots to individual surgical services or individual surgeons. Allocation of operating room slots is usually based on historical data of usage of the according discipline. This allocation is reviewed and adjusted on a regular basis as workload of some specialties declines and others rises.

If these OR rules are respected, then scheduling of single surgical procedures in the allotted time slot can be accomplished by the individual surgical services or surgeons or their secretaries. Some hospitals have opted for a centralized office for booking of individual surgical cases, managing all the required paperwork for individual patient scheduling.

While the overall goal of OR planning should be to minimize cancellation of elective surgical procedures on the day of surgery due to a late-running OR schedule, sometimes the dilemma arises that an OR is overrunning and there are remaining cases. If the cancellation of an elective case is the result of an emergency surgical procedure, then it is easier to accept, but institutions with a high proportion of emergency cases understand the need to plan their elective cases accordingly.

If cases do run late, there are three options to consider, used in the following order:

1. Staff are asked to work overtime until elective cases are finished.
2. The emergency team takes over the late-running elective cases.
3. The last elective case is cancelled.

If late-running elective cases are the exceptions rather than the rule, then staff are generally prepared to work overtime and finish the cases. However, in centres where tardiness has become the norm, this policy is unsustainable. Using emergency teams is always problematic due to their commitment to other, emergency, cases.

On the other hand, if allotted surgical time is not used on some lists, the local OR rules usually allow defining a time point at which the unused time slot is released to other surgical services. This mitigates against late running and cancellation.

Bottlenecks and Pressures within the System

Bottlenecks can be found in different areas, depending on the hospital setting. Institutions with elective cases exclusively are the easiest to manage and to eliminate bottlenecks, and downstream resources such as access to PACU/ICU beds and ward bed capacity have to be aligned with the caseload coming from the OR. However, quantitative algorithms for how to achieve such alignment are absent, and decisions are made on qualitative judgements.

It is a different story in hospitals with variable caseload and trauma centers. Trauma centers usually set aside OR slots during the day and night to accommodate emergency cases. Some trauma centers with a significant seasonality in emergencies, such as those situated close to a winter sports area, usually adjust their time slots accordingly, offering more emergency slots in the high season. PACU beds are usually not the bottlenecks in Switzerland, but rather ICU beds in major hospitals with surgeries relying on postoperative ICU treatment can be rate-limiting. Because there is a trend to ever-shorter duration of hospital stay, beds on the ward are usually also not the bottlenecks of the system.

The most pressing problem in the context of theatre management in Switzerland is certainly the shortage of staff, especially in OR nursing. It is not uncommon that hospitals are not able to run all the scheduled operating theatres due to lack of staffing.

The percentage of non-Swiss nationals working in the healthcare business is high, with nurses and with doctors, which is not only due to staff shortages but also due to higher salaries paid in Switzerland, compared with many surrounding EU countries.

The second-most-pressing problem is the lack of managerial resources for the important task of management and coordination of the OR activities. There are far too many institutions in Switzerland that do not have dedicated OR management. In 2016 a group of interested anaesthesiologists and OR managers founded a society for OR management in Switzerland to bring together people with diverse backgrounds but sharing a common interest. It is too early to say whether this society is able to advance its goal of increasing the knowledge and application of OR management in this country.

A third problem probably lies with the reimbursement system itself. The fee for service system in the ambulatory setting for most procedures is much less favourable than the reimbursement system for inpatient services. As a consequence, the shift to a higher proportion of ambulatory procedures as happened in many countries has not yet materialised in Switzerland

to the same extent, and to this extent the situation resembles that in Japan (see Chapter 10).

In terms of solutions to these problems and pressures, perhaps most important would be the introduction of formal or professional OR management that puts the focus on the objective, rational coordination of all activities in the OR to increase efficiency. Ideally this would be coupled with more effective information and data management systems.

In turn this would make important the need for standardisation, not only in terms of material and medications or procedures but also in terms of measurement of processes and outcomes. Standardisation has a positive impact on productivity as well as on safety and should therefore be on any task list of hospital administration. Many of the chapters in this book therefore offer a way forward to achieve this goal.

A third step to increase overall theatre efficiency would be centralisation of services in Switzerland, with the closure of smaller hospitals, which would allow cost savings to be made, as well as allow improved emergency surgical facilities with round-the-clock coverage for wider parts of the population.

Appendix 11A: Short Case Studies of Some Common OR Management Problems in Switzerland

Example 1

A surgeon schedules an elective case at 2 pm, despite his available operating theatre slot starting at 11 am. He argues that a rescheduled meeting would not allow him an earlier start. Starting the case at 2 pm would keep the operating theatre with all its personnel idle for 3 hours.

The OR management is able to use the local policy to dictate the choices that (a) the procedure should be done at the correct time of 11 am by this surgeon (e.g., the surgeon could send a substitute to the meeting), (b) at the correct time of 11 am by another surgeon (e.g., of the same team) or (c) the case would have to be cancelled and the list offered to another specialty service.

Example 2

The hospital administration questions the performance in operating theatres due to excessively long turn-over times between cases.

The OR management team performs an in-depth analysis using principles outlined in Chapters 2 and 3). They conclude that (a) efficiency (assessed by ε; Chapter 2) is acceptable, with good utilisation and few overruns or cancellations, even with the putatively long turnovers; (b) significant additional investment will be needed to reduce the turnover times (e.g., additional portering staff, extending hours of work for ward staff); (c) although turnover times would be reduced (but not eliminated), the time saved would be insufficient to include an additional case. In other words, productivity (as measured by Φ; Chapter 3) would not be increased. All that would result is early finishes, which, although welcome, would be unnecessary.

Moreover, attempts to schedule additional cases would then likely result in overrun with attendant increased overtime costs, or cancellation on the day of surgery.

The OR management in this way successfully challenges the interpretation of its performance.

Bibliography

Dexter F, Abouleish AE, Epstein RH, Whitten CW, Lubarsky DA. 2003. Use of operating room information system data to predict the impact of reducing turnover times on staffing costs. *Anesthesia & Analgesia* 97: 1119–26.

Dexter F, Wachtel RE, Epstein RH. 2016. Decreasing the hours that anesthesiologists and nurse anesthetists work late by making decisions to reduce the hours of over-utilized operating room time. *Anesthesia & Analgesia* 122: 831–42.

Ehrenfeld JM, Dexter F, Rothman BS, et al. 2013. Case cancellation rates measured by surgical service differ whether based on the number of cases or the number of minutes cancelled. *Anesthesia & Analgesia* 117: 711–16.

Fong AJ, Smith M, Langerman A. 2016. Efficiency improvement in the operating room. *Journal of Surgical Research* 204: 371–83.

Macario A, Vitez TS, Dunn BA. 1995. Where are the costs in perioperative care? Analysis of hospital costs and charges for inpatient surgical care. *Anesthesiology* 83: 1138–44.

Meeusen V, van Zundert A, Hoekman J, Kumar C, Rawal N, Knape H. 2010. Composition of the anaesthesia team: a European survey. *European Journal of Anaesthesiology* 27: 773–9.

Overdyk FJ, Harvey SC, Fishman RL, Shippey F. 1998. Successful strategies for improving operating room efficiency at academic institutions. *Anesthesia & Analgesia* 86: 896–906.

Chapter 12

Operating Theatre Management in Australia

André Van Zundert

Introduction

Australia is a very large island continent consisting of six states and two territories. Each of these has their own healthcare system, within a very federalised structure; hence, to talk about theatre management 'in Australia' is a necessary generalisation. Most people (84%) live in state/territory capital cities, i.e., generally within 50 km of the coast. The total population is ~25 million, which includes an indigenous Aboriginal and Torres Strait Islander people (totalling ~700,000) who have their own specific health problems. Notably, as many as one in four residents of Australia have been born overseas (that number is even higher for the parents of currently resident Australians).

There are some ~ 110,000 doctors with ~5,000 anaesthetists, intensivists and pain physicians). There are ~753 public hospitals and ~573 private hospitals. The majority of beds are in hospitals in the more densely populated areas with the largest public hospital having >1,000 beds (e.g., Royal Brisbane and Women's Hospital [RBWH]), but over 70% of hospitals have <50 beds; some states like Queensland have a large number of facilities with <10 beds.

The public expenditure on health services stands at ~AUS$ 42 billion (about £24 billion or ~3% of gross domestic product, or about ~AUS$ 2,000 per person). Hospital spending has been increasing faster than inflation at ~5% each year between 2004 and 2009.

The staffing mix in private hospitals is somewhat different from that in public hospitals because most medical services are not provided by hospital employees (but rather by specialist staff with practising privileges), and the range of services provided is different.

Public and private hospitals are funded from a range of different sources, reflecting the types of patients they treat and the services they provide. Governments mainly fund emergency department and outpatient services, whereas elective patient services are commonly funded by private (nongovernment)

sources, as well as by government sources. It is important to emphasise between the *original* sources of funding versus *immediate* sources. The Australian government makes indirect contributions to public hospitals via the Australian Health Care Agreements, via funds provided to state and territory governments for their spending on public hospitals. The Australian government is also regarded as the source of funds for contributions to private hospitals via the private health insurance premium rebates, although immediate sources of funding are the health insurance funds of their members. Some patients pay directly due to gaps in insurance coverage or because of no insurance at all.

Private funding of health services completely independent of government constitutes only ~5% of the market. Even in private hospitals, ~40% of funding is ultimately via government sources.

From the patients' perspective, all citizens and eligible residents (i.e., permanent visa holders) are covered by Medicare, which provides care free at the point of delivery in public hospitals and for emergency care. Or, patients can opt for private insurance care packages, giving them a wider choice of hospitals and services.

Staff (surgeons and anaesthetists) are paid a regular salary in public hospitals, but operate on a fee-for-service basis in the private sector. Staff members in the public sector are allowed to work part-time in the private sector, although the details of how these arrangements work can vary across the country. Often, staff may work privately 'in their own time' but sometimes need the permission of their primary employer to do so. Very rarely some private, nonpublic hospitals directly employ staff (including part-employment of staff otherwise committed to the public sector). Some major public hospitals (and rarely some private hospitals) include the role of an academic/university hospital and have integrated teaching and research programs, often in partnership with a university. Incentives are provided for nonclinical time for teaching, research and organisational duties through university appointments.

There are ~8.5 million episodes of admitted patient care annually in Australian hospitals, ~ 60% in public and ~40% in private hospitals, some two-thirds of these being same-day episodes. About a fifth of these are surgical episodes.

The growing role for private hospitals in Australia's health system has been supported by the Australian government through measures such as the Private Health Insurance Rebate and reflected in the inclusion of private hospitals in national performance monitoring initiatives such as those of the National Healthcare Agreement, the National Health Priority Initiative (see: www.aph.gov.au) and in the Performance and Accountability Framework of the National Health Reform Agreement (see Council of Australian Governments, COAG, at www.coag.gov.au).

Private hospitals are generally grouped into those hospitals that provide services on a day-only basis (free-standing day hospital facilities, or 'day hospitals') and those that provide overnight care (referred to here as 'overnight hospitals'). This distinction reflects that, under state and territory regulatory arrangements, overnight care requires the provision of 24-hour qualified nursing care that permits a broader range of medical and surgical procedures to be undertaken. Some hospitals offering overnight care also provide same-day services.

Private hospitals are those that are owned and managed by private organisations, whether for-profit or not-for-profit. Private hospitals can fall into several 'ownership' types according to whether they are for-profit or not-for-profit (the latter being charitable or religious foundations).

In many instances, public and private hospitals do not operate in isolation from each other, but instead provide healthcare services in a coordinated manner. Interactions between public and private hospitals include contracted care arrangements, colocation and resource sharing and private-sector involvement in hospital infrastructure development for public patients. More details on these arrangements are provided in the next section. In some circumstances, hospitals provide care to admitted patients through interhospital contracted care arrangements, in which the care is organised and paid for by one hospital but provided by another. *Ad hoc* arrangements between hospitals can also exist (e.g., agreements to share equipment, which does not require actual payments for each instance).

Individual patients can also use their private insurance policies within the public sector.

Private-Sector Funding

The Australian private reimbursement system is complex. Medicare is Australia's federal-funded insurer, and doctors are offered financial rebates for private-sector services in line with a complicated 'relative value', unit-based Medicare Benefits Schedule. Doctors receive 75% of the government-determined schedule fee from Medicare, with another 25% at least being provided by the patient's own separate private insurer (if they have one). Australian private insurers provide 'no-gap' or 'known-gap' schemes, which offer rebates in excess of the government's Medicare Benefits Schedule fees when certain criteria are met (e.g., including limiting fees to the insurer's own limits). Doctors can charge more than the published fees and ask for shortfall payments direct from their patients, but this is common only in major cities. Naturally, doctors have been critical of the government's failure to increase reimbursement rates.

The Patient Pathway

Generally patients first consult a general practitioner, who makes a referral as appropriate to a public or private surgeon, subject to the patient insurance status. In the public sector patients are placed on a waiting list for an outpatient appointment and in turn, depending on need for surgery, on a surgical waiting list (Figure 12.1).

In the private sector the pathway depends entirely on the surgeon to whom the referral is made as to how long the patient needs to wait and what happens. Some private hospitals do not take any emergency or complex patients (as funding for critical care may not be provided by insurance) and factors such as these can dictate the ultimate pathway the patient enters.

Tactical Management in Theatres

Generally there is an operating room (OR) manager, who is responsible for the smooth running of lists. This may vary substantially from a major role to a minor role, depending on the size of hospital, the local agreements in place or the state/territory in which the hospital is based, and also roles may differ in private versus public hospitals. Quantitative information is available on key statistics like the arrival

Preoperative   Intraoperative   Post-operative

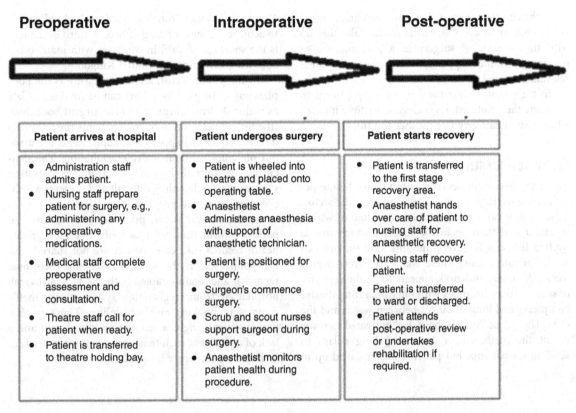

Patient arrives at hospital	Patient undergoes surgery	Patient starts recovery
• Administration staff admits patient. • Nursing staff prepare patient for surgery, e.g., administering any preoperative medications. • Medical staff complete preoperative assessment and consultation. • Theatre staff call for patient when ready. • Patient is transferred to theatre holding bay.	• Patient is wheeled into theatre and placed onto operating table. • Anaesthetist administers anaesthesia with support of anaesthetic technician. • Patient is positioned for surgery. • Surgeon's commence surgery. • Scrub and scout nurses support surgeon during surgery. • Anaesthetist monitors patient health during procedure.	• Patient is transferred to the first stage recovery area. • Anaesthetist hands over care of patient to nursing staff for anaesthetic recovery. • Nursing staff recover patient. • Patient is transferred to ward or discharged. • Patient attends post-operative review or undertakes rehabilitation if required.

Figure 12.1 Typical patient pathway in Australian hospitals (adapted from the Queensland Public Hospital Operating Theatre Efficiency Report, 2016).

time of the patient, the start of anaesthesia, start of surgery, WHO time-out procedure, surgery finish time, anaesthesia finish time, patient leaving theatre time, etc. There is a requirement for the OR manager to make an annual report to the hospital board. Thus efficiency is well understood at operational level (see Appendix 12A). An efficient OR is generally regarded as one in which a prebooked list of patients is known in advance to the whole team (surgeons, anaesthetists, nurses), who can then plan in advance (e.g., for special equipment/radiology). The OR manager's planning in this regard is assisted by an overall 'floor coordinator' in operating theatres (planner), who oversees and seeks clarification from the operating surgeon if there are any doubts.

Theatre nursing staff receive a list of operations, according to a specific specialty – with surgeons allocated to that list, with special requirements (special table, X-rays, special equipment), and particular information about the patient (name, hospital number, gender, age, DOB, ward, admit type, class, operation code, operation descriptors, special equipment, surgeon, allocated anaesthetist, type of anaesthesia).

In the public sector, the large volumes of cases require a weekly program to be made up in advance, and 'hot spots' are identified/addressed by different specialties. However, as the Queensland Operating Theatre Report (Queensland Audit Office, 2016) makes clear, the success of these existing organisational arrangements leaves much to be desired, much as in the UK NHS (see Appendix 12A).

In the private sector, usually, a list is allocated to a particular surgeon for that day or a half day. In small units and the private sector, cases may be booked individually by surgeon (as in 'a typical US list' discussed in earlier chapters).

In the public sector, the norm is that if a list overruns, the allocated anaesthetist completes the case. However, the OR floor coordinators do cancel cases as dependent on the availability of nursing staff's, surgeons', or anaesthetists' ability to stay late. Other options provide an anaesthetist-on-duty to cover the emergency list. If a surgeon repeatedly over-books lists, then the OR manager can take this up with the director of surgery as a performance or behavioural issue. Appendix 12A illustrates some relevant data and statistics.

In the private sector there is naturally a norm to complete the whole list, regardless of the time it takes, which may mean very late finishes to ORs.

Current Pressures

There are several bottlenecks within the system, especially for a tertiary hospital. First, in the public sector, patients wait both for the initial consultation with a specialist and then again for surgery, which means waiting lists can be several months long (in contrast to the private sector, where waits are rarely over a week). Another bottleneck appears to be the very size of some tertiary hospitals with huge operating theatre complexes and long distances between wards and the ORs. The use of 'holding bays' has mitigated to some extent the inefficiencies caused by long delays in sending for patients, but patients can be called up to 45 min in advance from the ward to the holding bay to achieve smooth running of lists. A third bottleneck is the shortage of staff, in common with many other countries, including the United Kingdom.

In the public sector, another pressure is the poor planning of surgical lists. Lists can be finalised as late as within 24 hr of surgery, and for 'urgent bookables' (the list agreed upon to operate patients the following day) it frequently happens that adjustments are made out of hours, without wider consultation. The deficiency of overall hospital electronic registration systems make scheduling difficult and presents a technological barrier to progress.

In the private sector, pressures include 'silos' of patient information, with lack of integrated private health records (i.e., case records are not shared with the public sector; the specialist keeping their own records), and again coupled with the lack of overall hospital electronic registration system means inefficiencies in booking and scheduling. There is also, perhaps surprisingly, a reliance on casual staff and a lack of equipment such that equipment often needs to be loaned from larger hospitals.

Appendix 12A: Data from Queensland Audit Office

In 2016 the State of Queensland produced a comprehensive report on operating theatres (see Bibliography). Almost all the themes reflect chapters in this book, relating to the problems of balancing the following: utilisation, cancellation, overrunning, cost, staffing, etc. However, the report offers few if any solutions and has several important shortcomings, in the sense of not reflecting existing literature. For example, there is no academic paper referred to, and the report lacks a reference list, giving the false impression that the arguments in the report are entirely novel or created de novo. Some comparative data for New South Wales and Victoria are presented, along with the main measures they aspire to for theatre performance. This underlines the federalised (i.e., state/territory) nature of the Australian health system and also reflects how different localities prioritise different things.

Critique of the Report

Efficiency and Productivity

While the report correctly makes a distinction between 'efficiency' and 'productivity' (along similar lines explained in Chapters 2 and 3), it wrongly suggests there is no definition of efficiency (overlooking details of Chapter 2 and efficiency measured as ε). Rather, the report seeks to define efficiency as (a) starting on time, (b) reducing gap times, (c) maximising utilisation and (d) minimising cancellation. We have already seen in previous chapters of this book that both starting on time and reducing gap times should only rarely be the prime focus of investment or corrective action; rather, both these things, if awry, are to be best regarded as symptoms. Indeed, the report's own data show that mean gap times between surgeries are generally 15–10 min, which in fact does not seem excessive. Reducing cancellation rates is unobjectionable (the Queensland data suggest on-the-day cancellations running at up to ~7%), but

maximising utilisation as a goal fails to appreciate the detrimental effects of late finishes.

Starting on Time

Another shortcoming is that the reference point for the definition of 'starting on time' is taken as the patient being 'wheeled into theatre'. As we have already seen in Chapter 2 any 'start time' is by definition arbitrary, and what is really needed to make progress is displaying the data on the distribution of start times (see Figure 2.12 in Chapter 2). An omission is that the report does not countenance the possibility that some theatres in Queensland may have started early. Put simply, assigning 'wheeling in time' as the start time automatically means that those cases needing long anaesthesia times (i.e., long cases where invasive monitoring lines, epidurals for pain relief, difficult airway cases) are all starting 'late'.

Much of the tone of the report, reflective as it is of current theatre management thinking in Australia, resembles the dilemmas faced in the UK NHS. There are several other interesting points to note from the report, discussed next.

Staffing Policies

Hospitals assign anaesthetic and nursing staff to theatres using one of two approaches: (a) in teams linked to a specialty, allowing staff to develop rapport and skill sets within a single theatre team and (b) random approach, based on staff availability, with focus on ensuring staff have broad skills to be used flexibly.

Managing Theatre Costs

Theatres costs AUS$ 2.039 billion per year with 504,000 hours of theatre capacity budgeted; making theatre costs ~AUS$ 67/min (£39/min), which is perhaps a little higher (but not unreasonably wider than) than the estimate of £16–20/min often used for the United Kingdom. As shown in Chapter 7, budgeting

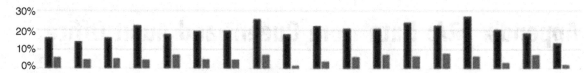

Figure 12.2 Data from one Queensland hospital. The *y*-axis is the percentage of operating lists exhibiting a serious overrun of >60 min of the scheduled time (black bars). Also shown (grey bars) is the proportion of these that started late. Each block represents one month of data 2015–16. Plot redrawn from data in the Queensland report (see Bibliography).

of theatres is complex, and the Queensland figure might include factors not generally included in the United Kingdom, but the difference is relatively small.

It is particularly interesting that the description of the Queensland Efficient Price (QEP) as an arbitrary tariff to help drive efficient practice so closely resembles the Payment by Results system (PBR) in the UK NHS, described in Chapter 7. That chapter explained how PBR was not, in fact, rewarding efficient practice, and correspondingly the report highlights that only five of sixteen hospital services in Queensland provide surgical services at or below the QEP. The concern arises that (as for the UK tariff), the Queensland tariff as it is calculated will not cover theatre costs.

In an example given in the report, it is stated that a gall bladder operation (known mean duration 90 min, plus ~10 min of gap time) will accrue income according to the formula of AUS$ 3,736 for the operative time component. However, if theatres cost AUS$ 67/min then even when a gall bladder is performed efficiently it will cost AUS$ 6,700; i.e., almost twice as much. This difference – even by the example given for a common operation – is huge. And even if the lower figure of approximately half the theatre cost estimate is used, to bring calculations in parallel with the United Kingdom, calculations only just break even. In other words the analysis of Chapter 7 would seem valid for Queensland.

Some Data Patterns

Although the bulk of the Queensland report focuses on underused theatre time, Figure 12.2 confirms that for a very large proportion of operating lists in fact the main problem is persistent overrunning (which as we have seen is predominantly due to overbooking rather than unpredicted overruns). Moreover, it is only a small percentage of these overruns that are associated with a late start (i.e., as we discussed in Chapter 2, prompt starts may not guarantee a finish to time). By contrast, data from this same hospital shown in Figure 12.2 showed that 10–20%

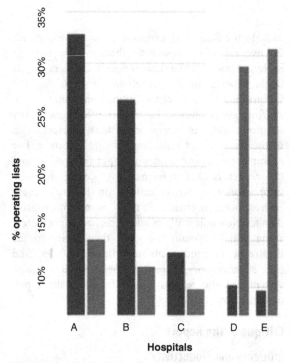

Figure 12.3 Data from three hospitals (A–C) in Queensland over one year showing that the proportion of lists overrunning by >60 mins (black bars) greatly exceeds those underrunning (grey bars). Note, however, that there is considerable variation in this outcome: two further hospitals D and E (smaller units) show the reverse pattern.

of lists underran by >60 mins (i.e., fewer than overran; Figure 12.3)

Bibliography

Australian Government. 2009. Medicare Benefits Schedule. Available at: www.health.gov.au/internet/mbsonline/publishing.nsf/Content/Downloads-200911.

Australian Government. 2009. Productivity Commission. Public and Private Hospitals: Productivity Commission Research Report. Available at: www.pc.gov.au/__data/assets/pdf_file/0015/93030/hospitals-report.pdf.

Ben-Tovim DI, Bassham JE, Bolch D, Martin MA, Dougherty M, Szwarcbord M. 2007. Lean thinking across a hospital: redesigning care at the Flinders Medical Centre. *Australian Health Reviews* 31: 10–5.

Cegan PC. 2005. The easiest cut: managing elective surgery in the public sector. *Medical Journal of Australia* 182: 605–6.

Lawrentschuk N, Hewitt PM, Pritchard MG. 2003. Elective laparoscopic cholecystectomy: implications of prolonged waiting times for surgery. *Australian and New Zealand Journal of Surgery* 73: 890–3.

McIntosh C, Dexter F, Epstein RH. 2006. Impact of service-specific staffing, case scheduling, turnovers, and first-case starts on anesthesia group and operating room productivity: tutorial using data from an Australian hospital. *Anesthesia and Analgesia* 103:1499–516.

Queensland Audit Office. 2015–2016. *Queensland Public Hospital Operating Theatre Efficiency*. Brisbane: Queensland Audit Office.

Schofield WN, Rubin G, Piza M et al. 2005. Cancellation of operations on the day of intended surgery at a major Australian referral hospital. *Medical Journal of Australia* 182: 612–5.

Winch S, Henderson AJ. 2009. Making cars and making health care: a critical review. *Medical Journal of Australia* 191: 28–9.

Wu R. 2005. Cancellation of operations on the day of surgery at a major Australian referral hospital. *Medical Journal of Australia* 183: 551.

Operating Theatre Management in the United States

Emily B. Goldenberg and Alex Macario

Introduction

Healthcare in the United States is a complicated and expensive effort provided by a number of organisations, both public and private. According to 2016 data 36% of Americans received healthcare via one of several publicly funded programs (see Kaiser Family Foundation, 2016). Medicare covers adults >65 years of age, people with qualifying disabilities and those with end-stage renal disease. Medicaid aims to provide coverage for low-income adults, children, pregnant women and those with certain disabilities. It is the single largest source of coverage in the United States. The Veterans Health Administration (VHA) serves nine million American military veterans. There are other government health programs in the United States including the Military Health System, providing healthcare to active duty military personnel and their dependents, and the Indian Health System, serving Native American tribes and Alaska Natives. The majority of the private health insurance coverage in the United States is employer-sponsored. It may cover employees, their spouses and their dependents. The premiums are shared by the employer and the employee. Depending on the employer, there are typically a variety of health insurance options, including a more expensive but more flexible preferred provider organisation (PPO) plan and a more affordable but slightly more restrictive health maintenance organisation (HMO) plan. Approximately 7% of Americans purchase their own private, nongroup coverage (Kaiser Family Foundation, 2016).

Before 2013 when the Affordable Care Act (ACA) began to take effect, >44 million Americans lacked health insurance because they did not qualify for public insurance or could not afford the private options available to them. The uninsured rate decreased from 16% to ~10% after the inception of the ACA, largely due to expansion of Medicaid coverage in certain states (Antonisse et al., 2017). Despite improving access to insurance coverage, US healthcare spending continues to rise. In 2015, healthcare spending reached almost $10,000 per person (National Health Expenditure Accounts Fact Sheet, 2018).

The majority of hospitals in the United States are community hospitals. This category includes general facilities as well as those that offer specialty care such as obstetrics and gynaecology, otolaryngology, orthopaedics and rehabilitation. Academic medical centers and other teaching hospitals are usually considered community hospitals: ~59% are non-profit organisations, whereas ~21% are for-profit. The remaining ~20% are state or local government community hospitals. A much smaller proportion of hospitals are psychiatric, long-term care or federal hospitals, which are typically military hospitals, not open to the general public (see Fast Facts on US Hospitals, 2018).

Surgical-Anaesthetic Costs and Practise Structures

It is difficult to quantify the cost of surgery in the United States because charges are often divided into hospital expenses, physician payments and postsurgical care costs. In addition, these charges vary based on geographic location of the hospital. Data from the Blue Cross and Blue Shield Association (an insurance provider that covers ~33% of Americans) reported that the average price for knee replacement surgery was ~$30,000 in 2015. Yet in Dallas, Texas, the price varied between $17,000 and $62,000 depending on the hospital (Millman, 2015). Medicare and Medicaid reimbursements are fixed, whereas private insurance companies generally negotiate their fees in advance. The discounts to hospital charges will vary based on these negotiations. Amounts will differ for people who pay out-of-pocket, without insurance coverage.

Generally there are three practise options for anaesthesiologists in the United States: (a) academic practise at a teaching hospital, (b) private practise or

(c) practise as an employee of a healthcare system or hospital. Pay structures vary depending on the practise.

Anaesthesiologists in academic practise are often employees of a group comprised of either the entire department or all faculty physicians practising at the institution. Billing and collections for services rendered are negotiated by the hospital, and predetermined salaries are paid either as a negotiated dollar amount or based on volume (Eichhorn & Grider, 2013). At some academic institutions, faculty may also receive an academic salary, which attempts to compensate for nonclinical pursuits such as teaching and/or research endeavours.

In private practise, anaesthesiologists may practise completely independently by making themselves available to surgeons on an individual basis and awaiting requests for anaesthesia services. Billing and collections may be done by the individual physician or by contracting with an outside billing service. Nowadays this individual model is less common. Most anaesthesiologists in private practise belong to a private group that has agreements with community hospitals and/or outpatient surgery suites. Billing and collections are managed by the group's administrative staff; clinical assignments and call responsibilities rotate among members of the group. Take-home pay varies based on case volume. Junior members of the group often forgo a percentage of their earned billing to the group's more senior partners. Junior physicians may or may not have the option of buying into the group to become a partner after a few trial years. Depending on the state or region of the country, anaesthesiologists may work alone caring for one patient at a time or cover multiple operating rooms by supervising nurse anaesthetists and/or anaesthesia assistants. In any event, the responsibilities are nearly all clinical with little time or financial reward for nonclinical work.

More recently, independent private practise anaesthesia groups have seen significant changes to their structures. Many groups have merged with other practise groups in their geographic areas, while others have partnered with regional or national companies, often tied to private equity investment firms. In doing so partners usually receive a large upfront payment in exchange for their ownership stakes. Future growth may result in increased profit-sharing among members of the group. As they grow and become more influential providers in the healthcare market, these groups may be able to arrange more favourable contracts with

payers. The administrative responsibilities can be efficiently managed by a central office, and information technology (IT) infrastructure can be shared. Having a larger pool of anaesthesia providers results in greater flexibility and the ability to adapt to staffing needs at multiple facilities. While some anaesthesiologists may benefit from these changes, others have left their old groups before or soon after large takeovers. Physicians have cited decreased income, less flexibility and lack of appreciation when part of such a large group.

A third practise option exists. As an employee of a healthcare system or hospital, anaesthesiologists generally negotiate a salary or agree to what is offered to their colleagues. In return for a consistent income, benefits (health insurance, paid vacation, retirement contributions) and a more predictable schedule, the employer can guarantee the availability of anaesthesia services (Eichhorn & Grider, 2013). In the United States, anaesthesiologists may be employees of Veterans Affairs (VA) hospitals, health maintenance organisations (HMOs) such as Kaiser Permanente or a local government community hospital such as Los Angeles County Medical Center.

Billing for anaesthesia services is based on 'units', which account for both time and case complexity. Every surgical procedure that requires anaesthesia is associated with a base number of units. Beyond the base, additional units accrue for each 15-minute interval in which the anaesthesia provider is involved in patient care. Additional units are added for higher-acuity patients, in other words for American Society of Anesthesiologists (ASA) physical classification 3 or higher or emergency procedures, as well as for invasive procedures such as arterial lines, central lines or regional blocks for post-operative pain control. The dollar value of a unit varies widely across the country. Based on this complicated billing mechanism, charges are submitted to insurance companies. Public payers such as Medicare pay at set, nonnegotiable rates, whereas private insurers may negotiate payments with individual hospitals or groups. It is feasible that any charges not covered by the insurer ultimately become the patient's responsibility.

Place of Academia and Training

Academic medical centers in the United States train resident and fellow physicians, conduct research and provide clinical care to improve the health of the communities they serve. Medicare is the largest financial supporter of graduate medical education (GME), and the amount of Medicare GME payments a teaching hospital receives depends on the number of the hospital's inpatients who are Medicare beneficiaries (see Association of American Medical Colleges, 2013). Other grant programs from the VHA, Department of Defense, Medicaid and the Public Health Service provide some support, but the majority of the cost of graduate medical education lies with the academic medical center itself.

The ten highest-rated hospitals in the United States, according to the most recent *U.S. News & World Report* rankings, are all academic medical centers with very similar missions. In addition to providing the highest-quality patient care, all of these institutions value education and research as essential components of their overall missions. Continuing to provide quality care and making new discoveries in scientific research and clinical practise depends on educating and training new scientists and physicians. These institutions, as well as other US academic medical centers, understand the significant roles they play in caring for the communities they serve and the intangible value of prioritising education and research (Table 13.1).

The Patient Pathway

At an academic medical center with a well-established preanaesthesia clinic, patients are referred by their surgeons prior to surgery. Some hospitals have policies in place by which all surgical patients must be evaluated by the preanaesthesia clinic before surgery. However, most institutions leave this decision to the discretion of the surgeons. As many studies have shown that preoperative clinics decrease operating room cancellations, it is clearly to the surgeons' advantage to refer patients to the preoperative clinic. There they are evaluated by a physician, nurse practitioner and/or registered nurse depending on how the clinic is staffed. Based on each patient's comorbidities and proposed surgery, additional studies may be needed. Blood tests, electrocardiograms (ECG), chest x-rays and other imaging may be obtained during a preanaesthesia clinic visit. Some institutions will have the ability to obtain studies conducted outside the institution, so as to avoid repetition. Patients who have established care with specialists in their communities may be referred back to their cardiologists, pulmonologists or endocrinologists, for example, for additional testing or medication management when deemed appropriate by the preanaesthesia clinic. If additional testing such as echocardiograms, cardiac stress testing or pulmonary function testing is deemed necessary, the patient may be referred to the appropriate specialists within the institution. Once all the necessary testing has been obtained and reviewed, the patient is ready for the procedure. Hopefully the preanaesthesia assessment does not delay scheduling the surgery. Wait times for procedures vary by institution, but generally higher-acuity cases such as oncologic

Table 13.1 The ten best hospitals in the United States.

Mayo Clinic	Rochester, MN
Cleveland Clinic	Cleveland, OH
Johns Hopkins Hospital	Baltimore, MD
Massachusetts General Hospital	Boston, MA
UCSF Medical Center	San Francisco, CA
University of Michigan Hospitals and Health Centers	Ann Arbor, MI
Ronald Reagan UCLA Medical Center	Los Angeles, CA
New York Presbyterian Hospital	New York, NY
Stanford Health Care	Stanford, CA
Hospitals of the University of Pennsylvania – Penn Presbyterian	Philadelphia, PA

Adapted from Comarow A, Harder B. 2017–18 Best Hospitals Honor Roll and Overview. *U.S. News & World Report*. 8 Aug 2017 At: https://health.usnews.com/health-care/best-hospitals/articles/best-hospitals-honor-roll-and-overview). The columns show the centre name and the state location.

surgeries have a much shorter wait than purely elective ones such as orthopaedic or cosmetic procedures.

A standardised patient pathway is much less well-defined in the private setting, especially at smaller community hospitals. Many surgeons understand the need for proper preoperative assessment, but without a dedicated preanaesthesia clinic, preparation for surgery falls to primary care physicians in the community. Surgeons will generally instruct patients to obtain medical 'clearance' for surgery. Testing such as blood tests and ECGs are obtained by the patient's primary care physician. The need for additional testing such as echocardiogram or stress testing is at the discretion of the community physician. The information may be sent to the surgeon's office, the hospital where surgery is scheduled to occur, or the patient may bring this information with them to the hospital on the day of surgery. The anaesthesiologist assigned to the case evaluates the information available on the day of surgery when meeting the patient for the first time. Ultimately it is up to the anaesthesiologist to determine if the information provided is enough to proceed with the case safely. Production pressures may force an anaesthesiologist to take poorly prepared patients or patients with insufficient preanaesthesia evaluations to the operating room. In some situations, however, surgeons will send their patients for unnecessary batteries of tests to lessen the chance of cancellation on day of surgery. Redundant and/or unnecessary testing is expensive and clearly a poor use of healthcare resources.

After having met with the surgeon who has determined that the patient meets the criteria for surgery, the case may be scheduled. While some hospitals track the time between the decision for surgery and the day of surgery (DOS), others track the time from when the case is booked until the DOS. This is an important distinction because there may be a significant lag, 7–10 days at some US institutions, between the decision for surgery and the booking date, which reflects cumbersome administrative processes.

Regardless of which duration is being measured, there are many factors that influence it. Patients or their families may prefer to wait for time that is mutually convenient to schedule elective procedures. For example, parents may wait until there is a break in the school year for their child to have an orthopaedic or otolaryngology procedure. For patients electing to have a joint replacement surgery with a particularly busy, well-regarded orthopaedic surgeon, the understood wait time may be 4–6 months. Cardiac surgery, which tends to be more urgent in nature, may take place within a week to 10 days of the booking date. Because there is such a varied mixture of insurance payers in the United States, it is possible that the financial authorisation needed prior to surgery may delay a case or prolong the wait time. At one academic medical center in California, the average times between the booking date and the day of surgery showed enormous variation: less than 10 days for cardiac surgery, just under 14 days for gynaecologic oncology and colorectal surgeries and approximately 4–6 weeks for elective gynaecologic, general and vascular surgeries.

Historically anaesthesiologists in the United States have had very little involvement in the care of surgical patients in the post-operative period. It has been the surgeon's responsibility to coordinate immediate post-operative care, either sending the patient to an intensive care unit with its dedicated specialists or consulting a general practitioner to manage comorbid conditions post-operatively. In recent years with the development of the perioperative surgical home (PSH) concept and the implementation of enhanced recovery after surgery (ERAS) protocols, anaesthesia providers are becoming more involved in the continuum of surgical care. Anaesthetic choice and medication selection have implications in how quickly patients ambulate after surgery and how long they need to recover in the hospital before being discharged home or to a rehabilitation facility (Cannesson & Kain, 2014). As the trend in reimbursement shifts from fee-for-service to bundled payments, how patients recover in the immediate and subacute post-operative periods is a reflection on all of the physicians involved in their care. Anaesthesia providers are ideally suited to help develop and implement these protocols to benefit patients, not only intraoperatively but also post-operatively.

According to most anaesthesiologists, the typical bottlenecks in the patient pathway tend to occur in the immediate perioperative period. At our institution where, on average, <8% of patients scheduled for elective procedures are expected to recover in an intensive care unit (ICU), this is still a major bottleneck. Patients are funneled to the ICU not only from the operating room (OR) or the recovery room but also directly from the emergency room, from the lower level of care beds in the wards and even as transfers from other hospitals requiring higher levels of care. It is a challenge to determine which patients will require post-operative ICU care and what their anticipated length of stay in the ICU will be. However, this information is vital to ensure that demand for such an expensive resource will not exceed its capacity. Many hospitals will regulate how cases are scheduled within a surgeon's block time in order to prevent a heavy load of ICU admissions at one time.

Ryckman et al. (2009) redesigned the ICU flow at Cincinnati Children's Hospital Medical Center in order to improve patient access and safety. By limiting elective surgical ICU admissions each day (theirs was a maximum of five cases per day) they avoided diverting elective surgery ICU patients to other ICUs, having to hold patients in the post-anaesthesia care unit (PACU) longer than planned or having to delay or cancel future cases due to lack of ICU bed availability.

Another bottleneck frequently encountered involves PACU bed availability, which may be due to physical space limitations in the PACU or the number of nurses available to care for the patients destined to the PACU. Dexter et al. (2005) suggest several strategies for OR managers to mitigate delays in admission to the PACU. Nurse schedules can be adjusted monthly based on times of day when peak workload is expected. Similarly, smaller adjustments to PACU nurse staffing can be made one day in advance once the final schedule for the following day's cases has been published. Changes can be made to the order of cases in the OR such that there is not a surge of PACU admissions at one particular time of day (Marcon & Dexter, 2006). Inefficiencies in the PACU process should also be examined. If, for example, a patient undergoes a 15- to 30-minute cataract extraction with intraocular lens placement, their PACU recovery time should be equally as brief. For these and other patients who receive minimal anaesthesia (sedation, regional blocks) or recover quickly from a short, outpatient procedure under general anaesthesia, there should be processes in place to fast-track patients through the PACU and/or discharge home. Some hospitals may see a delay in getting patients transferred from the PACU to their hospital beds, which might result from nursing staffing issues on the floor or even lacking environmental services staff to clean a room after another patient has been discharged from the hospital.

Theatre Efficiency

There are several factors to consider in order to evaluate OR efficiency. Excess staffing costs, both underutilised and overutilised OR time, are important. If staff are scheduled to work from 7 am until 5 pm (a 10-hour shift) yet their operating room finishes at 3 pm, 2 out of the 10 hours (20%) that they were supposed to work were not utilised. On the other hand, if staff are scheduled to work the same 10-hour shift but instead of finishing early the cases in their OR finish at 6 pm, they are overutilised by an hour. The extra 1 hour they work is more costly than the contracted hours of work (i.e., overtime is always more expensive).

Extra time also results in decreased staff morale due to unexpected schedule changes and being asked or forced to work late. A well-managed OR should limit excess staffing costs to <10% of its staff budget. One study has shown that when wait time for surgery >14 days, it is easier to schedule cases appropriately to keep excess staffing costs down (Macario, 2006). In other words, very short wait times for surgery may lead to unpredictable lists, which results in short-notice changes to staffing, making overtime payments more likely.

Another factor to consider is on-time starts for the elective cases per OR per day. Some hospitals may track on-time first case starts only. But it may be more efficient to evaluate the timeliness of *every* case with respect to its scheduled/expected start time. When tardiness totals <45 minutes per 8-hour OR day, it means the OR director is able to determine when patients should arrive prior to their surgeries such that they are not waiting too long or arriving too late. Appropriate delays between successive cases may be scheduled, if needed. If other resources allow, cases can be shifted from one OR to another, and cases can be appropriately sequenced for each surgeon (based on both predictability and length; Macario, 2006).

An efficiently run OR should have a low cancellation rate on the day of surgery: <10% is good, <5% is ideal. It is understood that last-minute cancellations may result from factors outside any single entity's control. For example, a full intensive care unit, changes to a surgeon's availability, inclement weather or incomplete financial approval may result in an unanticipated cancellation. Having an organised and thorough preoperative screening process will likely catch the issues directly related to the patient well in

Table 13.2 Some causes for cancellation (NBM - nil by mouth).

Category of cancellation	Examples
Patient-related	Patient did not follow NBM guidelines; Patient did not discontinue anticoagulation medications as instructed
Unanticipated event	Upper respiratory symptoms; Car accident on way to hospital
Patient's clinical condition changed	Deterioration between preanaesthesia assessment and day of surgery
System error	Laboratory or other test results not reviewed ahead of time; Surgeon scheduling conflict
Financial reasons	Insurance clearance/preauthorisation not obtained

Adapted from Vlessides M. Preop Trip to Anesthesia Evaluation Clinic Lowers Surgical Cancellations. *Anesthesiology News*. 16 Feb 2016 (At: www.anesthesiologynews.com/Clinical-Anesthesiology/Article/02-16/Pre-op-Trip-to-Anesthesia-Evaluation-Clinic-Lowers-Surgical-Cancellations/35150/ses=ogst)

advance of the surgery date (Table 13.2; van Klei et al., 2002; Ferschl et al., 2005).

Admission delays to the PACU can also affect OR efficiency. At our institution we measure the percentage of workdays with at least one delay of 10 minutes or more because the PACU is full. PACU nurse staffing can be adjusted based on anticipated OR admissions, but the number of available PACU beds is usually a fixed resource. Whether the PACU and its staff can be used to care for 23-hour observation patients or ICU-destined patients depends on space, staff and expected continued OR admissions. These sorts of delays are so frequent and difficult to avoid in a busy OR suite that we determine that 10–20% of workdays having at least one PACU delay can be regarded as 'good', and <10% is 'excellent'.

Many surgeons and some hospital administrators see turnover (gap) times in the OR as the most important indicator of OR efficiency. While turnover times are a factor, clearly they are only one of several measures to consider. Turnover represents the time between a patient leaving the OR when cleanup may begin and setup for the following case. If turnover is to be used as a metric to judge theatre performance, it should not include other unrelated delays such as the surgeon being unavailable (surgeon contribution to delay), the patient not being ready (ward contribution to delay) or the anaesthesia team's scheduled lunch break (contractually imposed delay). In the United States, an efficient OR suite will complete its turnovers in <25 minutes; 25–40 minutes between patients is adequate but >40 minutes of turnover time is regarded as inefficient. It is understood that a

thorough cleanup after certain cases such as a multilevel spinal fusion will take significantly longer than the cleanup after less-invasive cases such as a tympanoplasty. Likewise, the setup for some cases is much more involved and time consuming than it is for others. Fewer than 10% of turnovers in an efficient OR should last >60 minutes.

Rather than tracking utilisation, we consider the financial perspective important: the contribution margin per hour of OR time used as a measure of efficiency. Consider the revenue generated by the hospital minus the labour and supply costs needed to generate this income. Slow teams will increase labour costs; selecting expensive implants or opening superfluous equipment will increase supply costs, thus decreasing the overall contribution margin. As discussed earlier, the hospital revenue generated will depend on the insurance or payer mix. At a hospital operating with a fixed annual budget, such as a VA hospital, maximising contribution margin per hour of OR time occurs when the variable costs are minimised. Those hospitals with a mean contribution margin of $1,000–2,000 per hour are doing well, whereas true fiscal efficiency results when more than $2,000 is generated per hour.

The final factor to consider when evaluating OR efficiency is prediction bias. When comparing the estimated duration of a case to the actual duration of a case, is the estimate consistently too high or too low? The prediction bias in a truly efficient OR should be <5 minutes per 8 hours of OR time (i.e., very accurate prediction); anything >15 minutes may be regarded as inefficient. In certain settings, this is a

Table 13.3 Summary of efficiency metrics discussed in text.

Metric	Needs improvement	Adequate	Efficient
Excess staffing costs[*]	>10%	5–10%	<5%
On-time starts (i.e., average tardiness of start time vs scheduled start time for all elective cases per OR day)	>60 minutes	45–60 minutes	<45 minutes
Cancellation rate on day of surgery	>10%	5–10%	<5%
PACU admission delays (i.e., % of workdays with ≥ 1 delay ≥ 10 minutes)	>20%	10–20%	<10%
Turnover/gap times	>40 minutes	25–40 minutes	<25 minutes
Prolonged turnovers (i.e., % of turnovers > 60 minutes)	>25%	10–25%	<10%
Contribution margin per OR hour	<$1,000/hour	$1,000–2,000/hour	>$2,000/hour
Prediction Bias (i.e., estimate vs actual case duration per OR day)	>15 minutes	5–15 minutes	<5 minutes

* Of total OR staff spending.
Adapted from Macario, A. Are Your Hospital Operating Rooms 'Efficient'? *Anesthesiology* 2006; 105(2): 237–40.

difficult measure upon which to improve. If a large hospital has a large number of surgeons, many of whom are new to the staff or do not operate frequently, it is difficult to predict case durations. If surgeons struggle with scheduling all of their cases, they may purposefully shorten their estimates in order to accommodate patients when (what they consider is) an inadequate amount of time is allotted to them. Historical data may provide baseline guidance to predict case duration, but this is something that all OR managers struggle with on a daily basis.

Summary of Efficiency Metrics

Based on the preceding discussion, we propose some efficiency metrics in Table 13.3.

OR Scheduling

Having a reliable scheduling algorithm is the means to achieve scheduling accuracy. Once accurate predictions can be made to estimate anticipated case durations, accurate and reasonable daily operating room schedules can be created. One of the biggest challenges faced is how to predict the duration of any surgical case. The two most important factors to consider are the case being performed and the particular surgeon who will be operating.

At any institution there may be several surgeons who do laparoscopic cholecystectomies. Dr A may complete her case in 45 minutes while Dr B, a less-experienced surgeon, may take 90 minutes. Is Dr B also routinely taking liver biopsies and/or performing intraoperative cholangiograms, which increase the duration of his cases? It is important that each case, including all the possible related procedures, be designated accurately such that the appropriate accommodations can be made when scheduling. To regard the cases as equivalent when in fact they are not, will lead to inaccuracies.

While we can evaluate historical data for procedures based on the case and the surgeon, doing so does not necessarily improve scheduling accuracy. If there is historical data, do you rely on the mean, the median or the longest iteration to estimate future events? Case duration for a particular procedure can vary significantly, and the statistical distribution of these case times is not a normal, bell-shaped one. The curve tends to be right-skewed, and the longer cases will have a bigger effect on the calculated average. Do you exclude both the bottom and the top 10% to eliminate outlier data? Oftentimes there is very little historical data on which to base future predictions (Macario, 2009). Do we use the surgeon's own estimate? Does this estimate represent in-room time to out-of-OR time, or is it simply incision to closing time? Is the surgeon purposely underestimating case durations to fit more cases in his or her scheduled block time? Or is the surgeon overestimating his or her case

Table 13.4 Summary of the START method of scheduling.

Scheduled procedure analysis: compare the scheduled procedures to see what procedure the surgeon plans to do versus what has been booked for them to do.

Time stamp assessment: define the data (in-room to out-of-room times work best) and then track it.

Actual procedure analysis: review what procedures are being done by the surgeon, and compare this to what was scheduled, such that the time stamps accurately correspond to the procedures being done.

Review of the algorithm: what tools and calculations are used to predict case duration?

Timely feedback and continuous improvement: making progress to increase efficiency depends on collecting feedback and consistently reevaluating the process initially created.

durations in order to reserve the remainder of the block time in the event that a new case appears? Some institutions will use a combination of both the surgeon's estimate and the available historical data at their particular institution in order to create a new estimate. Additionally it may be prudent to adjust the estimate such that case or patient complexity (for example, morbid obesity) is taken into consideration.

Ye et al. (2017) described a general method to evaluate and improve surgery scheduling accuracy called 'START'. They suggest critically examining each potential component separately (Table 13.4). In essence this is a continuous Plan-Do-Study-Act (PDSA) type cycle in which different specific tools may be used, adapted as information is used for learning to modify and improve a fluid process.

There are three systems commonly used to manage the daily scheduling of procedures and allocate OR time. These are termed: 'any workday', 'reasonable time' and 'fixed hours'. These have been presented in a different way with different terminology in Chapter 4.

Using the any workday system, a patient agrees with his or her surgeon the desirable date for surgery. This request is sent to the scheduler, who will accommodate the request assuming the resources to complete the case safely will be available on that date. While scheduling using the any workday system might please patients and surgeons, there may be large downtime gaps in the daily schedule for any given operating room. Staff may end up working beyond their scheduled shift if a case is scheduled outside of prime OR hours. Most ambulatory surgery centers (ASC) in the United States use the any workday system for scheduling (Pash et al, 2014). The cases performed in an ASC tend to be shorter in duration and have less variability. Therefore, the types of cases being performed fit more reliably into an allocated OR day.

The reasonable time system is more beneficial for the scheduler who is able to arrange when cases will happen in order to maximise productivity during regularly scheduled hours. With this system, the hospital guarantees that a surgeon will have time to perform the case within a certain time period (for example, 3 months) of booking it. The scheduler then books the case and notifies the patient and the surgeon of the surgery date. This is an unpopular method of scheduling in the United States because it affords very little flexibility to the patient. It may be feasible for the patient and the surgeon to go elsewhere or the patient may select a different surgeon who is able to accommodate his or her needs better.

In the fixed hours or block time system, OR time is allocated to a surgeon or surgical service. In other words, there is a beginning and an end time on a specific day or days of the week that comprises block time. This system is very close to the 'typical UK NHS list' described in Chapter 2. The surgeon or service is able to schedule cases that will reasonably fit into their dedicated block of time. For example, an orthopaedic surgeon may have one room designated from 7 am until 5 pm every Tuesday. Another surgeon, perhaps a newer otolaryngologist, will have one room from 1 pm until 5 pm every other Monday until his practise grows. The urology division may be have two operating rooms allocated to their group from 7 am until 5 pm every day of the week, and they are expected to divide this block time among their eight surgeons. Unused block time can be released in advance such that other surgeons or specialties can make use of this valuable commodity.

At a busy, academic medical center where physical OR space is a limiting factor and not all surgeons can be allocated 'sufficient' block time, some of these surgeons will say that the bottleneck is getting OR time in the fixed hours system. They may have patients scheduled for elective procedures 6 months in advance because they cannot easily accommodate their patients into their allocated OR time. But if they were given more time, they would use it, increasing their productivity and caring for more patients.

From the OR management perspective, utilisation is reviewed monthly in order to ensure that OR time is divided in an equitable and profitable manner. However, not every operating room will be allocated for all of the prime OR time. Certain operating rooms are designated as 'flexible' or 'urgent' rooms such that the emergency and urgent cases that come in through the emergency room, clinics or inpatient beds can be completed in a timely fashion. Depending on daily case load and the number of add-on cases, urgent and especially emergency cases may have to displace scheduled elective cases if OR room availability is limited. This is an ongoing issue for the OR manager at a busy, academic medical center.

Quite frequently cases are delayed. At some institutions, especially those operating on fixed budgets such as a VA hospital, delayed cases may have to be rescheduled. But in general, patients are not cancelled when the operating room falls behind its daily schedule.

If a case can be transferred to a different OR that has finished earlier than expected, the OR manager and/or charge nurse will work to shift the case. Occasionally staffing becomes an issue after allocated prime OR time (5 pm at our institution). There may be a sufficient number of anaesthesia and nursing teams on call who can cover the late-running operating rooms. However, noncall staff may be asked or, more unfortunately, told to work late in order to cover a larger number of late-running operating rooms that the call teams alone cannot cover. The delay of scheduled cases may be even more prolonged if nursing and/or anaesthesia staff is unavailable to safely cover another operating room. More often than not, it is to the hospital's financial benefit to complete surgeries after scheduled hours. In comparison to the enormous overhead of running a hospital and the other fixed costs related to the procedure, the increase in variable cost, overtime pay for staff, is quite minor.

When a particular surgeon or service consistently overruns its block time, the OR manager should closely investigate the reasons. Are the cases being done the same as the cases being scheduled? Is the time allotted for each case reasonable or is the estimated duration grossly inadequate? How long are the turnover times between cases? Are there other delays

between cases? Is the staff assigned to these rooms appropriately trained to assist in these sorts of cases? The list of possibilities is endless.

The utilisation of allocated OR block time is constantly reviewed. If surgeons or services are not making efficient use of their allocated time, it will probably be reassigned to a busier surgeon or service. When unexpected cancellations occur and block time becomes available at the last minute, other surgeons in that same group may use it or it may be used to offload urgent or elective add-on cases depending on what is already in the queue.

Ongoing Challenges

It is often difficult to safely staff late-running ORs with nursing staff and/or anaesthesia providers when there is an unexpected number of ORs running late. Many institutions will recruit volunteers to work late, earn overtime and complete the cases. However, at some hospitals there will not be any volunteers, and management may force unwilling staff to stay. This predicament reflects back on how staff is treated: if employees are appreciated and well compensated for their efforts, it is more likely that they will be willing to work late when requested. But when staff are mistreated or their needs are ignored, it is unlikely that they will decide to contribute beyond the minimum expectations set for them. One progressive clinical OR manager decided to create a 'flexible late nurse schedule' such that OR nurses can volunteer to stay later on certain days. In return, efforts are made to relieve these nurses earlier from their shifts on the day prior to and the day following their flexible late days.

While there is a significant amount of literature regarding OR management, it is often difficult to apply these principles in reality. In some cases, hospitals fail to recognise that the application of these proven measures may increase OR efficiency and, therefore, revenue. While some institutions have invested in information technology (IT) and electronic medical records (EMR) systems, this is not universally true nationwide – IT may be fragmented, antiquated or nonexistent. When it is difficult to gather past data to evaluate a potential problem it is even more challenging to collect data prospectively to make improvements and evaluate implementation. A data-driven platform to improve OR efficiency in terms of utilisation and contribution margins would greatly assist in OR management. Anaesthesiologists are well suited to serve as fundamental contributors to the OR managerial system, thus helping to create a transparent governance structure involving surgery, nursing and anaesthesia.

In the United States, as reimbursement shifts from fee-for-service to bundled payments, how we budget for the perioperative cost center is becoming increasingly important. Strategic planning to cover high cost areas such as the OR and the interventional suites is key. Applying the basic OR management principles more consistently may potentially achieve significant cost savings for an institution. Not only do institutions need to plan to update and replace expensive equipment, but they also need to recognise and appreciate the staff who allow them to succeed. It is necessary to recognise the intangible benefit that training, developing and supporting staff can bring to an institution. The culture of an institution, which may reflect the personalities comprising the OR leadership, plays an important role in how change is effected and how progress is made.

Appendix 13A Vignette of a Practical Solution to an OR Problem

An interventional pain physician had many procedures (30 on average) scheduled between 7 am and 5 pm. Some of these cases required sedation while others could be done safely under local, without an anaesthesia team needed.

The scheduler had booked the cases without regard to the type of sedation requested. As a result, many cases requiring anaesthesia care were booked back to back. The problem was that the preoperative preparation on the day of the procedure took longer than the procedure itself. One case would finish but the patient scheduled to follow would not be ready for the OR. This resulted in an unused OR time and longer wait times for patients during prime OR time.

Another issue that was encountered repeatedly was that the caseload ran beyond its allocated block time, as the anaesthesia team would be forced to wait to do the final sedation cases interspersed among the last local cases.

After many frustrating evenings, changes to case sequencing were made such that the sedation cases were preidentified and scheduled with at least one, preferably two, local cases in between. This way, completing anaesthesia preoperative paperwork did not cause delays or waste valuable OR time. Additionally, the sedation cases could be scheduled earlier in the day so that when the cases ran late, the overutilised time was limited to the nursing staff rather than nursing and anaesthesia, which in turn was less expensive.

Further issues relating to scheduling issues are discussed in Pash et al. (2014).

Bibliography

Antonisse L, Garfield R, Rudoqitz R. 2017. The Effects of Medicaid Expansion under the ACA: Updated Findings from a Literature Review. At: www.kff.org/medicaid/issue-brief/the-effects-of-medicaid-expansion-under-the-aca-updated-findings-from-a-literature-review-september-2017.

Association of American Medical Colleges. 2013. Medicare Payments for Graduate Medical Education: What Every Medical Student, Resident, and Advisor Needs to Know. Association of American Medical Colleges, Jan 2013. At: https://members.aamc.org/eweb/upload/Medicare%20Payments%20for%20Graduate%20Medical%20Education%202013.pdf. Accessed 7 Sept 2017.

Cannesson M, Kain Z. 2014. Enhanced recovery after surgery versus perioperative surgical home: is it all in the name? *Anesthesia & Analgesia* 118: 901–2.

Dexter F, Epstein RH, Marcon E, de Matta R. 2005. Strategies to reduce delays in admission into a postanesthesia care unit from operating rooms. *Journal of Perianesthesia Nursing* 20: 92–102.

Eichhorn, JH, Grider, JS. 2013. Scope of Practice. In Barash PG et al. (eds.). *Clinical Anesthesia*, 7th edn. Philadelphia, PA: Lippincott, Williams, & Wilkins. 29–60.

Fast Facts on U.S. Hospitals. 2018. The American Hospital Association. At: www.aha.org/research/rc/stat-studies/fast-facts.shtml#community.

Ferschl MB, Tung A, Sweitzer B, Huo D, et al. 2005. Preoperative clinic visits reduce operating room cancellations and delays. *Anesthesiology* 103: 855–9.

Kaiser Family Foundation. 2016. Health Insurance Coverage of the Total Population. At: www.kff.org/other/state-indicator/total-population/?currentTimeframe=0&sortModel=%7B%22colId%22:%22Location%22,%22sort%22:%22asc%22%7D.

Macario, A. 2006. Are your hospital operating rooms 'efficient'? *Anesthesiology* 105: 237–40.

Macario, A. 2009. Truth in scheduling: is it possible to accurately predict how long a surgical case will last? *Anesthesia & Analgesia* 108: 681–5.

Marcon E, Dexter F. 2006. Impact of surgical sequencing on post anesthesia care unit staffing. *Health Care Management Science* 9: 87–98.

Millman, J. 2015. A knee replacement surgery could cost $17K or $61K. And that's in the same city. *Washington Post*, 21 Jan 2015. At: www.washingtonpost.com/news/wonk/wp/2015/01/21/a-knee-replacement-surgery-could-cost-17k-or-61k-and-thats-in-the-same-city/?utm_term=.d10644222ea1.

National Health Expenditure Accounts (NHEA) Fact Sheet. 2018. Centers for Medicare and Medicaid Services. At: www.cms.gov/research-statistics-data-and-systems/statistics-trends-and-reports/nationalhealthexpenddata/nhe-fact-sheet.html.

Pash J, Kadry B, Burgrara S, Macario A. 2014. Scheduling of procedures and staff in an ambulatory surgery center. *Anesthesiology Clinics* 32: 517–27.

Ryckman FC, Yelton PA, Anneken AM, Kiessling PE, et al. 2009. Redesigning intensive care unit flow using variability management to improve access and safety. *Joint Commission Journal on Quality and Patient Safety* 35: 535–43.

van Klei WA, Moons KG, Rutten CL, et al. 2002. The effect of outpatient preoperative evaluation of hospital inpatients on cancellation of surgery and length of hospital stay. *Anesthesia & Analgesia* 94: 644–9.

Ye I, Macario A, Kadry B. 2017. START makes a good case for greater scheduling accuracy. *OR Manager* 33: 1–5.

Safety in the Operating Theatres

Meghana Pandit

Introduction

Almost all the preceding chapters in this book have focussed on managing the technical aspects of operating theatres, as explained in the Introduction at tactical level (Chapter 1). This has been primarily a focus on numerical aspects of performance, and the concept of efficiency has been introduced. However, a very important aspect of theatre management is governance and safety; that is, to ensure that while teams aspire to achieving efficiency and high productivity, the absolute priority must be that patients – and staff – are safe.

Safety in theatres is predicated on having a 'safety culture' across the whole organisation and not just in theatres. Theatres are a multiprofessional environment, and all staff need to recognise the contribution they make to promote safe practice. In order to understand safety, it is required that we define 'harm'.

Defining 'Harm'

Harm is categorised as 'no harm, low, moderate, severe harm and death' by the UK's National Patient Safety Agency (NPSA; Table 14.1).

Recommended Safe Practices

Safe practices would prevent such harm incidents from occurring. It is possible to think of what steps are required to be taken to ensure safe practice in theatres.

Appropriate Planning of Surgical Lists

Appropriate planning and safety are intimately linked. It is extremely common, in analysing of what went wrong, to find that an unnecessarily pressurised environment underpinned an event that led to harm. In the United Kingdom and Ireland, the 5th National Audit Project of the Royal College and Association of Anaesthetists reported that overbooked theatre lists,

where staff were under pressure and rushing, was a contributory factor even in the phenomenon of 'accidental awareness during general anaesthesia'. Intuitively one might not imagine these two things as related, but they clearly are.

Harm can also arise as a result of last-minute cancellations on the day of surgery. This can be physical harm because the underlying disease that led to admission is not then treated, and there is delay. There can also be psychological harm: patients have prepared themselves for surgery, which is then suddenly cancelled, leaving them with feelings of distress, concern or frustration. These feelings can extend also to family members who are offering the patient support.

The importance of Chapter 4 ('Case Scheduling') and also to an extent Chapter 5 ('Capacity Planning') is therefore not only in the domain of achieving theatre efficiency, but also in the realm of patient safety. Problems such as wrong side surgery, drug errors, failure to adhere to checklists, etc., are all less likely to occur in a calm, well-ordered environment.

Requirement of All Necessary Equipment Including Blood Products Is Anticipated and Is Available

This follows on from the first point. Only where an operating list is planned in advance will it be known exactly which equipment is required (including need for special investigation such as C-arm X-rays or blood salvage or blood products). The team must undertake a risk assessment for each case and prepare the equipment needed for safe completion of all procedures. This avoids any potential delays to cases and prevents frustration and workarounds on the part of the theatre team. In turn this requirement also means that, where equipment highlighted from the outset as essential is in fact unavailable, this might require cancellation of the case (as being the safest measure)

Table 14.1 Definitions of types of harm, adapted from NPSA.

No harm:
(a) Impact prevented – any patient safety incident that had the *potential* to cause harm but was prevented, resulting in no harm: diathermy pad applied wrongly but recognised and changed prior to surgery starting.
(b) Impact not prevented – any patient safety incident that ran to completion but no harm occurred: drug A prescribed and drug B administered with both drugs having same properties.

Low: Any patient safety incident that required extra observation or minor treatment and caused minimal harm: A patient rolled off the table during positioning and did not suffer any injuries

Moderate: Any patient safety incident that resulted in a moderate increase in treatment and that caused significant but not permanent harm: return to theatre from recovery for haemorrhage

Severe: Any patient safety incident that appears to have resulted in permanent harm: wrong site surgery such as removal of the wrong fallopian tube for ectopic pregnancy (also classified as a Never Event)

Death: Any patient safety incident that directly resulted in the death

rather than proceeding under suboptimal circumstances. This is a question of risk assessment.

WHO Safe Surgical Checklist

Simple interventions can have profound safety impact. The WHO checklist is a mandatory step prior to the start of theatre lists. Most organisations have locally adapted versions of the WHO checklist. However all checklists include a Team Brief, Time Out and Sign Out. Organisations need to audit compliance with the checklists and ensure the presence of the entire team for each part of the checklist, for each procedure. Lack of engagement with this simple safety measure is an indication of poor prioritisation of patient safety, and therefore, any refusal or resistance to undertake the checklist must be managed in a robust manner by the organisation's highest leadership. It is difficult to imagine any member of staff who does not engage with this important checklist, of whatever seniority or ability, being allowed to practice within an organisation.

Consistency of Staff within and between Cases

Operating room teams who work together regularly know each other's practices and anticipate surgical and anaesthetic events quicker and react appropriately. Most important is the fact that within such ideal teams, hierarchical barriers are absent, and as a result there is greater freedom to point out an impending calamity resulting from an error. Of course, keeping exactly the same team is impossible (due to staff leave,

sickness, etc.), and individual members will have multiple skill sets that require their presence at other sites or teams at times. There is also a need to retain skill mix and prevent 'silo working'. However, consistent training will help ensure both the optimum skill mixes and the ability to cross-cover where needed.

Unfortunate practices – to avoid – include changing shifts or giving staff breaks at enforced times even if inappropriate (e.g., half way through a complex surgical procedure). Chapter 6 ('Staffing and Contracts') underlines some of these key principles.

Debrief at the End of the List

Every day at the end of the routine theatre lists, a debrief helps assimilate good practice across theatres and points to the risks and deficiencies that occurred during the day. This debrief could follow a prescribed pattern and should involve all staff. It is an excellent way to promote teamwork. Comments and feedback need to be recorded and disseminated to promote learning.

Clear Accountability

Operating theatres should have a clinical director with whom ultimate accountability for the function of theatres rests. This could be the generic 'theatre manager' described in Chapter 1. Many organisations will have a triumvirate structure with (a) an administrative (nonclinical) manager and (b) a matron/nurse manager (to direct the nonmedical staff) supporting (c) the clinical director. Operating theatres constitute a complex environment with multiple professionals, and it is imperative that professional silos do not emerge. Where accountability for safety in theatres is devolved to a single practitioner, rotating across the specialty groups on a daily basis, it empowers staff groups, breaks down cultural barriers and delegates authority across professional boundaries.

Clinical Competence and Audit

It goes without saying that all those who work in theatres should be competent and trained. However, these things apply especially where new procedures and techniques are to be used. It is seen all too often that new anaesthetic and surgical procedures are introduced in operating theatres without adequate training of the entire team. This introduces risks to patient safety. Organisations are advised to introduce guidance that prevents such poor practice, whilst facilitating innovative practice. A continuous audit of new procedures/techniques is also recommended with up-to-date literature on patient information and consent.

Techniques That Promote Safety

A number of techniques will help achieve the aforementioned recommended practices.

Human Factors Training

As defined by the UK's Health and Safety Executive, human factors are the *organisational, environmental* and *cultural* factors, as well as *individual* and *group* characteristics that influence behaviour at work.

People don't choose to do the wrong thing. When things do go wrong blaming doesn't help. Reminding or retraining only helps in some instances, and then is rarely the only solution needed. Human factors is about fixing the system, not the worker. Human factors can also be used proactively to examine how people work. An understanding of human factors enables teams to question practices, recognise risks and suggest alternatives before the incident occurs. It also helps to break down hierarchical barriers that often exist in operating theatres. Human factors training should be offered to all theatre teams proactively rather than as a reaction to significant events.

Application of 'Lean' Principles

The Introduction (Chapter 1) made the point that much of the book does not directly mention 'Lean'.

It also correctly summarises the limitations of Lean in the context of operating theatres. However, the realm of patient safety is one where Lean can have a distinct contribution to make. Lean is a set of concepts, principles and tools used to create and deliver maximum value from the patient's perspective whilst using the fewest resources and fully using the knowledge and skills of the staff.

One tool available in Lean management is '5S' (standing for: sort, simplify, standardise, self-discipline and sustain). This focuses on making the work environment mistake-proof and helps prevent process problems. It can be used to huge benefit in theatres applied to drug cupboards, resuscitation trolleys and theatre instrument trays. Applying 5S to drug cupboards helps prevent drug errors, (e.g., as drugs with antagonistic actions are presented in very similar looking packaging). Standardising where and how drugs are stored in anaesthetic rooms is important so that the person reaching for a drug in an emergency finds the correct one. Equally, resuscitation trolleys being cluttered or kept away from places where they might be required in an emergency or kept poorly stocked can only result in chaos in an emergency. Again, 5S is a tool that helps practitioners obtain the correct device promptly and aids safe practice.

Learning to Improve Quality of Care

Safety can only be improved or sustained through continuous learning. One way to achieve this is by using a 'scorecard' approach. A scorecard can be used prospectively to record all surgical complications at surgeon and patient level. This would enable analysis of trends and themes by teams and thereby improve quality of care, by putting in place any required changes to surgical practice. It also enables a meaningful preoperative discussion with patients and facilitates adequate consent by providing hard, quantitative data about complication rates.

How Can It Go Wrong?

One of the biggest challenges to safety in theatres is poor organisational culture and leadership. Culture is 'how we do things here'. Culture is too often determined by historical events and embedded hierarchies. Instead it should be built upon values. Staff should display behaviours that demonstrate the subscribed values. This, of course, has to be modelled by the leadership of the organisation at all times. Another important and critical point to make is appreciation of those that do, and accountability for those who don't demonstrate behaviours is a must. Without this, organisational culture is unlikely to be one of continuous learning, compassion and improvement.

Certain styles of leadership can promote a positive culture and help create an ability to adapt and adopt improvement methodology, with innovative practice and change. The theatre manager should try to embrace an adaptive leadership style; i.e., one that could be 'directive' in an emergency situation and also be 'facilitative' at a scheduling meeting.

We learned earlier that multiple professionals interact in theatres, and whilst most organisations have a triumvirate leadership structure, overall accountability often rests with a single clinical director. This person needs to operate in this complex environment with the highest regard for a 'distributed leadership'. This is a model of leadership when the traits of the individual leader are less important than other factors. The leader has to be collaborative and inclusive and understand the context of the situation within an organisation. Operating theatres are an appropriate environment for practice of distributed leadership due to the multiprofessional diverse workforce and competing demands on various groups.

To achieve their goals, the leader should be a strong proponent of patient safety principles and enforce all policies that deliver patient safety without regard for individual power amongst or between the various staff groups. Equally, the leader needs to facilitate an open discussion about change and innovation, where staff are given opportunities to engage in discussions so that they can make suggestions concerning changes to their own work practices. The leader should also constantly review emerging evidence of new practice: this requires them to be familiar with principle of critical appraisal, where they weigh sometimes conflicting lines of evidence.

What to Do When Things Go Wrong?

Adverse incidents are inevitable. The most important thing is to investigate incidents and learn from them such that the incident does not occur again. Most important, there must be no blame when mistakes occur. Staff must be encouraged to be open to learning, and this is only possible in a truly blame-free culture. When there is fear of blame, incidents won't be reported, and there will be no learning.

Daily *safety huddles* can promote a reporting culture and enable a discussion of low or no harm incidents (Table 14.1). These important 'near misses' are important substrates for learning. Analysis of these incidents can help put changes in place that prevent their occurrence. Staff engagement at safety huddles is empowering and facilitates feedback to reporters and encourages suggestions from front-line staff to improve safety. Such suggestions often 'stick'.

In the United Kingdom, the 'duty of candour' is a legal duty on a hospital to inform and apologise to patients if there have been mistakes in their care that have led to moderate or severe harm. The apology need not be an admission of guilt but an empathetic acknowledgement that something has gone wrong. Under this guidance, doctors, nurses and midwives should:

(a) speak to a patient, or those close to them, as soon as possible after they realise something has gone wrong with their care;

(b) apologise to the patient – explain what happened, what can be done if they have suffered harm and what will be done to prevent someone else being harmed in the future;

(c) use their professional judgement about whether to inform patients about near misses – incidents that have the potential to result in harm but do not and

(d) report errors within an organization at an early stage so that lessons can be learned quickly, and patients are protected from harm in the future.

A patient safety response team is a team that responds to any incident that has resulted in moderate or severe harm (Table 14.1). The team can consist of a senior doctor, senior nurse and a trained quality officer. Upon receiving a briefing about the incident, the team visits the site of the incident, speaks to the patient or relatives and staff. The team undertakes a debrief and commences an investigation. Staff involved in the incident should find such an approach very supportive – and definitely not a vehicle used to assign blame.

Fundamental to the team's approach is root cause analysis and learning (termed 'RCA'). Everyone, including involved staff and patients or relatives contributes to the RCA evidence base in an open and neutral way. There are various ways of undertaking a RCA, and the details of the different ways is not detailed further in this chapter. However, the common principles applicable to all RCAs include the following:

(a) The RCA is not a vehicle for assigning blame.

(b) In the main it is systems failures and not individual failures that lead to harm.

(c) Learning must be organization wide and not specific to any department.

(d) Any learning should be effectively disseminated.

This last can be achieved in the form of *safety messages*, discussed at quality meetings and at 'grand rounds' (organization wide meetings where a range of staff get together). There needs to be a *learning hub* in each organization, i.e., a resource that is easily accessible by all staff.

Conclusions

A focus on production pressure must never override or detract from an emphasis on safety. Regardless of how superficially 'productive' is an operating theatre, it is useless if it is unsafe. Sound organisation of operating theatres (e.g., rational planning of lists and staffing and equipment) creates an environment in which there are few if any production pressures, and this is a basis for a safe system. Or, expressed differently: operating theatres consistently described as 'busy' are likely to be unsafe. The chapters in this book indicate how to achieve that good level of organisation.

Safety (or lack of it) is not measured crudely by the number of adverse incidents; larger hospitals or busier theatres will always have more incidents. Rather, safety is engendered by the approach the organisation takes to incidents, especially its approach to near misses, and how and whether it demonstrates learning from the incidents (therefore evidenced by a gradual decline in the number of incidents).

An operating theatre suite can be regarded as well managed if:

1. There is a clear management structure with an identifiable OR manager.

2. There is collection of key data especially timing of surgical operations.

3. This timing data is used (focussed on mean/median *and* a measure of variance like standard deviation) to plan operating lists, assess demand and capacity and organise staffing.

4. Overall performance is measured using balanced measures such as efficiency, ε, and not on individual measures (such as start times, utilisation or cancellation rates) alone.

5. Safety measures such as WHO checklists are well embedded in theatre processes and analysed for compliance.

6. Critical incidents and near misses are logged and appropriately analysed using RCA methodology, with evidence of learning from these.

The chapters in this book explain clearly how these goals can be achieved.

Bibliography

Hill MR, Roberts MJ, Alderson ML, Gale TC. 2015. Safety culture and the 5 steps to safer surgery: an intervention study. *British Journal of Anaesthesia* 114: 958–62.

Hovlid E, von Plessen C, Haug K, et al. 2013. Patient experiences with interventions to reduce surgery cancellations: a qualitative study. *BMC Surgery* 13: 600.10.1186/1471-2482-13-30.

Ivarsson B, Kimblad PO, Sjöberg T, Larsson S. 2002. Patient reactions to cancelled or postponed heart operations. *Journal of Nursing Management* 10: 75–81.

Leonard M, Graham S, Bonacum D. 2004. The human factor: the critical importance of effective teamwork and communication in providing safe care. *Quality and Safety in Health Care* 13, Suppl 1: i85–i90.

Moppett IK, Moppett SH. 2016. Surgical caseload and the risk of surgical Never Events in England. *Anaesthesia* 71:17–30.

Pandit JJ. 2016. Deaths by horsekick in the Prussian army – and other 'Never Events' in large organisations. *Anaesthesia* 71: 7–11.

Pandit JJ, Andrade J, Bogod DG, et al. 2014. 5th National Audit Project (NAP5) on accidental awareness during general anaesthesia: summary of main findings and risk factors. *Anaesthesia* 69: 1089–101.

Sevdalis N, Hull L, Birnbach DJ. 2012. Improving patient safety in the operating theatre and perioperative care: obstacles, interventions, and priorities for accelerating progress. *British Journal of Anaesthesia* 109, Suppl 1: i3–i16.

Chapter 15

A Personal Overview

Peter H. J. Müller

Scope and Purpose of This Chapter

The focus of this book is to describe the processes in operating theatres in an objective analysis that leads to rational, data-led solutions. Chapters from Europe, Asia, Australia, New Zealand and the United States add different perspectives from a great variety of cultures in healthcare systems, as well as hospital and operating theatre organisations. The purpose of this chapter is to offer a reflection on the material, from my experience and knowledge as an operating theatre manager at a university hospital, and my thoughts on the extent to which – and how – the lessons and recommendations of the foregoing chapters can be applied in a practical context. This chapter also seeks to identify remaining gaps in the literature that are amenable to future research or audit. It is exciting to see such progress made in this field, and the principles enshrined in this book can be used to obtain more data and information to help pull some threads together.

Theatre Management Organisation

Chapter 2 correctly stresses the different patterns of assigning theatre time to surgeons or surgical specialties. In the United Kingdom, hospitals typically work with operating lists filled by one surgeon with a rather similar set of surgical cases (e.g., orthopaedic, vascular) in the form of a 'block time'. In many other countries, the block time (which may constitute a portion of a day's theatre schedule) is assigned to the surgical subspecialty and may be actually occupied by different surgeons (sometimes from day to day or week to week, or even within a single block time). This allows several surgeons from the same department or specialty to book cases into this block time, an advantage being that of cross-cover. However, a disadvantage is that the process relies upon timely arrival of each surgeon into their slot. Another potential disadvantage is that estimated timings for the

same procedure may vary substantially between surgeons, and this can lead to under- or overbooking. Furthermore the variety in the way even similar operations are conducted can be great, so theatre staff have to accommodate different surgeons' needs, which increases complexity.

Although this book is written primarily for a notional or hypothetical 'theatre manager', very few countries, perhaps with the exception of the German-speaking areas in Europe, distinguish the role of a theatre manager, who is not at the same time a practising consultant anaesthetist or surgeon (e.g., a head of the department, responsible for the efficient usage of the operating theatre complex of a specific hospital). In some hospitals in Switzerland, theatre managers can be physicians, nurses or even economists by primary training. However, most of them have additional qualifications, e.g., in form of a diploma or certification in operating room management (see: www.vopm.de/ger_zertifizierung/), Master's of Business Administration (MBA), Master's of Public Health (MPH) or similar. Associations of theatre managers have been formed to create networks of interested people and share recommendations and information in Switzerland (www.op-man agement.ch), Germany (www.vopm.de) and Austria (www.vopmoe.at). In the United States interested anaesthesiologists formed the International Consortium (iCORMET at www.cormetanes.org) in 2015, with a mission to develop a formal training curriculum in operating theatre management, ideally as obligatory for anaesthesia residents to advance anaesthesiologists as operating room leaders. Their goals also include to publish relevant papers and to collaborate with the American Board of Anesthesiology (ABA) to introduce this material into residency training, to try to ensure that no anaesthesiology resident graduated without understanding some basic concepts in operating room (OR) management. From

2018, iCORMET will be a section of the Association of Anesthesia Clinical Directors (AACD).

In this context this book forms a very valuable contribution in helping to internationalise these common aims, and if and when a curriculum is developed it will need to recognise an international perspective.

The Operating Theatre 'Black Box'

To many hospital executives, operating theatres are perhaps a 'black box'. Although it is widely known that at least 50% of any given hospital's revenue is generated by surgery, senior managers do not always know what is going on inside this 'surgical-anaesthetic box'. Surgeons themselves often claim that they are the 'workhorses of the hospital' by earning most of the revenue; however, what they tend to forget is that they are also the biggest spenders in this game. Staffing cost are reported to be at least 70% of the total expenses in operating theatres (the remainder includes 'housing', consumables, etc.).

As presented in previous chapters, data is sparse that might otherwise shed some light into this black box. In these circumstances, creating a formal branch of 'theatre management' can be difficult to justify in economic terms as essential and is instead often regarded as added value. In Germany, there is economic pressure on the healthcare system to operate efficiently, but it is very surprising to see that even in Switzerland, where the DRG system has been implemented since 2012 (see Chapter 11), accurate data recording the appropriate aspects of theatre performance remain sparse.

Therefore, a suggestion to any operating theatre manager with some interest in the efficiency or productivity of their department is to seek access to reliable and reproducible data of everything that is going on in their theatres. Make it simple in the beginning and then add more complex performance indicators whilst establishing periodic reporting (see later) of these data.

When publishing or disseminating the data to colleagues, it is important to be careful, as many indicators are subject to different interpretations or, at worst, if presented poorly can be meaningless. One example, as has been carefully discussed in Chapters 2 and 3, is the measure of 'utilisation' of operating theatres. Much beloved of many hospital or theatre managers, it also one of the least meaningful and most open to manipulation.

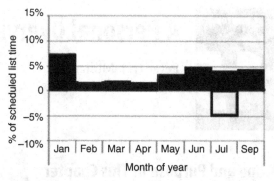

Figure 15.1 Example of data circulated by one UK university hospital to its senior staff on start times. Tardy (or early) starts are plotted (each bar is the mean for the month in question) against the month of a given year. Further explanation in text.

Figure 15.1 shows a poorly presented data set that was sent by one hospital to its consultant surgical and anaesthetic staff concerning start times. Notwithstanding the fact that start times are a poor way of measuring performance (Chapter 2), there are several serious problems with the data presentation here and how it might be interpreted. First, the hospital has chosen to use percentage of scheduled list time as its metric. This means that if a member of staff is consistently late to arrive by 15 minutes, then the impact of this will be far greater for a short list of 4 hours than a longer list of 12 hours. In other words, the metric is greatly influenced by list length and not independent of it. The tardiness is equal in both these hypothetical cases, but regarded differently, and this is not justifiable. Second, the blocks represent means; medians would naturally be better to prevent the effect of skew of one very late or very early start. Third, the monthly blocks show no error bars whose presence would better indicate the spread of start times over a particular month (i.e., apparent differences month by month may not be real). Fourth, and most bafflingly, is the data presentation for the month of July. This shows a mean late start of ~4% but at the same time a mean early start of ~5%, which does not make sense. What the hospital has (probably) done is to take all the late starts in the month and average them to produce the positive block (+4%); then it has taken all the early starts in the month and averaged those to produce the negative block (−5%). The missing data is, of course, the number of lists contributing to each block; we do not know if any given block represents the mean of just one list, or of many dozen.

Other than meaningful presentation of relevant data, a theatre manager can 'open up the black box', by correlating theatre metrics to the revenue generated. This is an approach that could increase the standing of the theatre management role within the hospital organisation. Hence, the issues discussed in Chapter 7, 'Theatre Finance') are useful not only for some aspects of day to day management, but more so for effective presentation to more senior managers.

Data Collection around the Patient Pathway

There is hardly any other area in a hospital continuously confronted with greater emotional challenge than the operating theatres. This is primary because here different groups have to work together successfully under high pressure, towards the common aim of bettering the health of the patient, whilst contributing economically to the hospital. Therefore the staff users, especially the surgeons, are generally always concerned if they have insufficient resources (in terms of quantity and quality) to be able to meet these goals. Emotions can run high, leading to conflict, inefficiency and lapses in safety. This is something increasingly recognised in the emerging science of 'human factors', which concerns in part how teams can more effectively work together.

One way of neutralising emotions involved is to have enough data available to measure the performance of the system and its parts. Many chapters already have discussed the importance of the availability of robust data. What is most striking is the fact that there are still very advanced countries, like Japan, with high technological resources, where little or no data are available. In countries where the healthcare system is completely funded by the government, a case needs to be made that more investment in information technology and obtaining the correct data will help manage costs. In other countries where private funding is meeting the costs of healthcare, a similar argument might be used to show that obtaining this data will increase profits.

Specific software tools are desirable, wherein patients can be booked for surgery, patients tracked on a daily (or hourly) basis and operating lists created in advance. Coding for procedures might then become more accurate, and this in turn has been shown to reduce costs (Palmer et al., 2017). Fully electronic patient records are nowadays very customary, and

ideally all software tools should be interconnected in a hospital information system (HIS). The greatest difference across hospitals is in the performance of the various HIS applications, including, for example, the availability of management tools for data collection and periodic reporting.

In our hospital in Switzerland we have a single dedicated software tool to manage the whole perioperative patient pathway, from the initial appointment, anaesthesia assessment, documentation of all test and consents, documentation of the procedure, discharge letters, etc. (and even the billing can be initiated from this system). Within this system the theatre manager, and all the controllers of the various departments involved, have access to all the data generated by this particular patient, including timestamps of all the perioperative processes. This enables us to prospectively determine the demand for theatre capacity in the future (as described in Chapter 5). The challenge is now prospectively to apply the principles contained in this book and harness the power of that data available to us.

Terms and Definitions

To be able to report and compare the data we have to establish a commonly accepted definition of roles, processes and performance indicators.

In Germany, for example, this was first published in 2008 and updated in 2016 (Bauer et al, 2016). It was conceived by a group of theatre managers, surgeons and anaesthesiologists and is now generally accepted by the academic associations of these groups. This glossary of definitions and performance indicators has proven to be a valuable tool for theatre managers and has recently also been fully accepted by the Swiss Hospital Group H+ (see www.hplus.ch/de/servicenav/ueber_uns/fachkommissionen/rechnungswesen_und_controlling_rek/rek_entscheide/). In the United States a similar approach was considered necessary as long ago as 1995 by the American Association of Anesthesia Clinical Directors (AACD) and published in 1997 (American Association of Anesthesia Clinical Directors, 1997). These glossaries define the terms and metrics to be calculated in the timing of procedures (e.g., what is meant by 'list time', 'surgical time', 'patient arrival time'). This process of normalisation is essential if different hospitals are to be compared. It is also essential to keep to the same definitions within any hospitals across teams.

Reporting and Benchmarking

Establishing the routine reporting of agreed performance indicators to the hospital executives, surgical departments and anaesthesiologists is a key mission for operating theatre managers. Each hospital has to define its own set of indicators reported, but here is a shortlist of useful data required and performance indicators:

(1) Theatre capacity (e.g., in minutes per day).
(2) Demand on theatres (in minutes per day as a case load for both elective and separately, emergency cases).
(3) Utilisation of theatre capacity (as a percentage of that available in (1) above. This might be further subdivided if needed into (a) surgical (cutting) time and (b) anaesthesia time (from start to end of anaesthesia) and (c) total procedure time (from patient arrival to departure from theatre).
(4) Overrun (minutes per theatre/day).
(5) Cancellation rate.
(6) Start times.
(7) Turnover or gap times.

What Chapters 2 and 3 have done in this book is to combine some of these essential measures into a composite index of efficiency (ε) and productivity (ρ). When these performance indicators are combined with specific goals, they become key performance indicators (KPI).

Most hospitals with an established reporting system can then benchmark against other similar hospitals, thus enabling them to bring their own results into line and improve efficiencies. What is useful to any given hospital to be included in their periodic reporting can also be used for comparison (Pedron et al., 2017). A good example here is turnover times of a specific surgical discipline. Even if the time is stable within the reporting period, it is possible that times are extremely slow compared with other similar hospitals. Then, the theatre manager can start to examine the underlying reasons for this departure from benchmark (Figure 15.2).

The 'Holy Grail' and 'Holy Trinity' of the Theatre Manager

As noted in Chapter 2, some of the potential KPIs listed earlier (1)–(7) can be conflicting. It can be described as a 'Holy Grail' to try to attain them all (in Dark Ages mythology, the Holy Grail was the cup that Jesus drank from at the Last Supper, and finding it said to be something of an impossibility). The concept of efficiency, ε, is an important means to acquire the Holy Grail.

The 'Holy Trinity' can equally be regarded as the three most important benchmarks that a hospital sets for itself to attain. There may not be three (I use the term because there are three in our centre), and they may be different for different hospitals. But the notion is an important one as a driver for improvement. Efficiency, as defined by the concept of ε (Chapter 2) is the first.

The second is starting on time. Although this is a poor measure of overall efficiency in isolation, it should be seen as would be a temperature measurement in a sick patient. Something is wrong when there is a pyrexia, but it is not the aim of treatment simply to bring the temperature down. Just as so many patients have perished normothermic, so too have so many operating departments disintegrated whilst nevertheless demonstrating perfect on-time starts. Probably the most important single factor for a delayed start in the morning is a change of order of the first patient on the list. If the new first case of the list is a different surgical procedure, then the necessary material has not yet been prepared. And if this was caused by bad planning, there will be much discussion and frustration, leading to further additional delay. This underlines the importance of psychology and human factors in the processes.

The third part of the Trinity is the reduction of turnover or gap times. Although these are generally modest, as discussed in Chapters 2–5, it is the focus on any *excessive* gap times that is relevant. In other words, there is little justification for trying squeeze down gap times to zero: as explained, this is hardly worth the cost. However, given that gap times are generally modest, then any outlier gap times should be regarded as significant, and efforts made to reduce them will likely yield important gains at little expense. We should also look at turnover times with respect to the additional cases that can be booked when time is saved by reducing any excessive gap times. (Again, trying to reduce already acceptable gap times to zero is pointless effort, as no extra cases can be added to the few minutes saved.) Reduction of gap times can also contribute to preventing overrun and so staff overtime.

Note also that turnover times are also important for capacity planning and should be taken into account in any such calculation.

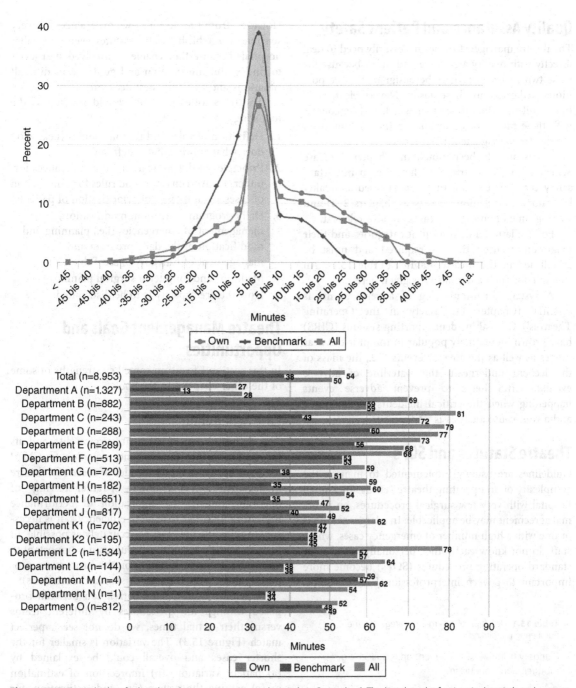

Figure 15.2 Example data for benchmarking across university hospitals in Switzerland. The benchmark of university hospitals and average of all hospitals are marked; the remaining line is the single hospital data. Left panel: Average delay of first case start, percentage of the time gap, all departments. Right panel: Average turnover time for individual surgical departments: each department is listed in order on the y-axis, with (for each department) the bars being in the order: average, benchmark, single hospital data.

Quality Assurance and Patient Safety

The theatre manager does not necessarily need to deal directly with quality assurance and safety because for these two issues there may be designated office positions dedicated to these tasks. Nevertheless, it is important that the theatre manager has close contact with these offices or contribute to the analysis from the theatre management perspective.

It has already been noted in Chapter 4 ('Case Scheduling') that overbooked lists are an important safety concern. Because they can be used as quality indicators, cancellation rates (see Chapters 2–4) and waiting time of emergency cases are also relevant.

For the latter, a definition of categories and their maximum waiting time is required and must be established in the theatre statutes (Table 15.1). An example for such a definition is given here.

A system for monitoring of adverse events is essential (Chapter 14, 'Safety in the Operating Theatres'). Critical incident reporting systems (CIRS) have grown increasingly popular to monitor the near misses as well as the adverse events (i.e., the mass of the iceberg underneath the waterline of adverse events). CIRS helps to prevent adverse events happening when the critical incidents are examined and a root-cause analysis is performed.

Theatre Statutes and SOPs

Guidelines are usually implemented to manage the complexity of an operating theatre setting. In a small hospital with very few surgical procedures, an informal agreement may be applicable. In a larger setting is or one with a high number of emergency cases, where staff do not know each other personally, statutes or standard operating procedures (SOPs) become more important to govern interprofessional relationships.

Table 15.1 Definition of emergency categories (the numbering is arbitrary)

Category 0: Immediate intervention required, e.g., ruptured aortic aneurysm

Category 1: Urgent intervention in < 2 h, e.g., bowel perforation

Category 2: Intervention necessary in < 6 h, e.g., acute appendicitis

Category 3: Intervention necessary in < 24 h, e.g., femoral neck fracture

However, from the author's own experience, it is very sensible to establish theatre statutes even in smaller hospitals because they enable all involved staff levels to find useful information and guidance in difficult situations and make the best decision.

Theatre statutes or SOPs should encompass the following:

1. Definition of roles and responsibilities (i.e., who does what and in what timeframe)
2. Principles of theatre planning (i.e., tolerances for under- or overrun or ground rules for cancellation of cases, or of lists; or of prioritisation of patients)
3. Daily program – creation, modification, management of emergencies (i.e., planning and modification of the daily program and management of Category 3; see Table 15.1)
4. Medium- and long-term surgical planning
5. How theatre capacity is to be distributed

Theatre Management Goals and Opportunities

In this section I focus on some key strengths of some of the other chapters in the book.

Case Scheduling

The definition of an efficient surgical list and its incorporation into the efficiency equation (ε; Chapter 2) encapsulates nicely the idea of successful theatre management: i.e., controlling – or rather steering – of operating theatres by application of performance indicators. In order to achieve efficiency ε, it is necessary to schedule the cases as accurately as possible. In turn, to achieve accurate scheduling, it is important to know the accurate timings for the procedures proposed (along with variance or standard deviations).

When we examine the correlation between proposed timings for procedures by different teams versus their actual times, we do not see a perfect match (Figure 15.3). The variation is smaller for the shorter cases and overall could be explained by (a) patient variation, (b) imprecision of estimation or (c) gaming the system (i.e., underestimation, for which Figure 15.3 does provide some evidence).

This type of data can be used in two ways: first, to adjust the surgeon-provided estimate according to the known variation, and second, to provide feedback to surgeons and itself set a benchmark or reward system for greater accuracy in estimation.

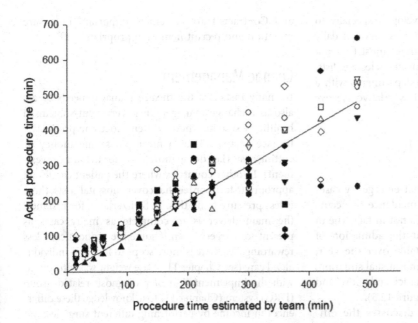

Figure 15.3 Plot of actual procedure time against estimated procedure time for unselected operations across fifteen teams. For each estimated procedure time, each symbol represents a different subspecialty team. The line of identity is shown. There is variation in the estimates, wider for the longer procedures, and some bias towards underestimating times.

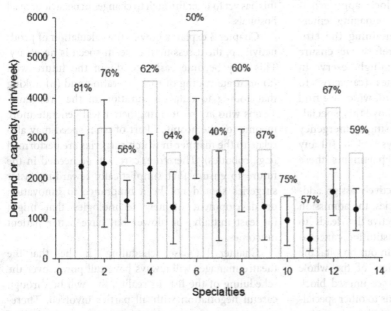

Figure 15.4 Capacity (in minutes/wk; bars) plotted for each of thirteen surgical specialties along with the demand (mean and 95% confidence intervals), which is the minutes/week of capacity actually used. It can be seen that, in accordance with the local philosophy to ensure there is always spare capacity and no accumulating waiting list, more time is provided to all teams that comfortably meets the demand. Only perhaps for Teams 1, 2 and 10 do the error bars come close to the top edge of the capacity bar, suggesting these teams have ~80% chance (rather than near-100% chance) of meeting their demand. The numbers show the minimum utilization for each team (and confirm the case for Teams 1, 2 and 10).

Matching Capacity and Demand

Patients' demands and surgeons' availability cause a variation in the usage of allocated theatre block times. On the other hand, anaesthesia services and availability of theatre personal are more stable throughout the year. This causes a mismatch between the two and a loss of efficiency in theatre performance.

With fifteen surgical specialties competing for twenty-three theatres and a high flexibility in

anaesthesia and theatre staff, our hospital is able to reallocate unused theatre capacity to other surgical disciplines in need, in the short term. The local philosophy is to guarantee that there is no accumulating waiting list for surgery, so using the principles outlined in Chapter 5 ('Capacity Planning'), capacity is set at levels that exceed the 95% confidence intervals of the estimated demand (Figure 15.4). In absolute terms, utilisation might be low, but this provides an additional safety-envelope, especially to accommodate emergency cases. There is anyway a daily dedicated emergency list that separates most (but not all) of the emergency cases from the elective lists. Therefore it is possible that some departments with a high load of emergencies have less relative elective capacity available.

Managing Emergency Cases to Maintain Efficiency

Intuitively it might be thought that emergency cases are unpredictable, both in their incidence of occurrence and their timings, but this is not in fact true in our experience. We observe that the admission of surgical emergencies is highly stable over the year, except for a very few days where an unusual situation, for instance due to traumas during ice and snow, and typically on a weekend, exists (Figure 15.5).

Appendix 2E of Chapter 2 discusses the efficiency of an emergency list. Our local approach is to recognize that appropriately managing emergency cases is important in maintaining the efficiency of the elective lists. Therefore we ensure that each surgical specialty has enough reserve in their allocated theatre block times (capacity) to manage a ~25% emergency case load, which we find is typical (Figure 15.5). Over and above this, specialties can compete for access to the single emergency list at any given time or can always seek to fill any unused theatre capacity of other departments, these being secondary strategies.

In many hospitals that do not actively assign additional theatre capacity for emergencies, the admission of a surgical emergency to an elective list leads to elective case cancellations. In our institution cancellation rates are maintained below 3%. In our hospital the theatre management has an overview of the whole theatre program for the day. If we see unused block time in one specialty, we reallocate this to other specialties to meet their current demand, with any waiting emergencies taking priority. We then try to balance the elective lists of other specialties by moving cases that are prone to cause overrun to unused theatre block times.

Again, this requires a high flexibility of anaesthesia and technical staff. If this flexibility is lost, for instance by high specialisation of anaesthetists or scrub nurses, then reallocation of unused block time becomes impossible and efficiency is reduced. Therefore the principles discussed in Chapter 6 ('Staffing and Contracts') are extremely important to ensure retention and recruitment of appropriate staff.

Change Management

In many instances the theatre manager needs to act also as a change manager. In government-subsidised healthcare systems, there is often a focus on productivity (see Chapter 3) as a means of saving money or cutting costs (i.e., doing more work for the same investment). In other countries where the patient carries an appropriate tariff or fee that covers hospital costs, there is less pressure to do this. In Switzerland, for instance, the main driver is to complete as many cases as present for surgery, even if some are economically less rewarding, i.e., there is more scope to focus on individualised care (see Chapter 11). Case weight was introduced with the implementation of a diagnosis-related group (DRG) system (Chapter 11) to acknowledge these differences in income by performing different surgeries, but this has yet to filter through to changes in behaviour at all hospitals.

Chapter 3 explains how in the calculation of productivity ρ, the assessment of team speed is necessary. This may become easier to do in the future with (a) accurate coding of each operation and (b) linking that coding to data on duration of the procedure. Teams who are performing better will generate more income for the hospital. Part of team speed may also relate to the manner in which surgeries are performed (e.g., robotics). Therefore, care will be needed in the future to ensure that simplistically rewarding faster surgeries should not be a hindrance to innovation or development of new technologies that might (at least initially) be slower but have better patient outcomes.

Chapter 4 ('Case Scheduling') implies that the theatre manager will always have full power over the scheduling of the list. In reality, this will be through careful negotiation with all parties involved. Therefore, theatre management involves a great deal of change management. The psychology, communication and human factors involved will become more and more important in the future.

Future Research and Other Areas of Activity

No book can comprehensively cover all aspects of the complex work in operating theatres. Also, any book is limited by the results of research currently available.

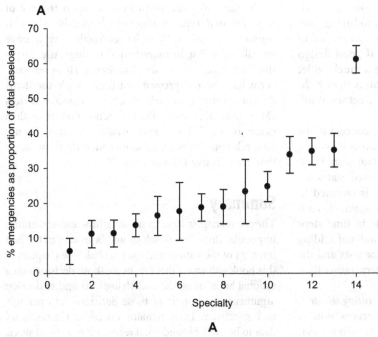

Figure 15.5 Plots of ratio of emergency cases as % (mean ± SD) of totals by (A) specialty and (B) totals across a calendar year. Note that in (A), although the ratio varies widely by specialty, the SDs are relatively modest and consistent. The variation across the year (B) is minimal.

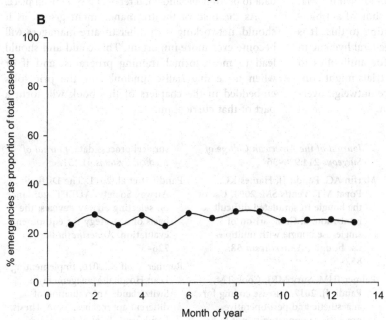

Certainly the principles in this book represent a state of the art that can be pragmatically applied to almost all operating theatres worldwide. Chapter 9 (New Zealand) is especially insightful into how the core principles are being used to good effect. Additional to the themes addressed in this book are the following.

The *architecture and design of theatres*, including geographical location of holding areas, recovery areas, access to the emergency department, radiology and intensive care. As there is increasing focus on the patient pathway, there is appreciation that physical barriers created by poor architecture can be impediments. In this regard, the introductory critique of Lean (Chapter 1) may need modifying over time, as one core principle of Lean is the removal of unnecessary elements in a pathway. If good design helps achieve that, then there will be a much wider application of Lean in operating theatres than hitherto imagined (Collar et al., 2012; Ruether-Wolf, 2016).

Perioperative patient pathways. The concept of the anaesthetist as a perioperative physician is emerging widely; in the United Kingdom the emphasis is on 'perioperative medicine' and in the United States the 'surgical home'. The patient pathway is outlined in Chapter 5 ('Capacity Planning'), and again, there is scope for Lean principles to eliminate in time steps that will be considered superfluous and not adding value (for example, performing baseline tests and the preassessment at time of booking surgery, rather than at some later visit).

Hygiene and infection control in operating theatres. One of the biggest public health concerns now is growing antibiotic resistance. It is not known to what extent the current norm of a 'single shot' of antibiotics for routine surgeries is contributing to this. It is also not known whether improved general hygiene in theatres could eliminate the need for antibiotics in some forms of surgery, or if future trials might conclude the risks of antibiotic resistance outweigh overall the risks of post-surgical infection.

In turn this discussion may relate to the use of *implants and consumables*, which can be a potent source of infection. There has correctly been a move overall (including in anaesthetics) to single use, rather than 'reusable after sterilisation' items. However, concerns have been expressed that these single-use items do not perform as well as older, reusable devices (Marfin et al., 2003). Poor functionality is both a cause of inefficiency and greater expense. Future research could better and sooner identify those items that are effective (Pandit et al., 2011).

Summary

Theatre managers have to make critical and sometimes unpopular decisions, which should be always in the best interests of the patient and the hospital. The chapters in this book will equip them to make those decisions on a rational basis, using the underlying facts and to develop arguments in support of those decisions transparently and objectively. There remains a need for the necessary data to be available and good reporting systems in place.

As the field of theatre management grows, as it should, networking with other theatre managers will become ever more important. This could and should lead to more formal training programs, and if or when these materialise, undoubtedly the principles embedded in the chapters of this book will form a part of that curriculum.

Bibliography

American Association of Anesthesia Clinical Directors. 1997. Glossary of times used for scheduling and monitoring of diagnostic and therapeutic procedures. *AORN Journal* 66: 601–6.

Bauer, M et al. 2016. The German Perioperative Procedural Time Glossary. A concerted recommendation of the German societies of anaesthesiology, surgery and operating room management. *Anaesthetist Intensivmedicin* 57: 669–83.

Collar, RM et al. 2012. Lean management in academic surgery.

Journal of the American College of Surgeons 214:928–36

Marfin AG, Pandit JJ, Hames KC, Popat MT, Yentis SM. 2003. Use of the bougie in simulated difficult intubation. 2. Comparison of single-use bougie with multiple-use bougie. *Anaesthesia* 58: 852–5.

Palmer JHM, Sury MRJ, Cook TM, Pandit JJ. 2017. Disease coding for anaesthetic and peri-operative practice: an opportunity not to be missed. *Anaesthesia* 72: 820–5.

Pedron, S et al. 2017. Operating room efficiency before and after entrance in a benchmarking program for

surgical process data. *Journal of Medical Systems* 41:151.

Pandit JJ et al. 2011. The Difficult Airway Society 'ADEPT' guidance on selecting airway devices: the basis of a strategy for equipment evaluation. *Anaesthesia* 66: 726–37.

Ruether-Wolf K. 2016. Implementing Lean Hospital Management in Switzerland: An evaluation of different approaches. MBA Thesis, Frankfurt School of Finance & Management, Frankfurt/Main, Germany.

Index

Printed in the United States
by Baker & Taylor Publisher Services

Printed in the United States
by Baker & Taylor Publisher Services